Current Cancer Research

Series Editor
Wafik El-Deiry

For further volumes:
http://www.springer.com/series/7892

Erle S. Robertson
Editor

Burkitt's Lymphoma

Springer

Editor
Erle S. Robertson
Department of Microbiology
Perelman School of Medicine
University of Pennsylvania
Philadelphia, PA, USA

Additional material to this book can be downloaded
from http://extras.springer.com

ISBN 978-1-4614-4312-4 ISBN 978-1-4614-4313-1 (eBook)
DOI 10.1007/978-1-4614-4313-1
Springer New York Heidelberg Dordrecht London

Library of Congress Control Number: 2012950585

Printed on acid-free paper

Springer is part of Springer Science+Business Media (www.springer.com)

Preface

The origins of this project began when I was approached by Beverly Griffin, who suggested that I put together a volume on Burkitt's Lymphoma, a problem which is still as dominant in Equatorial Africa as it was 50 years ago. Burkitt's lymphoma was first brought to the spotlight and recognized as a major cancer in the human population in the late 1950s to early 1960s by Dr. Denis Burkitt, a missionary surgeon in Equatorial Africa. The incidence of this disease can vary in different parts of Equatorial Africa, and is epidemic in proportion in this region of the African continent. It is quite concerning and disheartening that this treatable disease is still an epidemic in susceptible African children.

This project aims to bring together a spectrum of ongoing efforts by having a patient-oriented focus from physicians, to diagnostics and clinical implications of the disease as mostly seen in the Equatorial African setting. Importantly, the chapters cover the breadth of studies in Burkitt's lymphoma with some clues for the potential future of studies that can have therapeutic benefits for patients. A volume like this has not been previously completed; so this represents a unique text of its kind.

Additionally, we are grateful for the video documentary on Burkitt's lymphoma that is included in this volume as a compendium to the text. The documentary will give readers a real-life account of the clinicians' and scientists' fight against this deadly cancer, in areas of the world that have less access to first rate medical care. It is still heart breaking to know that in developed countries, where patients have access to the best medical care (if detected early), Burkitt's lymphoma is over 90% curable. However, in countries where access to good medical care is limited or non-existent, the survival rate is sometimes less than 50%. More tragic is the fact that the time period most affected is during early childhood where most of these patients are from families that are less capable of providing the best medical care. How do we deal with this devastating disease in this setting when we have the ability to enhance care and survival of these young patients? Developed countries in the West have a moral imperative duty to support efforts that substantially minimize and hopefully eliminate this disease in our world.

I'm dedicating this volume, in part, to Dr. Beverly Griffin who has been tireless in her pursuit to improving global exposure to Burkitt's lymphoma. She eventually convinced me that this project should be done, especially with a focus on highlighting the quest of clinicians and researchers in this field which would eventually bring better access to care and greater visibility to this devastating disease.

I would also like to thank the contributing authors who have provided insights and suggestions for topics that should be covered and to take time out of their hectic lives to contribute a chapter. I am grateful to all of them for their tireless pursuit to find therapies and develop vaccines to treat Burkitt's lymphoma.

I suspect that Denis Burkitt would be happy that his initial contribution continues to be pursued, although he may have more immediate questions as to why the available therapies are not available to the population most at risk. I hope that patients, physicians, and scientists are able to use the up-to-date information from this volume, and that it provides a helpful guide to novices including students, residents, and junior investigators who are now thinking about entering this field hoping that they may be able to have an impact.

Finally, a special thanks to Rosemary Rochford for her encouragements, Beverly Griffin for her efforts even during difficult times, and Harald Stein for working with Lorenzo Leoncini in completing their chapter even after having major difficulties which minimized his ability to use his hands. This was admirable and shows the enormous conviction of this group of individuals to one of the world's most devastating diseases affecting mostly children in Africa.

Philadelphia, PA, USA Erle S. Robertson

Contents

Chapter 1
An Introduction to Burkitt Lymphoma

Ian Magrath

The first description of Burkitt lymphoma (BL) was probably that of Albert Cook, the first missionary doctor in Uganda. He founded Mengo Hospital and subsequently Mulago Hospital, initially a center for the treatment of tuberculosis, which eventually became the University Hospital of Makerere University. Cook reported a child with a large jaw tumor who came to Mengo Hospital in 1910, and his illustration of the appearance in his meticulous clinical notes leaves little doubt that this was a case of BL [1]. In the first half of the twentieth century, a number of European pathologists working in equatorial Africa noted the high frequency of jaw tumors, or of lymphomas in children [2–6], but it was Denis Burkitt who provided the first detailed clinical description of the tumor in 1958 [7] while working at Mulago Hospital. He recognized a number of different clinical presentations of tumors in children, including jaw tumors and intraabdominal tumors, that could occur either alone or together, and it was this that led him to believe that many, if not all these children, had the same disease, although up until then girls with ovarian tumors were often diagnosed as having dysgerminomas, while other children were thought to have retinoblastoma, soft tissue, or even bone sarcomas. However, it should be remembered that at the time, pathologists also used the term "lymphosarcoma" such that the title of Burkitt's first paper, *A sarcoma involving the jaws in African children*, in which a brief description of the histopathology was given by Jack Davis, then the head of the pathology department at Mulago Hospital, may not have been as misleading concerning the origin of the tumor cells as would appear to be the case today.

Gregory O'Conor, an American pathologist working quite separately from Dennis Burkitt, recognized, with Jack Davis, around the same time as Burkitt's description that approximately half the cases in the childhood cancer registry that had been established

I. Magrath (✉)
International Network for Cancer Treatment and Research, Brussels, Belgium

Uniformed University of the Health Sciences, Bethesda, MD, USA
e-mail: imagrath@inctr.be

E.S. Robertson (ed.), *Burkitt's Lymphoma*, Current Cancer Research,
DOI 10.1007/978-1-4614-4313-1_1, © Springer Science+Business Media New York 2013

in the Mulago Hospital Pathology Department some 7 years earlier were lymphomas [8, 9]. The high frequency of BL observed in Africa, however, was not seen in Europe and the USA, leading to debate as to whether this disease was unique to Africa—many believed that it was, leading to the use of the term "African lymphoma"—but in the mid-1960s, several pathologists described lymphomas in Europe and the USA that were indistinguishable at a histological level, and also, for the most part, clinically, from African BL. This was doubtless because of the selection of children with jaw tumors that resembled those so characteristic of BL in African children, but regardless of this, these observations established that the tumor was not unique to Africa [10–12].

It was not until 1969 that a group of experts in the pathology of hematological neoplasms assembled under the auspices of the World Health Organization decided that the tumor should be defined purely on histological grounds [13]. While seemingly indicating that BL is a single disease, the high incidence in Africa, compared to the USA and Europe, led to the African variety (also common in Papua New Guinea) being referred to as "endemic" BL because of its higher incidence in these two regions. Tumors occurring elsewhere were referred to as "sporadic" although, unfortunately, these terms are often used in different ways such that they are not particularly helpful. In 1984 the observation that HIV infection predisposes to BL [14] led to the inclusion in the subsequently developed World Health Organization classification of hematological malignancies of a third variety of BL—immunodeficiency-related BL (see Fig. 1.1). The histological and immunophenotypic characteristics of BL are are described in detail in subsequent chapters.

Clinical Characteristics

Perhaps the most characteristic feature of BL in equatorial Africa (and New Guinea) is the occurrence of jaw tumors (Fig. 1.2) in young children (less than 5 years, and probably peaking at the age of 3). Why this should be the case is unknown, but the tumors arise predominantly around and within the developing molar teeth (often involving all four jaw quadrants, even if this is not always clinically apparent). Early clinical signs are loose teeth, and the earliest radiological sign is loss of the lamina dura surrounding the developing molar teeth with adjacent lytic lesions, all of which are readily detected by oblique X-rays of the jaws. These tumors tend to grow very rapidly, such that the teeth sometimes appear to be floating on top of the tumor, and although they may be lost, in some patients they settle quite quickly back into their sockets once treatment is begun. At this age, the jaw contains bone marrow tissue, and it is remarkable, therefore, that although the tumor cells infiltrate the marrow of the jaw, it tends not to spread to other marrow-bearing bones and diffuse bone marrow involvement is, therefore, uncommon (less than 10% in most newly diagnosed children). Although orbital involvement is also common at this age, and it has been suggested that orbital tumors arise from the maxilla, they are not necessarily associated with clinical jaw tumors and often do not seriously damage the eye, unless the ophthalmic artery or vein is compressed, or there is direct involvement of the retina—a very rare occurrence.

These characteristic jaw tumors have been described in other countries, even in Europe (at least, in the 1960s or so), and occur at somewhat higher frequency in

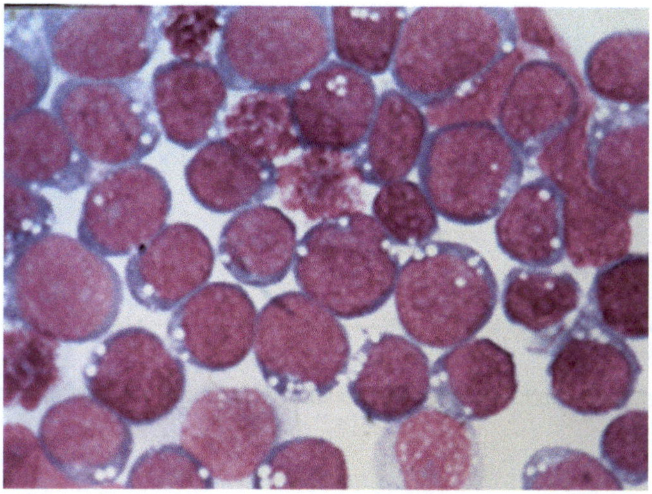

Fig. 1.1 Cytological appearance of BL showing the fenestrated nuclear chromatin with multiple nucleoli, and dark blue cytoplasm containing lipid vacuole. BL is a B cell lymphoma (i.e.,. derived from B cells, which are primarily involved in antibody production). BL expresses surface immunoglobulin, normally IgM, although sometimes IgG. It expresses other B cell markers such as CD20, CD22, CD79 and CD10 as well as proteins associated with very rapidly dividing cells – Ki67 (almost 100% of cells are positive). There is an indistinct dividing line between BL and diffuse large B cell lymphoma, which is reflected in tumors which have a molecular profile (gene expression pattern) that is intermediate between BL and DLBCL. Some of these intermediate tumors are probably derived from follicular lymphomas and have a more complex karyotype, occasionally expressing both the typical BLl MYC/Ig translocations (t8:14) and those found in follicular lymphomas, and some DLBCL, i.e., (t14;18). BL also has a typical gene expression pattern, although once again, intermediate patterns between BL and DLBCL are observed. The BL molecular profile is associated with a good response to intensive combination chemotherapy in countries where this can be given – with a higher survival rate than DLBCL, being in the range of 90–95%

some countries, such as Turkey, or Northern Brazil (and of course, New Guinea, where holoendemic malaria occurs in the river valleys). There is an impression that they were once more common, but today are vanishingly rare outside equatorial Africa and New Guinea. The reason for this is unknown. The high frequency of jaw tumors in young children is not the only difference in the clinical distribution of the tumor in endemic tumors versus tumors occurring elsewhere. In the former, frequent sites of disease include the salivary glands, ovaries, endocrine glands, and retroperitoneal structures, especially the kidneys [15]. Intraabdominal disease is the second most frequent site of involvement in African BL (Fig. 1.2) and the most frequent in all other world regions. Testicular involvement, extradural tumor causing cord compression, and malignant pleocytosis of the cerebrospinal fluid and cranial nerve palsies are also seen in a significant fraction of cases, but interestingly, peripheral lymph node involvement is uncommon as is involvement of the bone marrow or spleen, although splenomegaly is often present because of holoendemic malaria. In Dennis Wright's series of 50 post-mortem cases of BL, the most commonly involved organ was the kidney, and he clearly demonstrated the rarity of significant splenic involvement [16]. It was also possible to demonstrate, at post

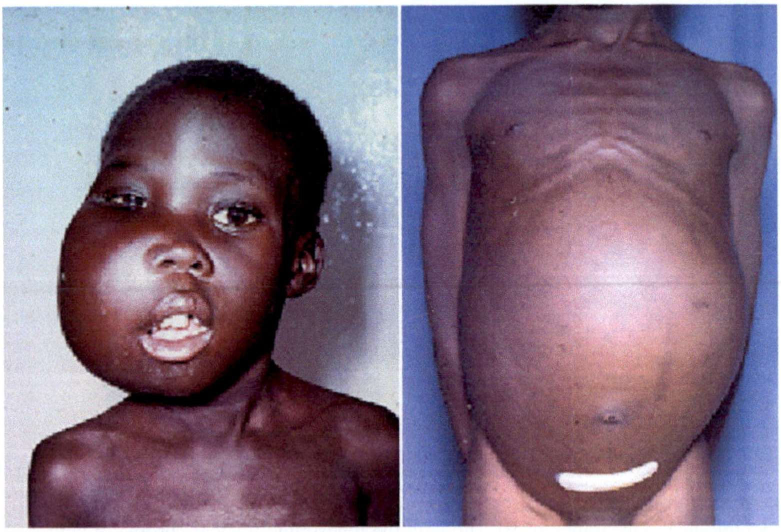

Fig. 1.2 The two most common sites of involvement in African BL—the jaw (*left*) and the abdomen (*right*)

mortem, that cranial nerve involvement was due to infiltration of the nerve by tumor cells—a situation reminiscent of Marek's disease in chickens, a diseases caused by a Herpesvirus. Bowel and mesenteric involvement is frequent (and lymph nodes in the mesentery adjacent to tumor sites in the bowel, most often the ileum may or not be invaded by tumor). Presentation with right-sided abdominal pain, suggesting appendicitis, or acute severe abdominal pain resulting from ileo-ileal intussusception appears to be much more common outside equatorial Africa, although occasional African cases have been described. Interestingly, involvement of the breast occurs particularly in pubertal girls or lactating women [17], suggesting that hormonal or growth factors are involved in creating an appropriate microenvironment in the breast for BL cells—the microenvironment probably also accounts for the high frequency of jaw tumors, and the differences in this respect between equatorial African and children elsewhere may well account for the observed differences in the sites of involvement of BL in different geographical regions. There can be little doubt, however, that at a global level, the abdomen is the most frequent site of involvement, sometimes accompanied by varying degrees of ascites, which can be massive, or involvement of other serous membranes such as the pleura or pericardium. In general, BL occurs particularly in areas where mucosal-associated lymphoid tissue is found and could be considered as a subtype of aggressive MALT lymphoma.

Epidemiology

Early estimates of the incidence of African BL in children (0–14 years) are quite variable, ranging from a few cases per 100,000 to as high as 18 per 100,000, but more recent figures suggest that the incidence in equatorial Africa is similar, in

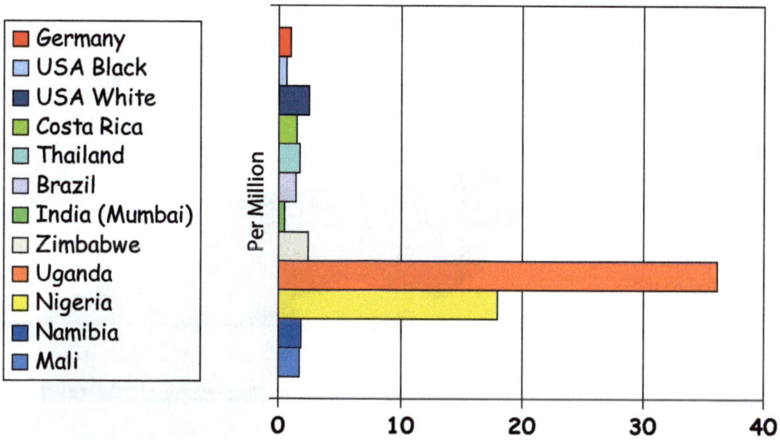

Fig. 1.3 Incidence of BL in selected countries. Data from the International Agency for Research on Cancer (1998)

children, to that of acute lymphoblastic lymphoma—the commonest childhood malignancy in European countries and the USA—probably of the order of 2–6 per 100,000 in children of 0–14 per year. However, case ascertainment is far from reliable, the quality of pathological diagnosis is variable and the incidence often varies within countries, possibly depending upon the local intensity of malarial transmission (see below). Good incidence figures are limited from most world regions, although in the USA and Europe, incidence is probably of the order of 1–3 per million—considerably lower than that of equatorial Africa (Fig. 1.3) [18]. Other world regions appear to have an intermediate incidence, although, once again, the paucity of population-based data, and the variable quality of the data must be taken into consideration in drawing such conclusions. This issue is further compounded by the definition of BL, since the use of microarray techniques does not result in precisely the same dividing lines between diffuse large B-cell lymphoma and BL as does pure histology. Nonetheless, there is no doubt that (a) BL is much more common in equatorial Africa than in other world regions and (b) the incidence varies throughout the world, probably due to differences in environment, and particularly, differences in exposure to particular infectious agents.

Because of its rarity outside Africa, Burkitt was curious with respect to the distribution of the tumor within Africa. He began to indicate on a map places where children with jaw tumors had been seen and sent 1,000 brochures to government and mission hospitals throughout Africa, using the information to plot the "lymphoma belt" shown in Fig. 1.4. Early publications had interested several research organizations in the tumor and Burkitt was given several grants, totaling £700, which enabled himself and two friends, Ted Williams and Cliff Nelson, both missionary doctors, to undertake a safari to define the southern limit of the high incidence zone on the eastern side of Africa. Burkitt and his coresearchers set off from Kampala on October 7, 1961 in a 1954 Ford station wagon and returned 10 weeks later, having visited some 57 hospitals in 8 countries and traveled 10,000 miles. In addition to

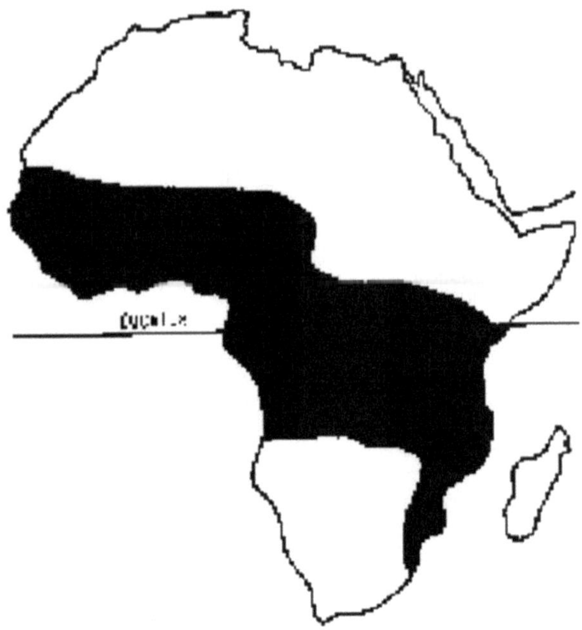

Fig. 1.4 The lymphoma belt extends across Africa approximately 15° north and south of the Equator, indicating a temperature and rainfall barrier to the occurrence of African BL, and suggesting that a disease transmitted by an insect vector predisposes to, or is causally related to the occurrence of BL

personal visits he and his colleagues had sent out a large number of leaflets showing pictures of the disease and to ask whether children with large jaw tumors and/or abdominal masses were frequently seen in that region. What came to be known as the "long safari" showed the southern limit of the high incidence region in the eastern part of Africa to be Lourenço Marques in southern Mozambique. As more information became available, it became clear that the "African lymphoma" had a high frequency in a broad band across equatorial Africa. At first, this was thought to be an altitude barrier, but later, it became clear that the height above sea level at which BL occurred became progressively lower as one moved either to the north or south of the equator, and that what appeared to be an altitude barrier was, in fact, a temperature barrier. Alexander Haddow, working in the Entebbe Virus Research Institute, also in Uganda, observed that the distribution was very similar to that of several virus diseases vectored by mosquitoes, such as yellow fever and various Arbor virus diseases, and it seemed quite likely that BL was caused by a virus vectored by an insect [19, 20]. Similar findings were reported by Booth from New Guinea, the other region where BL was known to have a high incidence [21]. However, Dalldorf proposed, in 1964, that malaria may well be implicated in the pathogenesis of the disease, since the distribution of BL corresponded not only to the distribution of malaria (not greatly different from that of other mosquito-borne infections) but also to the intensity of malarial infection [22, 23]. Subsequent observations have confirmed the relationship between the incidence of BL and the intensity of malarial infection

Malaria and BL

Among the many insect-vectored diseases in equatorial Africa, malaria (predominantly *Plasmodium falciparum*, the most severe form) has one particular and unique attribute, which provides a potential mechanism for its ability to predispose to BL—it induces B-cell hyperplasia. Equatorial Africa and New Guinea are holoendemic malarial regions (i.e., regions where essentially the entire population suffers from the disease). In holoendemic regions, >75% of children have splenomegaly and >60% of <5 years olds have parasitemia at any given time. Transmission is throughout the year (as opposed to hyperendemic malarial regions, where transmission may be limited in the dry season) and spleen and parasitemia rates are <70% in children less than 5 years. Most deaths from malaria occur in children <5 years, particularly in the first 2 years of life, and 75% of deaths from malaria occur in Equatorial Africa.

The particularly high frequency and severity of malaria in young children could explain the age distribution of BL in Africa. Malaria causes polyclonal elevation of immunoglobulins, IgM being elevated only in infants, but IgG being persistently raised thereafter, and also an increase in B-cell autoantibodies and an eventual loss of B-cell memory. In fact, malaria initially preferentially activates the B-cell memory compartment via a Plasmodium membrane protein known as cysteine-rich-inter-domain-region 1alpha (CIDR1α), expressed on the red cell surface. It can also induce virus production from such cells [24, 25]. This is almost certainly relevant to the increase in Epstein–Barr virus (EBV)-containing circulating B cells that occur in acute malaria [26, 27], which could be caused either by infection of other B cells by EBV or by inducing replication in the memory B-cell compartment . It is interesting that EBNA1 (see below) is only expressed in replicating memory B cells, not resting cells [28], creating yet another connection between malaria and BL, although by no means providing a definitive explanation for this relationship.

A Role in the Induction of Genetic Change?

In addition to its ability to cause B-cell hyperplasia, which could, on the basis of chance alone, increase the risk of a genetic change leading to BL, it is possible—even probable—that malaria has a direct role in the production of the chromosomal translocations associated with BL. This results from interactions with Toll-like receptors, which are part of the adoptive immune system. Toll-like receptors are expressed on a variety of cell types including monocytes/macrophages and mature B cells and are activated by T-cell independent, highly conserved antigens, such as lipopolysaccharide and CpG-enriched DNA that are present in a large number of microorganisms. The adoptive immune system is linked, via Toll-like receptors, to the adaptive immune systems, since Toll-like receptors are able to induce activation-induced cytidine deaminase (AID) in B cells, an enzyme which causes hypervariable region mutations and class switch recombination as well as B lymphocyte activation [29–31]. TLR9 receptors, for example, are expressed at all stages of

B-cell differentiation and ligand binding has been shown to result in the induction of AID, and in turn, class switching in all such cells regardless of the presence of VDJ joining. TLR9 agonists include hemozoin, produced by malaria parasites from hemoglobin, as well as CpG-enriched DNA. They bind to B cells in the course of acute malaria, leading to B-cell hyperplasia and class switching, regardless of the stage of differentiation of B cells. It is the ability of AID to cause DNA breaks between the heavy chain constant regions, an essential component of class switching, that leads occasionally, via erroneous re-ligation, to the genesis of chromosomal translocations or other genetic defects [32].

In primary B cells, the expression of the catalytically active form of AID has been shown to lead to *MYC*/Ig translocations, similar to those which occur in BL (see below) within a matter of hours [33]. These translocations are normally prevented by the tumor suppressor genes ATM, p19 (ARF) and p53, consistent with the ability of these genes to inhibit progression through the cell cycle and to initiate DNA repair or apoptosis in the presence of DNA damage, although the particular genes that protect against translocations varies with the translocation partner [34]. The development of translocations involving MYC is also inhibited by the pro-apoptotic genes PUMA, BIM, and PKCδ and enhanced by the anti-apoptotic genes BCL-XL and BAFF, while FAS-induced apoptosis is involved in the elimination of cells in which a functional class switch does not result. It is clear that inactivating abnormalities in protective pathways that normally induce cell cycle arrest and apoptosis in the presence of inappropriate regulation could lead to the persistence of chromosomal aberrations, including translocations. In this regard it is interesting that mutations in p53 are common in BL [35, 36]. There is also direct evidence, in mice at least, that the occurrence of MYC/IgH translocations similar to those occurring in B cell tumors is dependent on AID [37].

Finally, there is evidence for the induction of RAG1 and RAG2 in peripheral blood B cells in malaria [38], and although there is no definitive information that these enzymes, responsible for the normal rearrangement—and rearchitecture, e.g. in the case of autoreactivity, of the variable region of the immunoglobulin molecule [39]—are involved in the pathogenesis of BL, they may mediate at least some of the chromosomal translocations, particularly those occurring in the VDJ region of the immunoglobulin gene.

In spite of these experimental observations, there is no direct evidence that malaria is important to the pathogenesis of equatorial African BL. The most suggestive evidence is the correlation between the incidence of BL and the intensity of malaria transmission (Table 1.1) [40, 41]. This was first observed not long after the distribution of BL had been mapped in Uganda [41], and several investigators have confirmed these findings. Of particular interest in this regard are experiments of nature—the absence of BL in arid regions within the so-called "lymphoma belt" running across equatorial Africa, and alterations in the incidence of BL associated with the control of malarial infection. Thus, in the late 1960s, malaria had been essentially eradicated from the Zanzibar archipelago off the coast of Tanzania, and BL too, was noted by Burkitt to be essentially absent. Soon after, the eradication program was halted (it was felt that total success had been achieved), and BL

Table 1.1 BL is an aggressive B cell lymphoma with cells intermediate in size between diffuse large B cell lymphoma (DLBCL) and follicular lymphoma. BL cells typically have fenestrated nuclear

Malarial intensity	BL incidence rate	95% CI
Lake endemic	3.47	1.30–9.30
Endemic coast	1.67	0.56–4.27
Highland	1.22	0.46–3.17
Arid/seasonal	0.58	0.26–1.27
Low risk	–	–

Based on a 10-year retrospective review described in [40]

rapidly returned. Similarly, the administration of chloroquine prophylaxis against malaria to children in the North Mara region in Tanzania was associated with a reduction in the incidence of malaria, and a return to its previous incidence after cessation of the clinical study [42]. Some critics, however, noting a fall in the incidence of BL prior to the introduction of chloroquine have questioned the validity of these findings. More recently, malaria has again been eliminated from Zanzibar, and it would be of great interest to determine whether the incidence of BL has fallen correspondingly. It has also been known for some time that individuals with sickle cell trait and thalassemia are protected against severe malaria, such that it might be expected that individuals with these inherited hematological disorders would also be protected against BL. Although trends in this direction have been noted, statistical significance has not been demonstrable.

Epstein–Barr Virus

The distribution of BL in Africa suggested to Haddow, Burkitt and others that BL could be caused by an insect-vectored virus, a notion that was entirely consistent with the several animal tumors known to be caused by viruses at the time, although no human tumors caused, or even associated with a virus, had been described. In the early 1960s, following a lecture by Denis Burkitt on the African lymphoma in March, 1961 at the Middlesex Hospital in London, Epstein, a young microbiologist at the Middlesex Hospital, discussed with Burkitt the possibility of searching for virus particles in the tumor cells using the then quite recently developed technology of electron microscopy. Although no viruses were observed in fresh tumor cells, the delayed delivery of one particular sample was such that by the time it reached the United Kingdom, the tumor cells were growing as a continuous cell line in the media it had been sent in. When Epstein examined the cloudy medium, which he assumed was a result of infection, he saw that the cloudiness was caused by tumor cells freely floating in the tissue culture medium [43]. He examined the cells, which proved to be able to grow continuously in culture, by electron microscopy, and was able to rapidly establish the presence of an unusual type of Herpesvirus (unusual in that it appeared to be present in only a small percentage of the cells, and that the majority of cells appeared to be healthy).

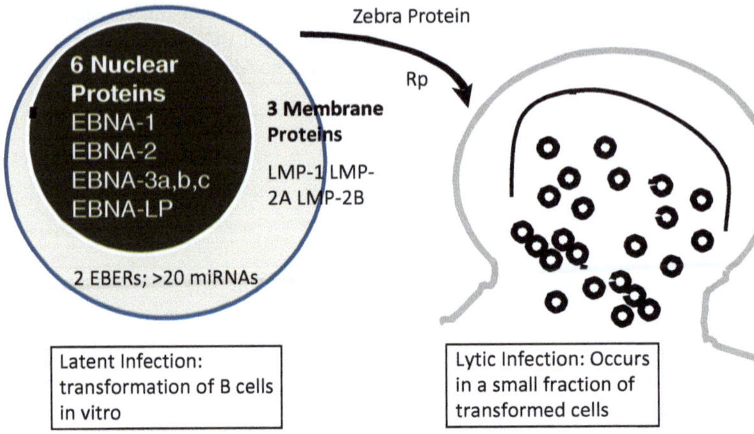

Fig. 1.5 Latent and lytic cycles of EBV showing expression of latent genes (six nuclear proteins and three membrane proteins) and viral non-coding RNAs—2 EBERs and more than 20 microRNAs. Viral structural proteins are not present in the latent cycle, but develop once the lytic cycle is initiated by expression of the Zebra protein, which is necessary and efficient, but is usually accompanied by the expression of other proteins such as "R"

It has subsequently become clear that all BL cells nearly always contain multiple EBV genomes [44] and that essentially all cells in culture express latent genes, i.e. either EBV nuclear antigens (expressed in the cell nucleus) or latent membrane proteins (expressed in the cell membrane) [45, 46]. EBV latent genes (Fig. 1.5) are necessary for the persistence of the virus in B cells (and possibly other cell types) throughout the life of the individual. The primary location of virus persistence is the memory B cell, and the latent genes can be thought of as ensuring that cells containing viral genomes are able to survive in situations in which uninfected cells would not. Normal B cells which do not make high affinity antibody undergo apoptosis when passing through the germinal center of lymphoid tissue, in order to hone the immune response, and ensure that only high-affinity antibody producing cells enter the memory B-cell pool. During this process, a large fraction of normal B cells undergo apoptosis because only those that make high affinity antibodies to the antigen that triggered their proliferation (functioning here as cell surface receptors) receive the necessary viability signals, including antigen and CD40 that are required for them to survive. It seems likely that EBV-infected cells, by virtue of the functions of their latent genes, can avoid undergoing apoptosis even if they do not make high affinity antibody, and thus EBV is assured of entering the B-cell pool, where it can persist in the individual for life. More detailed information regarding the functions of latent EBV genes and their role in virus persistence and the causation of a number of diseases has been published in numerous reviews [28, 46–48].

Persisting in the Population

The persistence of viral genomes in memory B cells is not enough, of course, to ensure survival of the virus in the human population. Virus propagation to other individuals requires the production of virus particles (in the viral *lytic* phase), which are released into the saliva, presumably largely from transformed cells present in pharyngeal lymphoid tissue—cells which may release their virus even as they die as a consequence of detection by T cells sensitized to various EBV latent antigens. Virus that is present in saliva can easily be passed on to other individuals. The switch from latent to lytic phase is triggered by the Z or Zebra gene (Fig. 1.5). It is probable that propagation via saliva leads to the earlier infection of individuals in lower socioeconomic groups in which exchange of saliva is more likely to occur. For example, in African populations, mastication of food by the mother during the weaning process is common, particularly in rural settings, where soft baby foods are not available or are prohibitively expensive. However, the production of virus particles during the "lytic cycle" results in cell death, and is, therefore, incompatible with neoplasia. Even the expression of the full range of latent genes, involved in the "transformation" of normal B cells, inducing proliferation of the infected B cells and expanding the virus pool in the infected individual, is a dangerous proposition since the uncontrolled proliferation of such latently infected cells would be the equivalent of neoplasia. Hence efficient immune responses develop shortly after primary infection against the latent EBV antigens, especially EBNA3a, 3b, and 3c, such that in the absence of mechanisms to overcome the immune response, cells transformed by the gamut of latent genes are rapidly destroyed by T cells [49]. In a number of inherited or acquired immunodeficiency states, the infected cells can, in fact, cause death from the quasi-neoplastic process (which may progress to true neoplasia) that can occur in such circumstances. Evidence has subsequently been acquired that the expression of other viral proteins (particularly the EB nuclear antigen 2) is likely to be detrimental to tumor cells, both because of their immunogenicity and because their expression appears to be inimical to *MYC* overexpression [50] (see below). The pathways to the immunodeficiency-associated neoplasms and classical Burkitt lymphoma appear, therefore, to differ considerably.

After the discovery of EBV, it soon became clear, as the result of a collaboration between Epstein and colleagues, and the virologists Werner and Gertrude Henle, working in Philadelphia, that antibodies to the virus capsid antigen (VCA) of this new virus (which was referred to as EBV by the Henle's, after the cell line in which it was first detected), were ubiquitous in human populations, although it tended to infect individuals of higher social class at a later age than children of low socioeconomic status [51]. A finding of particular importance was the approximately eightfold higher geometric mean titer of anti-VCA antibodies in patients with BL compared to controls [52]. The chance occurrence of infectious mononucleosis in a technician whose blood was frequently used as a negative control for the immunofluorescence tests that the Henle's developed (initially for VCA) led to the observation that the virus was the cause of a high fraction of cases of infectious mononucleosis [53]. Although of great interest, this finding did not shed light on a possible role for EBV in the genesis of BL, since infectious mononucleosis is nearly always self-limiting. Miller and others subsequently showed that EBV was able to transform circulating B lymphocytes and produce continuously growing cell lines in vitro [54]. This led to the hypothesis that EBV was the causal factor of BL and was responsible for driving proliferation of the tumor cells, although this hypothesis was short-lived for a number of reasons. For example, the latent genes induce a cytotoxic immune response that normally ensures that such an event does not occur. Moreover, the ubiquity of the virus indicated that other factors must be involved in the genesis of BL, since clearly, only a very small fraction of infected individuals develop BL. Further studies also demonstrated that the virus is not transmitted by insect vectors, and that none of the latent genes expressed in B cells transformed in vitro, except EBNA1, were expressed in fresh BL cells, although the majority of cell lines, grown in vitro soon revert to the expression of all six latent viral proteins and three latent membrane protein genes. As information accumulated, it became clear that the nuclear protein, EBNA1, was responsible for the persistence of EBV genomes in the form of intranuclear plasmids, and their equal distribution to daughter cells—thus ensuring the maintenance of the EBV genome in transformed cells. The expression of EBNA1 in BL suggested that the virus is required for the maintenance of the neoplastic state (although it could not be excluded that in some cases of EBV negative BL, the virus could have been lost from the cell after onocogenic genetic changes had occurred, thus rendering the presence of virus-derived molecules superfluous).

In fact, African cases are almost always EBV+ whereas only a small fraction of cases in Europe and the USA contain EBV, and a significant fraction of EBV cases are seronegative for EBV, suggesting that the patient had never been infected by EBV. It also became clear that in addition to EBNA1, in EBV+ BL, small untranslated RNAs including microRNAs from the BART and BHRF1 regions of the genome and the so-called “EBERs” are also present in tumor cells [55]. Thus, it seemed probable that EBV, and particularly early (i.e., at a young age) infection with EBV, predisposes to the development of BL, although it was not clear how. A much greater understanding of the survival strategy of EBV had been gained in recent years, however [47], and Thorley-Lawson, in particular, began to consider the possibility that BL might use its B-cell transforming ability to gain access to the immune system, then switch off all its protein products in order to avoid detection and elimination by T cells such that it could persist throughout the life of the individual “invisible” to the host, or at least, to T cells generated against EBV latent antigens [28]. Whatever the mechanism of avoiding detection by the immune system, it may well be relevant to the pathogenesis of BL. Support for this hypothesis was provided by the initial observation that only EBNA1 could be detected in circulating B cells (it subsequently became clear that some virus containing circulating B cells fail to express any viral antigens), and that EBNA1 is the sole protein expressed when such cells replicate (this would be essential to ensure the persistence of the virus in the cell clone). This pattern of latent gene expression was remarkably similar to that observed in BL, but even EBNA1 is immunogenic, such that its persistence in BL cells could result in elimination of the tumor.

The demonstration that EBNA1 contains a glycine–alanine repeat region which inhibits the expression of EBNA1 in the context of class I major histocompatibility antigens (which are also expressed at low levels in BL cells), and hence makes it difficult to for EBV-infected cells in the B-cell memory compartment to be detected by the immune system—even though EBNA-1 reactive T cells may be present, e.g., generated via antigen presentation after B-cell death by reticular dendritic cells. The blocking of the ability of CD8 cytotoxic T cells to react with EBNA-1 present in BL provided a possible explanation for how EBV-containing B cells can escape immunosurveillance. This has been further bolstered by the recent demonstration of the lack of an intereferon gamma CD4+ T-cell response against EBNA1 in Africa children with BL [56] even though in other circumstances, such CD4+ T cells can be detected [57]. This suggests a rather comprehensive impairment of the ability of immune cells to detect the presence of EBV in the context of BL cells [49] and raises the possibility that variable ability to generate immune responses against EBNA-1 could be one of the factors relevant to whether or not BL develops in a particular individual.

In an attempt to demonstrate that EBV is responsible for the pathogenesis of BL, Geser and colleagues undertook a large study in the West Nile district of Uganda, where they collected serum from some 42,000 children and stored it, assuming that some of these children would subsequently develop BL. In fact, 14 children did develop BL in the course of the next several years and all had higher anti-VCA antibody titers to EBV than did normal controls at the time their first serum was drawn, sometimes a few years prior to the development of BL [58]. This suggested strongly to the authors that EBV was likely to be the causal factor of BL, but although there can be little doubt that it is implicated in a high fraction of tumors around the world—being present, for the most part, in some 95%+ of equatorial African cases and more than half of the cases in most published series from outside the highest income countries (Europe and North America being exceptions), the mechanism whereby EBV predisposes to BL remains unknown.

The presence of typical somatic hypervariable region mutations in the antibody genes of EBV-containing memory B cells [28] strongly suggests that these EBV-containing cells have passed through the germinal center, where such mutations are induced by the enzyme AID [59]. Most probably, the route to the peripheral blood is predominantly via tonsillar or at least pharyngeal lymphoid tissue—the closest to its usual point of entry (via saliva) into the body. It seems probable that the ability of several EBV genes, and potentially untranslated RNAs, to prevent apoptosis ensures that the virus-containing cells are protected while passaging through the germinal center, whether or not they have encountered antigen, and thus avoid diversion into the apoptotic pathway that ensures the elimination of cells which produce lower affinity antibodies to the epitopes to which their immunoglobulin molecules are directed. However, this process would need to be associated with the switching-off of latent genes by the time the cell leaves the germinal follicle, since it would no longer be protected from apoptosis (or, indeed, immune destruction) in the periphery.

Persisting in the Individual

Traversal of the germinal center may be an absolute requirement, as suggested by Thorley-Lawson, for the entry of EBV-containing B cells into the memory cell compartment, where they are sheltered for the life of the infected individual, with only occasional need for replication to maintain the particular cell clone [28, 48]. If so, then the pattern of latent and lytic gene expression might well be: (a) infection of naïve B cells with initial expression of all latent genes, thus transforming the cells, increasing their numbers (and the numbers of virus particles), and protecting them from apoptosis as they pass through germinal follicles in order to enter the memory B-cell compartment (some may become plasma cells, which can produce virus). These cells will eventually reach the memory cell compartment and become small resting lymphocytes, whether or not they have been stimulated by antigen (which can be substituted for by LMP2a). What prompts their occasional replication to maintain numbers is unknown, but it is this replicating memory cell that expresses EBNA1. In (b) infection and transformation of secondary B cells results in cell lysis due to the action of antigen (and epitope) specific T cells, infection of more naïve B cells and also passage of virus into the saliva for transmission to other persons. From the perspective of neoplasia, the point is that the cells are protected from apoptosis whilst in the germinal center, where hypervariable region mutations and class switching occurs, such that aberrant ligations (that can result in tumorigenic chromosomal translocations) do not (always) induce apoptosis and can persist. This hypothesis is supported by the demonstration that several EBV genes, and potentially untranslated RNAs are anti-apoptotic [60].

An Alternative Latent Gene Expression Pattern in BL

Quite recently, a second pattern of latent gene expression in BL was observed by Rickinson and colleagues, who showed that as many as 20% of BLs in Africa express all the latent viral proteins except EBNA2, a gene critical to the transformation of normal lymphocytes [61]. This provides further evidence that EBV infection does not drive proliferation in BL cells, although why this alternative pattern of EBV latent gene expression, which includes the immunogenic proteins EBNA3a, 3b, and 3c should exist is a matter for speculation. Whether or not it is relevant to normal EBV biology is unknown, but the alternative latency pattern in BL also appears to be anti-apoptotic, and can, in the presence of appropriate genetic lesions, give rise to neoplasia [61]. But if EBV is not the driver of neoplastic proliferation, what is? There is little doubt that a major factor in the genesis of BL is the ectopic expression of MYC, caused by a chromosomal translocation resulting from aberrant immunoglobulin gene recombination between *MYC* on chromosome 8 and IgH t(8:14) or, more uncommonly, light chain immunoglobulin genes t(2:8) and t(8:22) or, rarely, other genes. The same pathophysiological impact, however, may, on occasion, be brought about by epigenetic regulation of *MYC* rather than a translocation, e.g., via the inappropriate expression of specific miRNAs. These gross cytogenetic changes result in a molecular profile that is specific for BL and clearly distinguishes it from diffuse large B cell lymphoma, although some intermediate patterns can also be observed.

AIDS-Associated Burkitt Lymphoma

Ziegler et al. described the increased incidence of non-Hodgkin's lymphomas (NHLs) in homosexual males in 1984 [62], and subsequently of BL [14]. Since then, the relationship between NHL and HIV infection has been confirmed in many parts of the world, including, for example, South Africa. It remains uncertain, however, how much HIV infection predisposes to BL in equatorial Africa. In fact, the relationship is tenuous at best, at least in children, since although a few percent of children with BL are HIV positive, this is similar to the frequency of HIV infection in children in the normal population. Similarly, although HIV infection is more prevalent in adults, the degree to which it predisposes to BL in equatorial Africa is uncertain [63]. HIV is known to alter the immune response to malaria, resulting in increased prevalence and severity [64], and this could, in turn, affect the probable influence of malaria on BL in equatorial Africa, although it would be expected, from the arguments discussed above, to result in an increased predisposition to BL. HIV infection also causes B-cell hyperplasia, and, like malaria, increases the proportion of circulating EBV-containing cells and results in the reactivation of EBV infection, thus increasing the EBV load in HIV-infected individuals [65–67]. However, the memory B-cell population is reduced in HIV infection, and other B cells may become the primary EBV reservoir [65]. Thus, even though HIV+ individuals have a higher EBV load than HIV-persons, the failure to see an obvious and marked connection between HIV infection and predisposition to BL in holoendemic malarial regions, as occurs in non-malarial regions, could possibly arise from the suggestive evidence that B-cell hyperplasia of the memory cell compartment is central to the pathogenesis of BL, and that the differences in the hyperplastic B-cell populations in malaria versus HIV infection could possibly explain differences in the relative proportions of EBV+ and EBV–BL.

It will be of interest to investigate the influence of highly effective antiretroviral therapy on the incidence of BL in Africa. Because BL in HIV+ patients is not associated with severe immunodeficiency, it is even possible that partial immunological reconstitution through the administration of antiretroviral drugs may eventually lead to an increased risk of BL or other forms of aggressive B-cell lymphoma, although this has not been reported to date. Meanwhile, the limited resources in equatorial Africa pose significant difficulties on studies of this kind [68], and it will be important to develop improved pathological diagnosis, better tumor registration as well as facilities for storing human tissues in order to further understand the relationship between HIV infection and BL in equatorial Africa.

Deregulation of MYC

In 1975, a characteristic chromosomal translocation, in which the *MYC* gene is translocated to the immunoglobulin locus, was discovered by Zech et al. [69]. Subsequently, variant translocations, in which the *MYC* gene is translocated to the light chain loci on chromosomes 2 (kappa) or 22 (lambda) were also indentified. Interestingly, *MYC* is not expressed in the majority of cells that reside in normal germinal follicles, indicating that MYC expression is ectopic in BL, assuming that its cell or origin is the centroblast of normal germinal follicles [70]. The presence of hypervariable region mutations in BL strongly suggests that BL cells have passed through the germinal center, as does their pattern of gene expression (at an mRNA level). Further, differences in the average number of hypermutations and small differences between the gene expression pattern of equatorial African and European Burkitt lymphoma suggest that there may be differences in the pathogenesis of these tumors [71, 72], although the most recent miRNA profiling data suggests that the three subtypes of BL are very similar to each other, while clearly differing from diffuse large B-cell lymphoma [73]. Regardless of these findings, there can be little doubt that BL cell proliferation is driven by *MYC* expression, which in turn is usually the consequence of a chromosomal translocation involving immunoglobulin genes (heavy or light) [74] and *MYC*. In fact, it could well be that the rarity of other genetic abnormalities in BL [75] results from the profound effect of ectopic *MYC* expression in germinal center cells. Rarely, an alternative partner to immunoglobulin genes has been identified, and even the absence of a translocation. In such cases, epigenetic lesions or the inappropriate expression of miRNAs) could also lead to ectopic *MYC* expression [76]. In otherwise normal cells, such a major abnormality would almost certainly lead to programmed cell death—indeed, inappropriate *MYC* expression has been known for many years to be capable of initiating the apoptotic pathway in a number of cell types, presumably to avoid inappropriate cellular proliferation, and more recent work indicates that this process is mediated by the pro-apoptotic protein BIM, which can be upregulated by MYC [77]. Point mutations in the *MYC* gene, which has been identified in BL, have been shown to deactivate this pathway, thus inhibiting a mechanism that protects against the genesis of MYC-driven neoplasia [76, 77]. Indeed, protection against apoptosis is required in normal cell types undergoing somatic hypermutation or class-switching, since, as discussed earlier, AID carries a risk of predisposing to chromosomal abnormalities via the production of double-strand breaks. Defects in this mechanism may be relevant to BL pathogenesis, since there is good evidence that AID is involved in the translocations that result in ectopic MYC expression in BL and the potential for MYC-driven neoplastic cell proliferation [78–80]. It has been suggested that the ability of both HIV and malaria to induce B-cell hyperplasia may also counterbalance the tendency of EBV containing B cells bearing *MYC* translocations to undergo apoptosis increasing the likelihood of their emergence as BL [81].

Although there is much to be learned regarding the relationship between potential environmental factors and the pathogenesis of BL, it seems highly probably that the *MYC* translocation is the driver of proliferation, but that other factors, related to environmental agents such as malaria and possibly HIV, both of which cause B-cell hyperplasia and interfere with immunity and control of the proliferation of EBV, thereby increasing the EBV burden, are important in allowing such genetically damaged cells to persist and may even increase the likelihood of them arising in the first place. The need to rearrange DNA, through a physiological recombinational process in order to generate a tightly binding variable immunoglobulin region and to allow class switching, and the need to prevent apoptosis from occurring during this process, creates a weak point that is likely to give rise on rare occasions to inappropriate recombinations, some of which have the potential to create a neoplastic cell. The experimental evidence supporting the role of AID in mediating chromosomal translocations favors this hypothesis. The details of the pathogenetic events may still need to be worked out, but there is little doubt that the germinal center, a location where apoptosis must be particularly carefully balanced against proliferation, is a critical region for tumorigenesis, precisely because of its importance in the differentiation of B cells. Passage through the germinal center seems to be critical to tumorigenesis in BL and probably also to the genesis of other lymphoid neoplasms, just as it may be to the establishment of a reservoir for EBV. In this case, tumorigenesis can be viewed as an aberration of physiological events, the likelihood of which is increased by the presence of environmental agents such as malaria and EBV, which exploit them for their own purposes, increasing the risk of an aberrant recombination, while removing the defense mechanism that should ensure that cells containing such aberrations (normally a consequence of an abnormal pathophysiological event) are destroyed. Yet the creation of a tumor is not in the best interests of the microorganism, and in comparison with the numbers of people infected with these agents, BL is a rare event indeed, demonstrating the degree to which these parasites have adapted to their human host.

Epidemiology: The Demonstration of Activity of Single Agents

BL was one of the first tumors to be shown to be curable by chemotherapy alone, thus providing critical support to pioneer chemotherapists who, at the dawn of the chemotherapy era, were often maligned for prolonging the misery of patients who were ultimately doomed to die, although occasional cases were cured by radiation or surgery. In the case of African Burkitt lymphoma, surgery was rarely an option although heroic surgery had, from time to time, been attempted when tumor appeared to be localized—for example, to a single jaw quadrant. These attempts invariably met with failure, and usually even more distress to the patient. Radiotherapy was not then available in equatorial Africa (even now, there are very few radiotherapy facilities in this region, and certainly those that do exist are grossly insufficient to provide for the needs of cancer patients), but in any event, radiation was later shown to be of essentially no therapeutic value. By the late 1950s, however, a number of chemotherapeutic agents had become available and several were known to be particularly active in childhood acute lymphoblastic leukemia (ALL). It was clearly of considerable interest to know whether Burkitt's lymphoma responded to chemotherapy in the same way. Investigators in Africa, such as Burkitt in Uganda, Clifford in Kenya and Ngu in Nigeria, aided by pioneer chemotherapists, including Oettgen and Burchenal from the Sloan-Kettering Institute for Cancer Research in New York, and Alexander Haddow and David Galton from the Chester Beatty Institute in London set out to examine the response of Burkitt's lymphoma to chemotherapy, supported by drug donations from companies such as Lederle, Asta Werke, Eli Lilly and Roche, as well as grants and other support from the Sloan-Kettering and Chester Beatty Institutions, and the National Cancer Institute in Bethesda, Maryland. While clinical trials at the time were performed in a rather haphazard manner, and treatment of most cancers resulted, at best, in transient tumor responses, in the case of BL, tumor regression of significant degree was observed within a matter of days (in fact, changes in the tumor, e.g., less stretching of the skin overlying jaw tumors could even be seen within 24 h).

In the course of the early 1960s, most of the available cytotoxic agents were explored. Although a significant fraction of patients was lost to follow up, the administration of a rather wide range of drugs in the course of time led to the clear demonstration that BL was highly chemotherapy-responsive, and Burkitt in Uganda, Clifford in Kenya and Ngu in Nigeria reported some astonishing apparent cures with minimal therapy (several years of disease-free survival after only one or two cycles of therapy) [82–84], although such impressive responses were much more often seen in patients with localized jaw tumors than extensive tumor, for example, in the abdomen. Of particular note was the rapidity of response—tumors would shrink within days, and in the case of jaw tumors, teeth, although sometimes lost, could even find their way back to the socket from which they had been displaced by tumor.

Much of the data collected in this first era of the chemotherapy of Burkitt's lymphoma was summarized in a meeting that was sponsored by the International Union Against Cancer (UICC) (now, the Union for International Cancer Control) that took place in Kampala, Uganda, in 1966. While diagnosis in the 1960s was not as accurate as today, in equatorial Africa a very high fraction of all lymphomas in children (over 80%) are BL, and the clinical features, particularly the presence of jaw tumor (some of the studies were carried out exclusively in patients with jaw tumors) is generally very distinctive. Thus, there can be little doubt that in the series described the diagnostic error rate was small.

Over the years, Burkitt collected a series of 88 patients with jaw tumors treated in Uganda (two relapsed with separate jaw tumors in other jaw quadrants and were dealt with separately, making a total of 90 jaw tumors). Many of these patients achieved long-term survival with only one or two doses of drugs [85]. A variety of doses and sequences of different drugs were used; for example, one and two doses of cyclophosphamide (60 patients were given 30–40 mg/kg IV, or the same dose given orally over 3–4 days), several days of methotrexate (17 patients received 1 mg/kg daily for 4–5 days), or one or two doses of vincristine (21 patients received 0.07–0.15 mg/kg). The period between drug doses regardless of the drug was 1–3 weeks. Among these patients, 36 had "total or virtually total tumor regression," another 38, "significant but only partial regression" and the remainder "little or no response." Thus 74, or 82%, of the 90 tumors had a clear response. How many of these patients had disease at other sites in addition to jaw tumor is not clear, although the jaw tumors were classified as small, moderate or large (grades A, B, or C). Complete, durable remissions were observed with all three agents and notably, all 10 patients with small tumors achieved complete remission. Since 16 of 40 patients with moderate tumors and 10 of 40 with large tumors also achieved excellent responses, this early data suggested a relationship between response and tumor size, although it was some years before this was verified, perhaps because some of Burkitt's patients had undetected tumor outside the jaw. Burkitt also noted that recurrent disease, whether at the same or different sites, did not occur after 11 months of remission—now a well-known characteristic of Burkitt lymphoma. Fourteen patients were known to be alive and well a year after treatment and were probably cured, but 38 patients were lost to follow up.

Interestingly, only four patients in Burkitt's series had received more than two doses of therapy and four had received only a single dose. It was also noted, however, that of 12 patients who relapsed after an essentially complete response, 6 developed central nervous system involvement, and many years of empiric approaches to its prevention were required before the predisposition to relapse in the CNS was overcome. In spite of this, as was demonstrated later by Ziegler et al. [86], that almost half of all patients with CNS disease, either at the time of relapse or presentation, could achieve long-term survival. This clearly indicated that CNS disease per se was not necessarily, as was believed in western countries, an obstacle to cure [87].

Ngu also noted that disease extent and site influenced the outcome of treatment. Patients with tumors localized to the facial bones had better responses than those with visceral or CNS involvement—the beginnings of a formal staging system. Patients with CNS involvement, not surprisingly, had a particularly poor response to intravenous cyclophosphamide, although extradural masses were seen to respond. Another observation made by Ngu was that serum uric acid levels were often raised in patients with extensive tumors, and sometimes became even more elevated following therapy. He described a patient who died quite probably from acute tumor lysis (serum uric acid on the day of death was 54 mg per 100 ml), and reported that this and other complications, such as perforation of the bowel, and in one unusual case, of the arch of the aorta, may ensue from rapid necrosis of tumor following therapy [88]. Indeed, in these early series, a significant fraction of patients died before any chemotherapy could be given—due, no doubt, to very advanced disease at the time of presentation, a problem that persists to the present day.

Clifford's observations regarding response to therapy were similar. Among 51 patients 8, 4 treated with cyclophosphamide and 4 with melphalan or orthomerphalan, achieved complete continuous remission, 3 for over 2 years, but 9 patients died from hematological toxicity (7 of these had received methyl hydrazine or mannitol myleran) and 5 from other treatment complications. In a later follow-up, Clifford reported 11 long-term survivors. All had been treated with either cyclophosphamide, or melphalan, sometimes with orthomerphalan in addition [83].

These early results laid the foundation for subsequent studies. Cyclophosphamide, orthomerphalan, melphalan, methotrexate and vincristine were effective drugs, all capable of inducing complete remission and potentially long-term survival. Chlorambucil, nitrogen mustard, vinblastine and several other drugs were much less promising, at least, at the doses used. Although there appeared to be an association of outcome with disease extent, documentation of disease sites was largely based on clinical examination, supplemented in some patients by bone marrow examination (at least in Clifford's series) and various X-rays, although not in a uniform manner. This may well account for the fact that while Ngu and Burkitt believed that tumor extent was a relevant factor in determining outcome, this was less apparent in Cliffords smaller series. In part, this relationship may have been obscured by the fact that a number of patients died from complications of treatment. Clifford did, however, observe that long-term survival was more likely in stage I patients. Because of the variability of dosage and route of administration, none of the authors were able to draw valid conclusions regarding the relationship between drug dosage and response rate. In part for this reason, as well as the observation of spontaneous remissions, and temporary remissions induced by the infusion of patient serum, an early attempt at immunotherapy, the notion that the host response was critical to success was widely accepted and Clifford, in collaboration with the Klein's and Stjernswärd reported a positive relationship between the presence of serum antibodies reactive with the membranes of BL cells in vitro and response to chemotherapy [89]. This appeared to indicate a "host-versus-tumor" effect, but since the nature of the antibodies is unclear and this data was not confirmed, it is not possible to interpret its significance. Additional studies of immunotherapy using BCG failed to show a clear effect on tumor response, in spite of augmented delayed hypersensitivity [90], and it must be concluded that there is presently no clear evidence of a role for the importance of a host response in the outcome of treatment for BL. In fact, there is considerable information, as briefly mentioned above, that the presentation of foreign antigens to the immune system by BL cells (e.g., EBV antigens) is impaired. With the development of improved staging systems, which probably largely reflect the tumor burden [91], there could be little doubt that outcome correlated with the extent of disease, although the latter, in turn, also influences the ability of the immune system to respond to foreign antigens [92].

The Evolution of Combination Chemotherapy

Denis Burkitt left Uganda in 1967, but his work was continued by means of an agreement between the National Cancer Institute of the USA and the University of Makerere in Kampala, Uganda, to establish the Uganda Cancer Institute. This led to more systematic attempts to improve the results of treatment, although interpretation is difficult in most of these studies because of their small size, limited staging studies and the fact that patients were almost certainly undertreated, such that recurrent disease sensitive to the same or different therapy was extremely frequent. Nevertheless, these early clinical trials were sufficient to extend the observations made previously in Uganda, Kenya, and Nigeria, and it is worth pointing out that even today, few African institutions are able to conduct clinical trials and there is limited collection of data of any kind. It is probable that most patients die for lack of any therapy, while others have inadequate therapy based only on what they can afford. Supportive care also remains inadequate except in a small number of elite institutions, usually in the private sector.

A number of randomized trials comparing treatment approaches were conducted in the 1960s and 1970s. Unfortunately, the numbers of patients randomized in each trial tended to be very smal, and, coupled to the limitations of the staging system used in early studies (stage III included patients with a broad range of tumor burdens, including some with completely resected disease), these studies left much to be desired. But it must be remembered that these were the early days of clinical trials, and in spite of their deficiencies, a number of interesting observations were made. An excellent response to therapy in patients with recurrent disease was often observed, particularly if the relapse occurred 10 weeks or more after the initiation of therapy (or the previous relapse) [93]. One patient had six relapses, including CNS recurrence, before achieving disease-free survival for 4 years. In these circumstances, the only realistic measure of success was overall survival, which, in spite of the difficulty of interpreting the studies, appeared to be better in patients who had received multiple drugs rather than cyclophosphamide alone, and responses were certainly seen to a combination of drugs including methotrexate, vincristine, and cytarabine (BIKE) in patients who has failed cyclophosphamide [86]. Of note was the fact that corticosteroids were not included in these regimens (which is a standard practice today in most treatment protocols), although there is one major exception—CODOX-M/IVAC, which gives similar results to other intensive regimens. Conversely, doxorubicin is a standard component of childhood B-cell lymphoma regimens, but its value is only now being tested.

In Ghana, similar results were achieved with either cyclophosphamide alone, or a drug combination that included vincristine and cytarabine [94]. The latter regimen, however, proved rather toxic. Among 103 patients who received cyclophosphamide as a single agent (two doses were given initially), 79 (77%) achieved CR. Two more patients achieved CR after VCR and MTX were added. Among those who achieved CR, 42 relapsed—very similar results to those obtained in Uganda. Patients who relapsed were given additional cyclophosphamide; 21 of 40 patients achieved a second CR following CTX alone, rather more among those who relapsed late (12 weeks or beyond) than those who relapsed early. These same 40 patients went on to receive the BIKE regimen designed in Uganda, and 9 achieved long-term survival.

Subsequently, Nkrumah and Perkins used a simultaneous combination of cyclophosphamide, cytarabine, and vincristine in patients with intraabdominal disease but without CNS involvement [95]. All patients received a single dose of intrathecal therapy with each course of combination therapy. Nkrumah and Perkins did not perform a randomized study, but included 42 consecutive patients admitted between April 1973 and September 1975, and compared them with a previous group of 44 patients with abdominal Burkitt's lymphoma treated between January 1969 and March 1973, who received cyclophosphamide alone, given at a dose of 40 mg/kg i.v. at 2–3 weeks' intervals for a total of 2–4 doses, but no intrathecal therapy. Of the patients treated with the three-drug systemic combination, 31 completed the 3 cycles of therapy (11 died during treatment), of whom 29 (94%) achieved a complete remission. In the preceding group of patients treated with cyclophosphamide alone only 2 died during therapy, and 34 of the remaining 42 patients (81%) achieved a complete response. Approximately twice as many patients (62% at 2 years) who received cyclophosphamide alone relapsed as those who received the combination of drugs (31% at 2 years), and more patients relapsed with CNS involvement in those who received cyclophosphamide without intrathecal therapy (19 patients, 4 during chemotherapy, and 4 with isolated CNS disease) compared with those who received the drug combination, which included intrathecal methotrexate (five patients, none during chemotherapy, one being confined to the CNS). This result was significantly different ($p<0.05$). Overall, although survival did not differ significantly between the two groups, it favored the combination regimen (41% compared to 33%). A high proportion of deaths in this group were from toxicity. These results strongly suggested that the combination regimen was superior in terms of disease control, including the control of CNS disease, but was sufficiently more toxic as to largely nullify its therapeutic advantage. Toxicity was clearly caused by neutropenia associated with septicemia in four patients, all during the first cycle of therapy. Subsequent courses were better tolerated.

The final clinical study conducted at the Lymphoma Treatment Center (LTC) consisted of multiple cycles of the same simultaneous combination therapy with cyclophosphamide, vincristine, and methotrexate (COM) [96]. The COM regimen was devised on the basis of the multiple responses seen with BIKE, in patients who had failed cyclophosphamide alone. In the randomized comparison of COM versus cyclophosphamide alone, 8 of 10 patients who recurred among the 21 who received COM were confined to the CNS, whereas 7 of the 8 recurrences among the 19 who received cyclophosphamide alone relapsed both systemically and in the CNS. Unfortunately, because of political problems, the trial was cut short and no final conclusion could be drawn, although it did appear that the control of systemic disease was more effective with COM than with cyclophosphamide alone.

At the time of this trial, effective intrathecal prophylactic therapy had not been defined, and in an attempt to prevent CNS disease, a simultaneous study of craniospinal irradiation was carried out at the recently installed radiotherapy unit in Nairobi immediately after the completion of chemotherapy. This study failed to show any benefit of radiation in the prevention of spread to the CNS [97]. Interestingly, a fraction of patients with isolated CNS recurrence were salvaged with subsequent intrathecal therapy and additional systemic therapy and in a later review of these patients, reported in 1980, there was a significant advantage to patients treated with COM+/− craniospinal irradiation, compared to CTX+/− craniospinal irradiation [98]. Because of the political unrest, a study in which intrathecal chemotherapy was to have been used to prevent CNS disease could not be conducted.

Intrathecal Therapy

In addition to the control of systemic disease, the ability to treat CNS disease, including malignant CSF pleocytosis, which had been reported earlier, was also studied in the early studies carried out by the NCI in conjunction with Makerere University, and it was soon found that excellent responses and even cure could be obtained with intrathecal MTX and/or cytarabine [99]. Prior to the trials conducted at the LTC, intrathecal therapy had not been tested (cyclophosphamide had been injected intrathecally in two patients without, not surprisingly, any benefit!). IT therapy has become a standard component of all treatment for BL except those with small volume disease involving the bowel—most of whom present with intussusception or a syndrome indistinguishable from appendicitis.

African Burkitt Lymphoma Is Curable in a Significant Fraction of Cases

Overall, these results confirm that a significant fraction of patients with Burkitt's lymphoma can be cured, and some by cyclophosphamide alone. However, there is little doubt, based on information from other world regions - see below - that the survival rate could be improved by using additional drugs, either per primum (which has the advantage of reducing the fraction of PRs) or following relapse. In the Kampala series of 192 patients treated with a variety of regimens between July 1967 and June 1973, which did not include patients treated per primum with COM, 72 (37%) were known to be alive and disease free in 1977–1978 (4–10 years of follow-up). In a subsequent review extending to July 1977, published in 1980 [98], 109 of 280 patients (39%) were known to be alive and well when last seen. Among patients treated with COM, 15 of 30 patients also treated without effective CNS prophylaxis were known to be alive after several years of follow-up (two patients were lost to follow up), and this figure might well have been higher had effective CNS prophylaxis been used. Data from Accra suggested that even a single dose of IT methotrexate delivered with each cycle of systemic combination therapy might prevent most of the CNS recurrences—in this respect, it may well be the *duration* of therapy that was inadequate rather than the number of doses delivered per course of IT therapy. The questions raised by these data remain today—how effective a regimen would COM plus intrathecal therapy be, using the same doses as used in the 1970s studies and how many cycles of therapy are optimal? The relative efficacy of CVA compared to COM also remains unknown—with improved supportive care results with CVA may have been much better.

Role of Other Therapeutic Modalities

Three other therapeutic modalities studied in Africa are worthy of mention—surgery, radiation, and immunotherapy. A retrospective study conducted in Uganda appeared to demonstrate a survival advantage to patients in whom the bulk (estimated to be at least 90%) of all abdominal tumor was resected prior to the commencement of chemotherapy [100]. This approach was particularly feasible in the setting of localized bowel involvement (a relatively uncommon occurrence in Uganda) or bilateral ovarian disease. Indeed, comparison of a small group of patients in whom both ovaries were resected, with a group in whom only one of two involved ovaries were resected (one was sometimes retained in the hope of preserving fertility—a critical factor to African families in arranging a marriage for their daughter) provided reasonable support for this notion. Obviously, even if bulk reduction by surgery is of benefit, such benefit is entirely dependent upon the efficacy of chemotherapy used after surgery. With modern event-free survival rates of 90% for the majority of patients treated in the most developed countries, surgical resection prior to chemotherapy is likely to be disadvantageous because of delays incurred in initiating therapy and the possible complications of surgery (including the increased likelihood of bowel perforation) rather than beneficial, but this does not exclude the possibility of benefit in situations in which only minimal therapy can be offered (as still applies to most equatorial African countries).

Radiation therapy was also studied in Africa, even though radiation was available only in Nairobi in the 1970s—a cobalt unit, as well as expert local supervision in the guise of Swedish radiotherapists, was installed in the Kenyatta National Hospital in Nairobi, Kenya [101]. Single daily dose radiation therapy was shown to be quite ineffective for the control of local disease (with remission occurring in only one of nine irradiated tumors), although hyperfractionation appeared to be of somewhat more benefit. No new evidence contradicting these data has been produced, either in Africa, or elsewhere [101, 102].

Early Therapeutic Studies Outside Africa

One problem that dogs any attempt to describe the history of the treatment of Burkitt's lymphoma outside Africa is the problem of diagnosis. Although a histological definition of Burkitt's lymphoma was established by expert hematopathologists under the auspices of the World Health Organization, in 1967 [103], which at least eliminated the need for the presence of EBV or the absence of bone marrow involvement for a diagnosis of BL to be made (which some pathologists insisted upon), histological definitions in those days were even less reproducible from one experienced hematopathologist to another than they are in the present. Coupled to variability in the preparation of histological material determining whether a non-African non-Hodgkin lymphoma was, indeed, a BL and comparison of the results of series from different countries could be hazardous. However, in spite of these difficulties, it was clear soon after the discovery of the disease, that BL occurred not only at a much lower incidence, but also accounted for a much smaller fraction of all NHLs in children outside Africa and Papua New Guinea. Moreover, prior to the growth of the pediatric oncology cooperative groups initially in the USA and Europe, most data was from single institutions, most of which could muster only occasional case reports. An exception to this was the National Cancer Institute

(NCI) of the USA. This institution had not only conducted early studies in Africa (by seconding clinical investigators) in what might be thought of as the second period of chemotherapy—the period in which the relative efficacy and optimal combinations of known active agents was examined—but continued to do so in what was known for some time as "American BL." Initially, treatment was very similar to that used in Africa—cyclophosphamide alone—and some patients did achieve long-term survival using this approach [104]. In addition, the danger of hyperkalemia due to renal obstruction from amorphous phosphates (caused by the tumor lysis syndrome) in patients with a high tumor burden was better defined and effective management with allopurinol and hyperhydration had been developed [105–107]. Following the introduction of combination chemotherapy in Uganda, slight variants of the COM regimen were introduced at the NCI, the methotrexate being given intrathecally on 2 of the 5 days of each therapy cycle in the US version and high-dose prednisolone (1,000 mg/m^2 daily for 5 days) and high-dose cyclophosphamide (1,600 mg/m^2 on days 1 and 2 in place of third cycle of therapy) being used in the variant regimen known as COMP [108, 109]. These regimens also initially included whole abdominal radiation, but this appeared to add toxicity without therapeutic efficacy and was eventually phased out. Although the numbers were small (a total of 54 patients were treated with COM or COMP), the survival rate was seemingly better than had been achieved in Africa, although this clearly resulted in part from the use of a very high-dose regimen including whole body radiation followed by autologous bone marrow rescue in patients who relapsed. This was the first documented use of autologous bone marrow rescue following high-dose therapy in patients with recurrent malignant disease. It resulted in prolonged survival in three patients who had developed recurrent disease [110].

Because all childhood non-Hodgkin lymphomas were often treated as acute lymphoblastic leukemia in Europe and the USA, these observations led to uncertainty as to whether all childhood NHLs should be treated as ALL or as BL, i.e., with COM or COMP-type therapies. Indeed, the significance of the by now well recognized different histological categories of childhood NHL (diagnosed according to the favored Rappaport classification scheme in the USA at that time) to the outcome of therapy was unknown. Accordingly, the Children's Cancer Study Group, becoming increasingly more active, conducted a randomized clinical trial in which all children with NHL (divided into two groups - lymphoblastic and non-lymphoblastic) were randomized to receive either COMP, a regimen similar to that used at the NCI, but with a lower dose of corticosteroid and intermediate dose methotrexate (500 mg/m^2), or the LSA_2L_2 regimen, which had been adapted from the LSA_1 treatment protocol used at Sloan-Kettering Cancer Institute for ALL. In both study arms, radiation was given to sites of bulky disease [111]. In view of the more prolonged duration of therapy given for ALL, patients were treated with 18 months of therapy.

While this study was going on, and in view of results achieved using high-dose methotrexate by Djerassi in relapsed patients with NHL, an NCI study was initiated in which high-dose methotrexate (2.7 g/m^2 given over 42 h) was given on day 10 of therapy cycles in which cyclophosphamide, adriamycin, and vincristine were given on day 1, and corticosteroid (at conventional doses) on days 1–5 [112]. In cycle 1 on day 1 cyclophosphamide was given as a single agent in an attempt to reduce the risk of tumor lysis syndrome. Initially, this therapy, which was referred to as protocol NCI 77-04, was not associated with intrathecal therapy, but in view of 4 isolated relapses in the CSF among the first 13 patients, all subsequent patients were treated with intensive intrathecal therapy, including both Ara-C and MTX. Again, given the strong influence of the therapy of ALL, treatment was continued for 15 cycles in all patients except those with completely resected disease or stage I or II disease, who received 6 cycles of therapy.

The results of both the CCSG and NCI studies in patients with BL, (initially combined with large cell lymphomas (B cell or anaplastic) and collectively referred to as non-lymphoblastic lymphomas in the CCSG study. BL (included in the non-lymphoblastic group by the CCSG) were similar, being approximately 50–55% EFS. However, an important finding in the CCSG study was that the ALL-like regimen, LSA_2L_2, was not nearly as effective in the treatment of non-lymphoblastic lymphoma as the COMP regimen, giving a prolonged EFS rate of only 27%. It was concluded that a "leukemia-like" therapeutic approach to BL and the lymphomas lumped together under the rubric of "non-lymphoblastic lymphoma", which were predominantly BL was inferior to the approach that had evolved from the treatment of BL in Africa.

Although at first site the results with COMP and NCI 77-04 appear remarkably similar to those obtained in Equatorial Africa in the late 1960s and early 1970s, it should be borne in mind that EFS in African patients was closer to 30%, an additional 20% of patients achieving long-term survival only after one or more relapses and treatment with MTX, VCR, and often Ara-C. Patients who relapsed in the USA generally had a poor prognosis, although a high fraction would respond temporarily to treatment with ifosfamide, etoposide, and high-dose Ara-C. This regimen (IVAC) was subsequently incorporated into the highly successful NCI 89-C-41 protocol (approximately 90% long-term survival) as an alternating regimen with an NCI 77-04-like combination (CODOX-M) for patients other than those with totally resected or localized disease (low-risk patients) [113, 114]. A total of only four cycles of therapy were given (two of each, starting with CODOX-M) for the high-risk patients, and three cycles of CODOX-M for low-risk patients, clearly demonstrating that longer duration therapy as in 77-04 provided no benefit. CODOX-M/IVAC like the similarly successful regimens developed around the same time in France (LMB protocols) [115] and Germany (BFM protocols) [116], that, like CODOX-M/IVAC were built on a backbone of cyclophosphamide, high-dose methotrexate and vincristine, but with significant variation in dose and schedule and additional drugs for higher risk patients (especially Cytostar, ifosfamide/mesna and etoposide) increased survival rates (albeit based on a retrospective comparison) by some 35%.

Of interest is the finding that adults with BL, at least up to the age of 60 years, had indistinguishable results from those observed in children in both protocols NCI 77-04 and NCI 89-C-41, and it is probable that these protocols are similarly effective for all ages, although the elderly may have comorbidities that reduce tolerance to full-dose therapy. Regimens used in adults have adopted the approaches developed in children and adolescents to good advantage, and intensive protocols of this kind appear clearly advantageous to the standard CHOP, and even R-CHOP [117, 118]. Continued evolution of the protocols has taken place in the context of the pediatric oncology groups, with improvements in triage of patients for different degrees of intensity—another important step designed to give each patient a maximum chance of cure with a minimal risk of toxicity and, particularly in the case of the French protocol, which in the last decade has undergone considerable simplification while maintaining the same excellent outcome.

One question that is important to answer is the role of rituximab in the treatment of BL. Most adult patients with BL, however, already receive rituxumab and there is some evidence to support its added value [119]. In children and young adults, while it may be possible to examine rituximab in particularly high-risk groups, and certainly patients who relapse (although these are very few), the only other approach is to use a phase II window to study efficacy—this has already been done and a positive result found [119]—or replacing a relatively toxic component of treatment with rituximab. Rituximab would probably be an excellent drug for low income countries because of its low toxicity profile, but its cost is likely to be prohibitive for some time to come.

Summary

This brief survey of the discovery, epidemiology, pathogenesis, and treatment of BL carries a number of lessons. Firstly, in Africa, where the disease was discovered some 60 years ago, BL arises from the combined effects of ubiquitous environmental agents. In effect, it results from pathophysiological errors associated with the immunological mechanisms that have evolved for protection against parasites or infectious agents in general, combined with the methods used by such infectious agents (EBV) to overcome immunological defenses against them. Functional variability in the numerous genes involved in these mechanisms (resulting from polymorphisms) doubtless influences the severity of the infectious disease and associated neoplasms, where they exist. Some infectious agents, over the course of millennia, have become adapted to these protective mechanisms to the extent that they can not only survive in the human host in spite of them, but have turned them to their advantage—such as the use of the memory B-cell compartment as a haven in which EBV can persist throughout the life of the individual. In this way, a once violent competition for survival, as is still the case with the much more recently evolved human pathogen, HIV, has, over the millennia, been turned into peaceful coexistence, although this has led to an increased risk of the occurrence of the molecular genetic changes capable of giving rise to neoplasia. In turn, this derives from the risk associated with breaking and relegating DNA strands or inducing mutations in human genes in order to create a more efficient "adaptive" or dynamic immunity that has been superimposed on the preexisting adoptive, or static immunity in the course of evolution. However, considering that the entire population is infected with EBV and malaria, the risk of neoplasia has been increased by only a small extent. Treatment of the extremely aggressive neoplasm first described as a clinical entity by Denis Burkitt has evolved in the course of approximately half a century from the single agents used by pioneer chemotherapists in Africa (surgery and radiation have little or nothing to offer), which produced long-term survival rates of the order of 20%, to intensive drug combinations making use of multiple active agents and capable of producing overall long-term survival rates in the region of 90%. Unfortunately, the complexity, toxicity, and cost prohibit the use of these approaches in the majority of patients who live in low- and middle-income countries, or, in the more technologically advanced of these countries, results in somewhat worse results because of the fact that medical and supportive care as well as the patient environment is suboptimal in these circumstances. The African experience, coupled to the subsequent clear demonstration that shorter, more intensive therapy is superior to less intensive therapy continued for over a year, clearly indicates that prolongation of therapy beyond a few months has no value, and indeed, is likely to be detrimental with respect to the added risk of acute and late toxicity. However, early studies in Africa with the COM drug combination suggested that simultaneous combination chemotherapy may be superior to sequential administration of single agents, and these three drugs may be thought of as the core upon which the modern drug regimens of the major cooperative groups in Europe and the USA have been developed. The need for CNS prophylaxis was quickly learned once a sufficient fraction of patients with systemic disease could be effectively treated, since CNS disease is a very frequent form of recurrence unless measures are taken to prevent it. Because CNS prophylactic therapy had to be developed empirically, it took some time to recognize the inadequacy, in this regard, of a single course of intrathecal therapy. Craniospinal radiation also proved ineffective in preventing CNS disease. The additional elements required to elevate the EFS rate to 90% or more include high-dose MTX and, depending upon the extent of disease (total tumor burden is probably the most important prognostic factor, and treatment is adapted to stage of disease), additional drugs, including ifosfamide, etoposide, and high-dose cytarabine, although the possibility that simpler therapies will be developed is high, e.g., by the replacement of some of the cytotoxic drug elements with rituximab or other targeted therapies, thereby resulting in a reduction of toxicity. At present, the cost of rituximab, although shown to be active in Burkitt lymphoma, is prohibitive in low-income settings such as BL in equatorial Africa, although it is routinely used in the treatment of adults with BL.

References

1. Davies JNP, Elmes S, Hutt M et al (1964) Cancer in an African community, 1897–1956. An analysis of the records of Mengo Hospital, Kampala, Uganda: Part 1. Br Med J 1(5379):336–341
2. Smith EC, Elmes BGT (1934) Malignant disease in natives of Nigeria. Ann Trop Med Parasitol 28:461–512
3. Davies JNP (1948) Reticuloendothelial tumours. E Afr Med J 25:117
4. Edington GM (1956) Malignant disease in the Gold Coast. Br J Cancer 10:41–54

5. Thijs A (1957) Considérations sur les tumeurs malignes des indigénes du Congo belge et du Ruanda-Urundi. A propos de 2,536 cas. Ann Soc Belg Med Trop 37:483–514
6. De Smet MP (1956) Observations cliniques de tumeurs malignes des tissus réticuloendothéliaux et des tissus hémolymphopoiétiques au Congo. Ann Soc Belg Med Trop 36:53–70
7. Burkitt D (1958) A sarcoma involving the jaws in African children. Br J Surg 46:218–223
8. O'Conor GT, Davies JNP (1960) Malignant tumors in African children with special reference to malignant lymphomas. J Pediatr 56:526–535
9. O'Conor G (1961) Malignant lymphoma in African children. Cancer. II. A pathological entity. Cancer 14:270–283
10. O'Conor G, Rappaport H, Smith EB (1965) Childhood lymphoma resembling Burkitt's tumor in the United States. Cancer 18:411–417
11. Dorfman RF (1965) Childhood lymphosarcoma in St Louis, Missouri, clinically and histologically resembling Burkitt's tumor. Cancer 18:418–430
12. Wright DH (1966) Burkitt's tumour in England. A comparison with childhood lymphosarcoma. Int J Cancer 1:503–514
13. Histopathological Definition of Burkitt's Lymphoma (1969) Bull World Health Org 40:601–607
14. Ziegler JL, Drew WL, Miner RC et al (1982) Outbreak of Burkitt's-like lymphoma in homosexual men. Lancet 2:631–633
15. Magrath IT (1991) African Burkitt's lymphoma: history, biology, clinical features, and treatment. Am J Pediatr Hematol Oncol 13:222
16. Wright DH (1964) Burkitt's tumour. A post-portem study of 50 cases. Br J Surg 51:245–251
17. Shepherd JJ, Wright DH (1967) Burkitt's tumour presenting as bilateral swelling of the breast in women of child-bearing age. Br J Surg 54:776–780
18. Orem J, Mbidde EK, Lambart B (2007) Burkitt's lymphoma in Africa, a review of the epidemiology and etiology. Afr Health Sci 7:166–175
19. Burkitt D (1962) Determining the climatic limitations of a children's cancer common in Africa. Br Med J 2:1019–1026
20. Burkitt D (1962) A children's cancer dependent on climatic factors. Nature 194:232–234
21. Booth K, Burkitt DP, Bassett DJ et al (1967) Burkitt lymphoma in Papua New Guinea. Br J Cancer 21:657–664
22. Dalldorf G, Linsell CA, Marnhart FE, Martyn R (1964) An epidemiological approach to the lymphomas of African children and Burkitt's sarcoma of the jaws. Perspect Biol Med 7:435–449
23. Morrow RH, Kisuule A, Pike MC, Smith PG (1976) Burkitt's lymphoma in the Mengo districts of Uganda: epidemiological features and their relationship to malaria. J Natl Cancer Inst 56:479–483
24. Chêne A, Donati D, Guerreiro-Cacais AO (2007) A molecular link between malaria and Epstein–Barr virus reactivation. PLoS Pathog 3(6):e80
25. Simone O, Bejarano MT, Pierce SK (2011) TLRs innate immunereceptors and *Plasmodium falciparum* erythrocyte membrane protein 1 (PfEMP1) CIDR1α-driven human polyclonal B-cell activation. Acta Trop 119(2–3):144–150
26. Moormann AM, Chelimo K, Sumba OP et al (2005) Exposure to holoendemic malaria results in elevated Epstein–Barr virus loads in children. J Infect Dis 191:1233–1238
27. Njie R, Bell AI, Jia H et al (2009) The effects of acute malaria on Epstein–Barr virus (EBV) load and EBV-specific T cell immunity in Gambian children. J Infect Dis 199(1):31–38
28. Thorley-Lawson DA, Allday MJ (2008) The curious case of the tumour virus: 50 years of Burkitt's lymphoma. Nat Rev Microbiol 6(12):913–924
29. Peng SL (2005) Signaling in B cells via Toll-like receptors. Curr Opin Immunol 17:230
30. Krieg AM (2002) CpG motifs in bacterial DNA and their immune effects. Annu Rev Immunol 20:709
31. Ruprecht CR, Lanzavecchia A (2006) Toll-like receptor stimulation as a third signal required for activation of human naïve B cells. Eur J Immunol 36:810
32. Edry E, Azulay-Debby H, Melamed D (2008) TOLL-like receptor ligands stimulate aberrant class switch recombination in early B cell precursors. Int Immunol 20(12):1575–1585

33. Ramiro AR, Jankovic M, Callen E et al (2006) Role of genomic instability and p53 in AID-induced c-myc-Igh translocations. Nature 440(7080):105–109
34. Jankovic M, Robbiani DF, Dorsett Y et al (2010) Role of the translocation partner in protection against AID-dependent chromosomal translocations. Proc Natl Acad Sci USA 107(1):187–192
35. Gaidano G, Ballerini P, Gong JZ et al (1991) p53 mutations in human lymphoid malignancies: association with Burkitt lymphoma and chronic lymphocytic leukemia. Proc Natl Acad Sci USA 88(12):5413–5417
36. Bhatia KG, Gutiérrez MI, Huppi K et al (1992) The pattern of p53 mutations in Burkitt's lymphoma differs from that of solid tumors. Cancer Res 52(15):4273–4276
37. Pasqualucci L, Bhagat G, Jankovic M (2008) AID is required for germinal center-derived lymphomagenesis. Nat Genet 40(1):108–112
38. Hillion S, Youinou P, Jamin C (2007) Peripheral expression of RAG in human B lymphocytes in normal and pathological conditions is dependent on interleukin-6. Autoimmun Rev 6:415–420
39. Wang YH, Diamond B (2008) B cell receptor revision diminishes the autoreactive B cell response after antigen activation in mice. J Clin Invest 118(8):2896–2907
40. Rainey JJ, Mwanda WO, Wairiumu P et al (2007) Spatial distribution of Burkitt's lymphoma in Kenya and association with malaria risk. Trop Med Int Health 12(8):936–943
41. Morrow RH Jr (1985) Epidemiological evidence for the role of falciparum malaria in the pathogenesis of Burkitt's lymphoma. IARC Sci Publ 60:177–186
42. Geser A, Brubaker G, Draper CC (1989) Effect of a malaria suppression program on the incidence of African Burkitt's lymphoma. Am J Epidemiol 129(4):740–752
43. Epstein MA, Achong BG, Barr YM (1964) Virus particles in cultured lymphoblasts from Burkitt's lymphoma. Lancet 1(7335):702–703
44. Schulte-Holthausen H, zur Hausen H (1972) Epstein–Barr virus DNA in human tumor cells. Zentralbl Bakteriol Orig A 220(1):47–51
45. Reedman BM, Klein G (1973) Cellular localization of an Epstein–Barr virus (EBV)-associated complement-fixing antigen in producer and non-producer lymphoblastoid cell lines. Int J Cancer 11:499–520
46. Young LS, Rickinson AB (2004) Epstein–Barr virus: 40 years on. Nat Rev Cancer 4(10):757–768
47. Thorley-Lawson DA (2001) Epstein–Barr virus: exploiting the immune system. Nat Rev Immunol 1(1):75–82
48. Roughan JE, Thorley-Lawson DA (2009) The intersection of Epstein–Barr virus with the germinal center. J Virol 83(8):3968–3976
49. Long HM, Taylor GS, Rickinson AB (2011) Immune defence against EBV and EBV-associated disease. Curr Opin Immunol 23(2):258–264
50. Pajic A, Staege MS, Dudziak D, Schuhmacher M, Spitkovsky D, Eissner G, Brielmeier M, Polack A, Bornkamm GW (2001) Antagonistic effects of c-myc and Epstein–Barr virus latent genes on the phenotype of human B cells. Int J Cancer 93(6):810–816
51. Musso A, Migliore G, Zuccolin G et al (1984) Epstein–Barr anti-viral antibodies in childhood in relation to social status. Minerva Pediatr 36(1–2):9–16
52. Henle G, Henle W, Clifford P et al (1969) Antibodies to EB virus in Burkitt's lymphoma and control groups. J Natl Cancer Inst 43:1147–1157
53. Evans AS, Niederman JC, McCollum RW (1968) Seroepidemiologic studies of infectious mononucleosis with EB virus. N Engl J Med 279(21):1121–1127
54. Miller G, Lisco H, Kohn HI, Stitt D, Enders JF (1971) Establishment of cell lines from normal adult human blood leukocytes by exposure to Epstein–Barr virus and neutralization by human sera with Epstein–Barr virus antibody. Proc Soc Exp Biol Med 137(4):1459–1465
55. Rowe M, Kelly GL, Bell AI, Rickinson AB (2009) Burkitt's lymphoma: the Rosetta Stone deciphering Epstein–Barr virus biology. Semin Cancer Biol 19(6):377–388
56. Ressing ME, Horst D, Griffin BD et al (2008) Epstein–Barr virus evasion of CD8(+) and CD4(+) T cell immunity via concerted actions of multiple gene products. Semin Cancer Biol 18(6):397–408

57. Moormann AM, Heller KN, Chelimo K et al (2009) Children with endemic Burkitt lymphoma are deficient in EBNA1-specific IFN-gamma T cell responses. Int J Cancer 124(7):1721–1726
58. Geser A, de Thé G, Lenoir G, Day NE, Williams EH (1982) Final case reporting from the Ugandan prospective study of the relationship between EBV and Burkitt's lymphoma. Int J Cancer 29(4):397–400
59. Pavri R, Nussenzweig MC (2011) AID targeting in antibody diversity. Adv Immunol 110:1–26
60. Kelly GL, Milner AE, Baldwin GS, Bell AI, Rickinson AB (2006) Three restricted forms of Epstein–Barr virus latency counteracting apoptosis in c-myc-expressing Burkitt lymphoma cells. Proc Natl Acad Sci USA 103(40):14935–14940
61. Kelly GL, Milner AE, Tierney RJ et al (2005) Epstein–Barr virus nuclear antigen 2 (EBNA2) gene deletion is consistently linked with EBNA3A, -3B, and -3C expression in Burkitt's lymphoma cells and with increased resistance to apoptosis. J Virol 79(16):10709–10717
62. Ziegler JL, Beckstead JA, Volberding PA et al (1984) Non-Hodgkin's lymphoma in 90 homosexual men. Relation to generalized lymphadenopathy and the acquired immunodeficiency syndrome. N Engl J Med 311(9):565–570
63. Parkin DM, Garcia-Giannoli H, Raphael M et al (2000) Non-Hodgkin lymphoma in Uganda: a case–control study. AIDS 14(18):2929–2936
64. Flateau C, Le Loup G, Pialoux G et al (2011) Consequences of HIV infection on malaria and therapeutic implications: a systematic review. Lancet Infect Dis 11(7):541–556
65. Richard Y, Amiel C, Jeantils V et al (2010) Changes in blood B cell phenotypes and Epstein–Barr virus load in chronically human immunodeficiency virus–infected patients before and after antiretroviral therapy. J Infect Dis 202(9):1424–1434
66. Bonnet F, Jouvencel AC, Parrens M et al (2006) A longitudinal and prospective study of Epstein–Barr virus load in AIDS-related non-Hodgkin lymphoma. J Clin Virol 36(4): 258–263
67. Adjei AA, Armah HB, Gbagbo F et al (2008) Seroprevalence of HHV-8, CMV, and EBV among the general population in Ghana, West Africa. BMC Infect Dis 8:111
68. Naresh KN, Raphael M, Ayers L et al (2011) Lymphomas in sub-Saharan Africa – what can we learn and how can we help in improving diagnosis, managing patients and fostering translational research? Br J Haematol 10, 1365–2141
69. Zech L, Haglund U, Nilsson K et al (1976) Characteristic chromosomal abnormalities in biopsies and lymphoid-cell lines from patients with Burkitt and non-Burkitt lymphomas. Int J Cancer 17:47
70. Klein U, Tu Y, Stolovitzky GA, Keller JL et al (2003) Transcriptional analysis of the B cell germinal center reaction. Proc Natl Acad Sci USA 100(5):2639–2644
71. Bellan C, Lazzi S, Hummel M et al (2005) Immunoglobulin gene analysis reveals 2 distinct cells of origin for EBV-positive and EBV-negative Burkitt lymphomas. Blood 106(3): 1031–1036
72. Piccaluga PP, De Falco G, Kustagi M et al (2011) Gene expression analysis uncovers similarity and differences among Burkitt lymphoma subtypes. Blood 117(13):3596–3608
73. Lenze D, Leoncini L, Hummel M et al (2011) The different epidemiologic subtypes of Burkitt lymphoma share a homogenous micro RNA profile distinct from diffuse large B-cell lymphoma. Leukemia 25:1869–1876. doi:10.1038/leu.2011.156
74. Magrath IT (1990) The pathogenesis of Burkitt's lymphoma. In: Klein G, Van de Woude G (eds) Recent Adv Cancer Res 55:133–270
75. Hummel M, Bentink S, Berger H et al (2006) A biologic definition of Burkitt's lymphoma from transcriptional and genomic profiling. N Engl J Med 354(23):2419–2430
76. Onnis A, De Falco G, Antonicelli G et al (2010) Alteration of microRNAs regulated by c-Myc in Burkitt lymphoma. PLoS One 5(9). pii:e12960
77. Richter-Larrea JA, Robles EF, Fresquet V et al (2010) Reversion of epigenetically mediated BIM silencing overcomes chemoresistance in Burkitt lymphoma. Blood 116(14):2531–2542

78. Casellas R, Yamane A, Kovalchuk AL, Potter M (2009) Restricting activation-induced cytidine deaminase tumorigenic activity in B lymphocytes. Immunology 126(3):316–328
79. Pasqualucci L, Bhagat G, Jankovic M et al (2008) AID is required for germinal center-derived lymphomagenesis. Nat Genet 40(1):108–112
80. Robbiani DF, Bothmer A, Callen E et al (2008) AID is required for the chromosomal breaks in c-myc that lead to c-myc/IgH translocations. Cell 135(6):1028–1038
81. Nagy N, Klein G, Klein E (2009) To the genesis of Burkitt lymphoma: regulation of apoptosis by EBNA-1 and SAP may determine the fate of Ig-myc translocation carrying B lymphocytes. Semin Cancer Biol 19(6):407–410
82. Burkitt D (1967) Long-term remissions following one and two-dose chemotherapy for African lymphoma. Cancer 20:756–759
83. Clifford P (1967) Long term survival of patients with Burkitt's lymphoma. An assessment of treatment and other factors which may relate to survival. Cancer Res 27:2578
84. Ngu VA (1965) The African lymphoma (Burkitt tumour) survivals exceeding two years. Br J Cancer 19:101–107
85. Burkitt D (1967) Chemotherapy of jaw tumours. In: Treatment of Burkitt's tumour. Monograph series number 8, International Union Against Cancer, pp 94–104
86. Ziegler JL (1972) Chemotherapy of Burkitt's lymphoma. Cancer 30:1534–1540
87. Haddy TB, Adde MA, Magrath IT (1991) CNS involvement in small noncleaved-cell lymphoma: is CNS disease per se a poor prognostic sign? J Clin Oncol 9:1973–1982
88. Ngu VA (1972) Chemotherapy of Burkitt's tumor at the University of Ibadan, Nigeria. JAMA 222(9):1166
89. Klein G, Clifford P, Klein E, Stjernswärd J (1966) Search for tumor-specific immune reactions in Burkitt lymphoma patients by the membrane immunofluorescence reaction. Proc Natl Acad Sci USA 55(6):1628–1635
90. Magrath IT, Ziegler JL (1976) Failure of BCG immunostimulation to affect the clinical course of Burkitt's lymphoma. Br Med J 1(6010):615–618
91. Magrath I, Lee YJ, Anderson T et al (1980) Prognostic factors in Burkitt's lymphoma: importance of total tumor burden. Cancer 45(6):1507–1515
92. Magrath IT (1974) Immunosuppression in Burkitt's lymphoma. I. Cutaneous reactivity to recall antigens: alterations induced by a tumour burden and by BCG administration. Int J Cancer 13(6):839–849
93. Ziegler JL, Bluming AZ, Fass L et al (1972) Relapse patterns in Burkitt's lymphoma. Cancer Res 32:1267–1272
94. Nkrumah FK, Perkins IV (1976) Burkitt's lymphoma: a clinical study of 110 patients. Cancer 37(2):671–676
95. Nkrumah FK, Perkins IV, Biggar RJ (1977) Combination chemotherapy in abdominal Burkitt's lymphoma. Cancer 40(4):1410–1416
96. Olweny CL, Katongole-Mbidde E, Kaddu-Mukasa A et al (1976) Treatment of Burkitt's lymphoma: randomized clinical trial of single-agent versus combination chemotherapy. Int J Cancer 17:436–440
97. Olweny CL, Atine I, Kaddu-Mukasa A et al (1977) Cerebrospinal irradiation of Burkitt's lymphoma. Failure in preventing central nervous system relapse. Acta Radiol Ther Phys Biol 16:225–231
98. Olweny CL, Katongole-Mbidde E, Otim D, Lwanga SK, Magrath IT, Ziegler JL (1980) Long-term experience with Burkitt's lymphoma in Uganda. Int J Cancer 26(3):261–266
99. Ziegler JL, Bluming AZ (1971) Intrathecal chemotherapy in Burkitt's lymphoma. Br Med J 3:508–512
100. Magrath IT, Lwanga S, Carswell W, Harrison N (1974) Surgical reduction of tumour bulk in management of abdominal Burkitt's lymphoma. Br Med J 2(5914):308–312
101. Norin T, Clifford P, Einhorn J et al (1971) Radiotherapy in Burkitt's lymphoma. Conventional or superfractionated radiation therapy in Burkitt lymphoma. Acta Radiol Ther Phys Biol 10:545

102. Norin T (1977) Radiation therapy in Burkitt's lymphoma. Long term results. Acta Radiol Ther Phys Biol 16:289–294
103. Berard CW (1985) Morphological definition of Burkitt's tumour: historical review and present status. IARC Sci Publ (60):31–35
104. Arseneau JC, Canellos GP, Banks PM, Berard CW, Gralnick HR, DeVita VT Jr (1975) American Burkitt's lymphoma: a clinicopathologic study of 30 cases. I. Clinical factors relating to prolonged survival. Am J Med 58(3):314–321
105. Arseneau JC, Bagley CM, Anderson T, Canellos GP (1973) Hyperkalaemia, a sequel to chemotherapy of Burkitt's lymphoma. Lancet 6(1):10–14
106. Brereton HD, Anderson T, Johnson RE, Schein PS (1975) Hyperphosphatemia and hypocalcemia in Burkitt lymophoma. Complications of chemotherapy. Arch Intern Med 135:307–309
107. Cohen LF, Balow JE, Magrath IT, Poplack DG, Ziegler JL (1980) Acute tumor lysis syndrome. A review of 37 patients with Burkitt's lymphoma. Am J Med 68(4):486–491
108. Ziegler JL, DeVita VT, Graw RG Jr, Herzig G, Leventhal BG, Levine AS, Pomeroy TC (1976) Combined modality treatment of American Burkitt's lymphoma. Cancer 38(6):2225–2231
109. Ziegler JL (1977) Treatment results of 54 American patients with Burkitt's lymphoma are similar to the African experience. N Engl J Med 297(2):75–80
110. Appelbaum FR, Deisseroth AB, Graw RG Jr, Herzig GP, Levine AS, Magrath IT, Pizzo PA, Poplack DG, Ziegler JL (1978) Prolonged complete remission following high dose chemotherapy of Burkitt's lymphoma in relapse. Cancer 41(3):1059–1063
111. Anderson JR, Wilson JF, Jenkin DT, Meadows AT, Kersey J, Chilcote RR, Coccia P, Exelby P, Kushner J, Siegel S, Hammond D (1983) Childhood non-Hodgkin's lymphoma. The results of a randomized therapeutic trial comparing a 4-drug regimen (COMP) with a 10-drug regimen (LSA2-L2). N Engl J Med 308(10):559–565
112. Magrath IT, Janus C, Edwards BK, Spiegel R, Jaffe ES, Berard CW, Miliauskas J, Morris K, Barnwell R (1984) An effective therapy for both undifferentiated (including Burkitt's) lymphomas and lymphoblastic lymphomas in children and young adults. Blood 63:1102–1111
113. Magrath I, Adde M, Shad A et al (1996) Adults and children with small non-cleaved-cell lymphoma have a similar excellent outcome when treated with the same chemotherapy regimen. J Clin Oncol 14:925–934
114. Adde M, Shad A, Venzon D et al (1998) Additional chemotherapy agents improve treatment outcome for children and adults with advanced B-cell lymphomas. Semin Oncol 25 (2 suppl 4):S33–S39
115. Patte C, Michon J, Frappaz D et al (1994) Therapy of Burkitt and other B-cell acute lymphoblastic leukaemia and lymphoma: experience with the LMB protocols of the SFOP (French Paediatric Oncology Society) in children and adults. Baillieres Clin Haematol 7:339–348
116. Reiter A, Schrappe M, Parwaresch R et al (1995) Non-Hodgkin's lymphomas of childhood and adolescence: results of a treatment stratified for biologic subtypes and stage—a report of the Berlin–Frankfurt–Munster Group. J Clin Oncol 13:359–372
117. Linch DC (2012) Burkitt lymphoma in adults. Br J Haematol 156:693–703. doi:10.1111/j.1365-2141.2011.08877.x
118. Mohamedbhai SG, Sibson K, Marafioti T et al (2011) Rituximab in combination with CODOX-M/IVAC: a retrospective analysis of 23 cases of non-HIV related B-cell non-Hodgkin lymphoma with proliferation index >95%. Br J Haematol 152(2):175–181. doi:10.1111/j.1365-2141.2010.08447.x
119. Meinhardt A, Burkhardt B, Zimmermann M, Borkhardt A, Kontny U, Klingebiel Berthold F, Janka-Schaub G, Klein C, Kabickova E, Klapper W, Attarbaschi A, Schrappe M, Reiter A (2010) Berlin–Frankfurt–Münster group. Phase II window study on rituximab in newly diagnosed pediatric mature B-cell non-Hodgkin's lymphoma and Burkitt leukemia. J Clin Oncol 28:3115–3121

Chapter 2
Diagnosis of Burkitt Lymphoma

Leona W. Ayers and Lynnette K. Tumwine

Clinical Presentation

Clinical presentation in extranodal and nodal sites of rapidly expanding masses in high-risk populations suggests Burkitt lymphoma (BL). Most patients present with advanced disease because of the rapid rate of tumor growth. BL cells have a remarkably short doubling time. Children in equatorial Africa and Papua New Guinea have endemic BL and present with facial tumors in the jaw or orbit, abdominal masses, enlarged gonads or bilateral massive enlargement of breasts, particularly if malignancy onset is associated with puberty, pregnancy, or lactation. Over 50% of such presenting tumors in the Burkitt Belt will be BL [1]. If the clinical presentation is an African adult with lymphadenopathy and suspected lymphoma, BL is less likely unless the patient is HIV infected. Longer standing HIV-associated lymphadenopathy can mislead clinical diagnosis away from BL which is classically associated with acute onset expansive tumor growth. BL is a common lymphoma subtype in HIV worldwide including regions of sub-Saharan Africa outside the Burkitt Belt where BL was previously uncommon [2]. The "jaw tumor" in equatorial Africa is the classic, most recognized BL clinical presentation but worldwide facial tumors constitute a small percent of BL and all presenting jaw and abdominal tumors are not BL [3, 4].

Sub-Saharan African diagnosticians expect that aspiration smears, tissue imprints, or tissue biopsies from most body sites can harbor BL. Figure 2.1 the diagnostic

L.W. Ayers (✉)
Department of Pathology, College of Medicine, The Ohio State University, Innovation Centre, 2001 Polaris Parkway, Columbus, OH 43240, USA
e-mail: ayers.1@osu.edu; Leona.ayers@osumc.edu

L.K. Tumwine
Department of Pathology, School of Biomedical Science, College of Health Sciences, Makerere University, Mulago Hill Road, PO Box 7072, Kampala, Uganda
e-mail: tumwinelynnette@yahoo.com

E.S. Robertson (ed.), *Burkitt's Lymphoma*, Current Cancer Research,
DOI 10.1007/978-1-4614-4313-1_2, © Springer Science+Business Media New York 2013

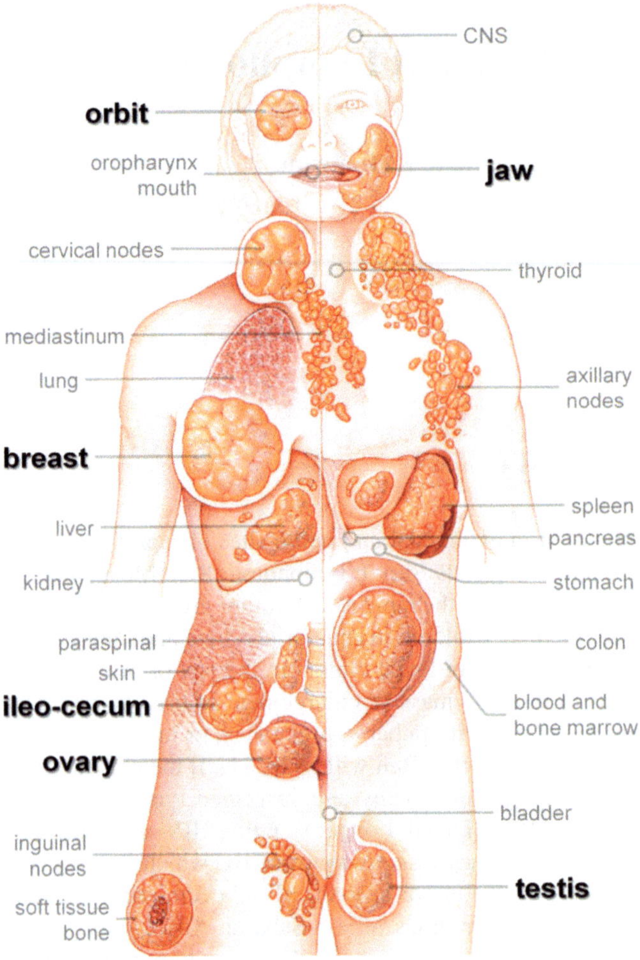

Fig. 2.1 Reported anatomical sites for Burkitt lymphoma primary presentation or extension, common and uncommon

challenge outside of BL endemic areas is to recognize sporadic BL in children and adolescence. BL is especially suspect worldwide in immune deficiency conditions such as HIV/AIDS, post solid organ transplants, and following chemotherapy for other malignant lymphomas [5]. The anatomical site of presentation in these non-endemic cases is unlikely to be facial and more likely to be abdominal. Ileo-colic intussusception may present as acute appendicitis even before an underlying BL tumor mass is clinically obvious [6]. BL may be primary in the stomach in association with *Helicobacter pylori* [7] and in gastric lymph nodes with erosion into the stomach [5]; primary in the wall of the colon [8] and in a variety of other abdominal organs, as primary or as part of multisite BL disease. The pancreas may be diffusely involved forming a deep abdominal mass along with involved periaortic lymph nodes. Symptoms of acute pancreatitis may be noted before the abdominal mass becomes obvious [9]. Pancreatic involvement can be uncovered during clinical evaluation of BL occurring in the oropharynx, a more common primary site [10]. Acute pancreatitis in an adolescent or young adult should raise concern for immune deficiency states including HIV/AIDS and post-transplant disorder. In transplant recipients it is important not to confuse other post-transplant lymphoproliferative disorders (PTLD) that are Epstein Barr virus (EBV) positive with the more aggressive BL-PTLD that is also likely to be EBV positive. Aggressive chemotherapy directed at BL-PTLD is more likely to be successful [11]. HIV-infected cases are more likely to have nodal presentation but also present with extranodal disease. Head, neck, oropharynx including tonsillar masses [10], thyroid nodules [12], pancreas [10], kidney with presenting gross hematopyuria [13] and acute renal failure [14], skin and soft tissue [15], breast, ovary [16], and testes can be the presenting site of disease. Diffuse large B-cell lymphoma (DLBCL) is the most common histological subtype of primary testicular lymphoma whereas BL has secondary involvement of the testis, particularly in relapsed BL where the central nervous system (CNS) or contralateral testicle is often involved. Bone marrow involvement is commonly present in late stage disease but circulating BL cells with leukemic signs and symptoms are rare [17].

Collection, Fixation, and Processing of Specimens

The appearance of tumor tissue and cytomorphology is adversely affected by faulty collection (crush trauma), delay in fixation, adverse fixative, and suboptimal processing temperatures and reagents. Morphology is altered or obscured by traumatic sampling causing disruptive bleeding or crush artifact. BL has relatively little supporting fibrovascular tissue and early necrosis so is susceptible to trauma during collection. Ninety-five percent alcohol for Papanicolaou smears and 10% buffered neutral formalin are the fixatives of choice. Buffering in formalin prevents acidification of the tissue over time and maintains the integrity of tissue antigens. Formalin in water or saline used in many parts of the world precludes reliable use of archived tissues for retrospective studies of tissue biomarkers. Proteins vary in sensitivity to adverse tissue management with mixed loss of antigenicity. Antibody staining (immunohistochemistry, IHC) for germinal center markers CD10 and BCL6 and proliferation rate using MIB-1 (Ki67) or in situ hybridization (ISH) for c-Myc (fluorescent in situ hybridization, FISH) may be weak or falsely negative in adversely managed tissues [18]. The method of fixation and processing may be excellent for specimens processed locally but for referred samples these factors may be unknown. Each histology laboratory processing biopsy or surgically removed lymphoma tissue should assure proper fixation for best diagnostic results.

Diagnosis

Aspirants and Imprints

Worldwide there has been growing interest in faster diagnostic methods than provided by tissue biopsy for obtaining diagnostic material for morphological, immunophenotypical, and cytological studies of malignancies [19]. Fine needle aspiration (FNA) which involves withdrawing cells from tumor masses by inserting a needle with attached syringe and drawing back to create a vacuum is widely deployed as a faster method. Early studies from sub-Saharan Africa by Magrath and others [20–22] all concluded that FNA was a safe, cheap and feasible method for obtaining material for diagnosis of NHL even though only one study [22] was sufficiently detailed to allow such a conclusion. Researchers from Malawi and South Africa have established that nurses trained in FNA can competently take FNA samples where quality is as good as that of cytopathologists [21]. This is a good example of task shifting [23] provided competency based training is implemented and maintained. This study was carried out in a research setting with diagnostic material being sent abroad for further ancillary tests not available in Malawi. Whether this approach can be replicated in other resource constrained settings remains to be seen.

Western literature regarding the diagnosis of BL using FNA yields conflicting results. FNA is well-established for the rapid and efficient diagnosis of cancer but use in the primary diagnosis of lymphoma is controversial. Suspicion of lymphoma on FNA cytology is often followed up by surgical biopsy to allow subgrouping by immunophenotyping. Use of FNA for diagnosis of recurrent lymphoma is less controversial. Cytopathologists, who endorse FNA, present impressive specificities and sensitivities [24–26]. Hematopathologists are more oriented to determine the NHL subgroup as proposed by the WHO 2008 classification which requires the addition of immunophenotyping in tissue samples to confirm NHL subtype [27]. While this is an important divide between two groups of medical specialists such issues do not exist in resource-limited countries where there is often preoccupation with finding sufficient resources for morphologic examination of tumors [18]. FNA has definite short-term advantages over surgical biopsy: cheap, safe, quick, and easy to perform [28, 29]. Relying on FNA aspirants for diagnosis of BL has specific challenges. Cytomorphology of tumor cells alone is limited by the skill and experience of those obtaining the aspirant and those interpreting the cytomorphology. Reliability for BL has not been established in studies specifically designed for this purpose. Additionally, there may be lost opportunity for future correlative studies requiring formalin fixed paraffin embedded (FFPE) tissue.

No matter whether the tumor sample is collected by FNA, Tru-Cut needle biopsy or surgical biopsy, once the tumor is in hand, the speed of BL identification can be augmented by immediate preparation of smears from aspirates or tissue imprints from tissue biopsies. Cell preparations should be air dried or fixed with 95% alcohol for cytologic examination and prepared for flow cytometry (FC), if available, to speed the diagnostic process. Morphology alone is error prone and not sufficient to

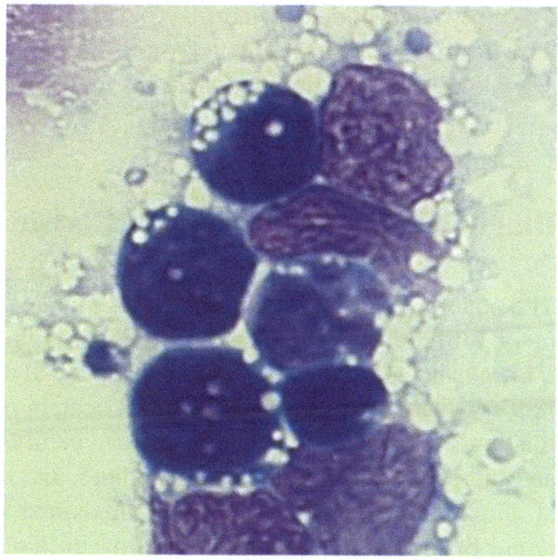

Fig. 2.2 Burkitt lymphoma, "touch prep," showing medium-sized, round, basophilic cells with numerous vacuoles (lipid) in their cytoplasm (Wright's stain)

establish an unequivocal diagnosis of non-Hodgkin's lymphoma (NHL) or establish a specific diagnosis of BL that can safely guide high intensity treatment [1].

Wright's stained air dried smears show BL cells of intermediate size, round with intensely basophilic scant cytoplasm, round to oval nuclei with multiple, small nucleoli per nucleus, and numerous clear vacuoles (Fig. 2.2). The background may be dirty because of necrotic debris and apoptotic bodies. Mitotic figures are usually prominent. In air dried cell preparations, the vacuoles retain the inclusion fat globules that can be stained with Oil Red O. The basophilic cytoplasm is caused by abundant polyribosomes.

Papanicolaou stained alcohol fixed smears of BL show numerous intermediate-sized cells, rounded nuclei with course chromatin and 2–5 nucleoli, scant cytoplasm with small vacuoles, apoptotic cells, mitotic figures, and scattered tangible body macrophages mixed with a dirty background of fine necrotic debris.

Flow Cytometry Cytometrics and Immunophenotyping

FC generated data for BL cells paired with characteristic cytomorphology from FNA smears provides acceptable diagnostic accuracy [24]. Other lymphomas without typical features or with overlapping features such as marginal zone lymphoma, high-grade follicular lymphoma, or DLBCL may be more difficult to classify. BL expresses monotypic surface immunoglobulin light chains and immunoglobulin heavy chain M and B-cell surface antigens such as CD19, CD20, CD10, CD43, and CD45. CD44 and CD54 may be added to improve the separation between BL and CD10-positive DLBCL [30]. Significantly, lymphoma can be excluded by FC if only polyclonal B cells or normal T cells are identified. Because false negative and false positive FC evaluations can occur, the two independent tests of FNA smear cytomorphology and FC immunophenotyping should be correlated for agreement [31].

Diagnostic Tissue Features of Classic Burkitt Lymphoma

The pattern of growth in tissue (Fig. 2.3) is usually diffuse within the tumor mass but is infiltrating as the BL cells move through adjacent tissues or metastasize and infiltrate distant tissue sites. If nodal, germinal centers may be involved early in the process or BL may colonize germinal centers metastatic from adjacent BL. A distinction between primary and secondary involvement with BL is difficult. BL cells are intermediate sized (10–25 um), round, and have a visible rim of cytoplasm that is amphophilic in hematoxylin–eosin-stained preparations. In over fixed tissue, tumor cells appear "squared off" against each other. This is a fixation artifact and is not a reliable criterion for diagnosis. Classic BL cell nuclei are round to oval, have a thick nuclear membrane, course or clumped chromatin, clear parachromatin and indistinct 3–5 paracentric, basophilic small nucleoli. Mitoses and apoptotic cells are numerous. Historically, morphologic variants designated as plasmacytoid or pleomorphic BL were included. The plasmacytoid BL variant was described as having eccentric basophilic cytoplasm containing immunoglobulin while the pleomorphic BL variant had nuclei with large, eosinophilic nucleoli along with binucleate and multinucleated cell forms. At the time of description of these BL variants, full descriptions of plasma cell tumors were not sufficient to assure differentiation from these BL variants.

A "starry-sky pattern" in smears and tissue section is a feature of BL. The perception of small points of light in a dark blue background occurs in BL because the

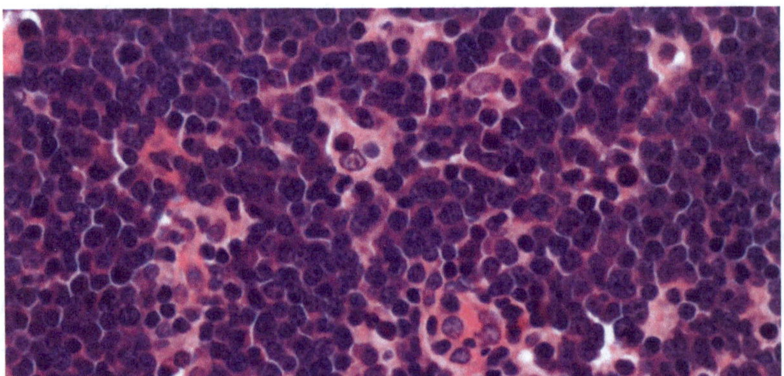

Fig. 2.3 Burkitt lymphoma diffuse pattern with grape-like clusters of medium-sized basophilic cells punctuated by few lightly colored macrophages (H&E stained tissue section)

monomorphic medium-sized tumor cells with basophilic cytoplasm in stained preparations are interspersed by lightly stained benign tingible body macrophages or necrophages, reminiscent of white stars in a blue sky. This is a nonspecific but useful observation reflective of the rapid rate of cell doubling with individual cell apoptosis and tissue necrosis. Other rapidly growing lymphomas and even other non-hematologic tumors composed of small round cells may have a similar "starry-sky" appearance. Lymphoblastic lymphomas (LBL) that occur in African children as well as in adults with HIV/AIDS [32], high-grade T-cell lymphoma, plasmablastic lymphoma (PBL), and some DLBCL have this *starry-sky pattern* in areas of diffuse growth. Lymphoma cells as well as non-lymphoid small blue cell pediatric malignancies lose the diffuse cell tissue patterns when they infiltrate normal tissues. Recognition of the "starry-sky" tissue pattern commonly associated with BL is useful in developing a working differential of likely malignancies and has general value in raising the possibility of BL but is of limited value in specific BL diagnosis. Beware too strong an emphasis on this BL feature.

A high cell proliferation index, usually >95% is a feature of BL. A proliferation index of >95% is a stable but not unique feature of BL. Since few other lymphomas present with such high proliferation rates, this feature is an important differential feature among non-Hodgkin's lymphoma subtypes. PBL and aggressive DLBCL can have cell proliferation markers (MIB-1) that are positive in 90% or more of cells. The common stain (IHC) used to detect proliferation, MIB-1, is sensitive but detection can be diminished or lost in inadequate tissue fixation and processing or technical staining failures [33]. MIB-1 does not have high inter-laboratory reliability so care must be taken not to overestimate the differential value of this feature. The proliferation index (MIB-1) has been used as a single test added to cytomorphology to improve the diagnostic accuracy for FNA smears in populations at high risk for BL [34].

Scant fibrovascular supporting tissue and necrosis are features of BL. Grape-like clusters of BL cells are rimed by delicate tumor vessels while individual tumor cells have little visible support. The rapid doubling of tumor cells appears to outpace this limited blood supply. Tumor cell degenerative changes and geographic areas of necrosis are common in BL. Biopsies from areas with degenerative cell changes or frank necrosis obscures typical morphology. Degenerative malignant cells from BL cannot be differentiated morphologically from degenerative cells of other lymphoma or plasma cell tumors. Cell aspirates or needle biopsies risk sampling such degenerative or necrotic areas within tumor masses thus providing limited, unrepresentative material for evaluation. Larger samplings of tumor such as surgical excisions offer better opportunity to select preserved tumor for diagnosis.

Epstein-Barr virus (EBV-Type 1 latency) in tumor cells is an important feature of BL. EBNA1 antigen is present in EBV-infected BL tumor cells. Endemic, sporadic, and immune deficiency variants differ in the percent of BL tumors that are EBV positive. In situ *hybridization* for EBV-encoded RNA (EBER) is positive in upward of 90% of endemic BL and variable from 20 to 40% positive in non-endemic variants (Fig. 2.4). Patients from non-endemic geographic regions with local high levels

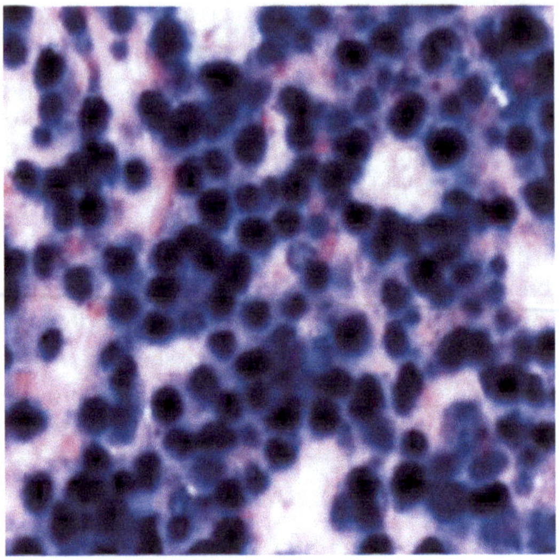

Fig. 2.4 Burkitt lymphoma with *Epstein-Barr virus (EBV-Type 1 latency)* demonstrated in BL cell nuclei (*blue*) by chromogenic in situ *hybridization* for EBV-encoded RNA (EBER)

of endemic Epstein-Barr virus infection [35] may have a higher prevalence of EBV-positive BL. EBV in tumor cells is a feature shared with some DLBCL and most high-grade extramedullary plasmacytomas (EMP) and PBL occurring in those immune deficiency populations also at risk for BL.

BL is a mature B cell lymphoma featuring germinal center origin. BL tumor cells express B-cell-related antigens and are positive for antibodies to B-cell antigens PAX 5, CD19, CD20, CD22, CD79a and germinal center origin antigens CD10 and BCL6. GCET1 (germinal center B cell-expressed transcript-1) mRNA protein is expressed heterogeneously in BL suggesting that BL is not exclusively derived from early centroblasts in lymphoid germinal centers [36]. A more heterogeneous origin within the germinal center might account for the presence of antigens such as the multiple myeloma antigen MUM1/IRF4 and BCL2 antigen that are rare in endemic BL, occasionally seen in sporadic but more commonly in immunodeficiency associated variants. Presence of the B-cell antigen CD20 is required for separation of BL from CD20-negative PBL which shares other BL features of "starry-sky," high proliferations rate, and EBER positive tumor cells. Confusion may emerge in separation of BL from gray zone BL/DLBCL because some DLBCL have similar B-cell and germinal center markers, tissue areas with "starry sky," EBV infection and high proliferation rates in tumor cells.

Immunophenotype (IHC) is a standard feature. NHL subgrouping of BL is facilitated by the use of antibody markers that demonstrate its B-cell and germinal center origin, high proliferation index, presence or absence of EBER, and other differential markers to avoid confusion with other lymphoma subgroups. Limited sets of antibodies have been proposed for economical immunophenotyping of BL for use with suspended cells from aspirates, blood, bone marrow, tumors aspirates, or tissue cell suspensions by FC or for IHC using 6 μ cut tissue sections (Fig. 2.5). BL has surface IgM and Ig light chain antigens, leukocyte antigens CD45, CD43; B-cell lineage

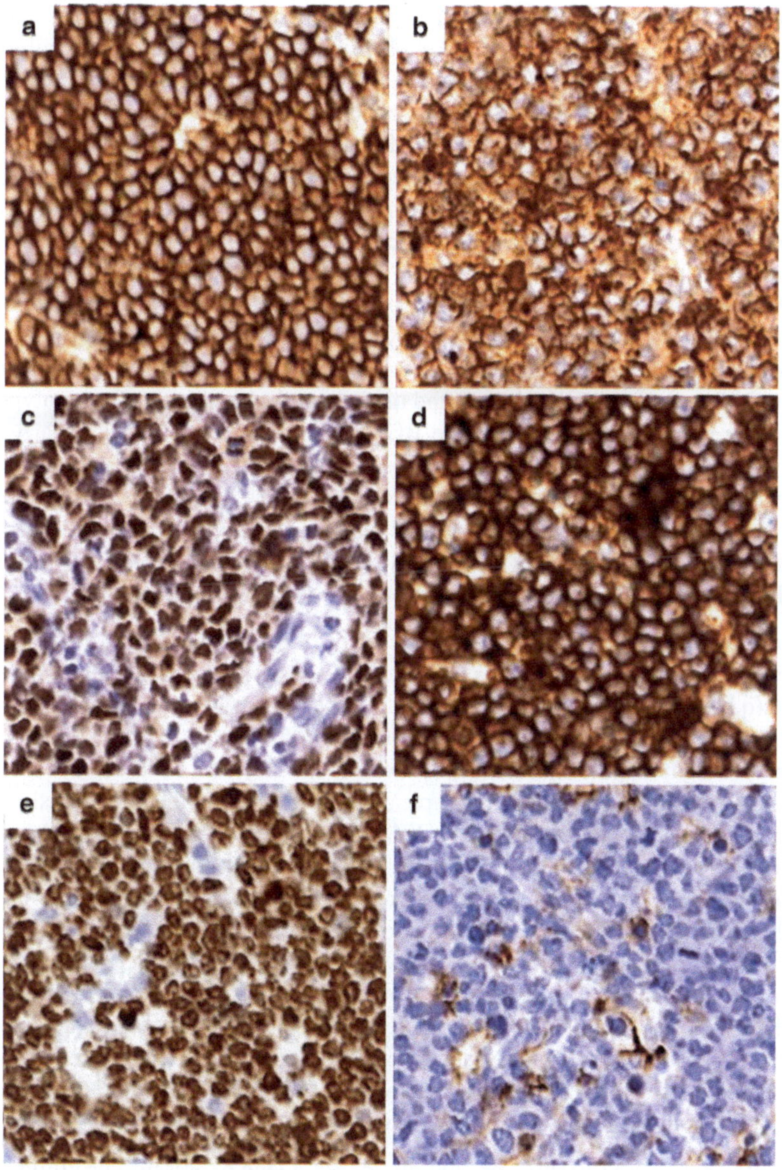

Fig. 2.5 Burkitt lymphoma immunophenotype (IHC) with (**a**) CD20+, (**b**) CD10+, (**c**) BCL6+, (**d**) CD38+, (**e**) MIB-1 (Ki67) >95% and (**f**) CD44−

antigens PAX5, CD79a, CD19, CD20, CD22; germinal center antigens CD10 and BCL6, plasma cell antigen CD38 but no T-cell antigens CD3, CD5, CD23, and absence of antigens CD44, CD138, TdT, cyclin D1, or CD34 specifically found in confounder lymphomas [37]. Classic BL morphology has been paired with abbreviated sets of antibodies or progressive algorithmic approaches to antibody use directed at the accurate identification of BL with specific emphasis of separation from gray zone BL/DLBCL and DLBCL [38]. A proposed tissue algorithm [39] uses tissue morphology of CD20-positive lymphomas plus expression of CD10 and BCL2, Ki67 (MIM1) proliferation index ≥95% and CD38+/CD44- phenotype along with the presence of rearrangements of Myc and Ig genes but the absence of BCL2 and BCL6 gene rearrangements for the specific classification of the BL subgroup. With this scheme *Phase One* uses morphology plus CD10 and BCL2 and reports to classify >80% of BL. *Phase Two* adds three stains, Ki67 (MIB1) and CD38+/CD44- and improves the BL diagnosis to >90%. *Phase Three* adds FISH determination of genetic rearrangements and translocations and completes the algorithm with few conflicts. However, what is made clear by all schemes and algorithms for the diagnosis of BL is that despite BL having a consistent, individual gene expression pattern, there is more variability in cell and tissue morphology as well as genotype than previously appreciated. Although the BL gene expression pattern is clearly separated from that of DLBCL, the two groups have difficulty in phenotypic separation. Some BL are CD10 negative, some are reportedly BCL2 positive and some lack Myc-Ig translocations where other pathogenic mechanisms perhaps related to microRNA expression are involved [40]. DLBCL and PBL with Myc and other translocations are similarly aggressive tumors with poor prognosis.

Chromosomal translocation features the MYC proto-oncogene on chromosome 8 and either the immunoglobulin G (IgG) heavy chain or K or λ light chain genes. The t(8;14)(q24;q32) is found in 80% or more of cases. Translocation may also be found at t(2;8)(p12;q24) in 15% and t(8;22)(q24;q11) in 5% or less of cases. Full genetic karyotypes demonstrate these translocations (Fig. 2.6) and have the advantage of easily verifying if the karyotype is simple or complex. Any of the three translocations found in BL can be demonstrated by FISH using break-apart fusion probes to the flanking regions of the MYC locus (Fig. 2.7). Myc translocations can reliably be demonstrated by break-apart probes where a split of the red–green signal indicates translocation (Fig. 2.8). MYC translocation is sensitive but not specific for BL and upward of 10% of apparent BL do not have a typical translocation [41]. PBL carries a Myc translocation as do some DLBCL but both usually have a complex rather than simple karyotype. Rare cases of multiple myeloma and follicular lymphoma may also have a Myc translocation. Analysis for Myc and for BCL2 and BCL6 translocations is useful to differentiate BL from gray zone BL/DLBCL and DLBCL confounders [42]. Ig-Myc translocation for BCL2 or BCL6 rules out BL.

Molecular expression profiles are unique for BL. Gene expression profiling (GEP) is a powerful tool in the classification of BL but has not become part of diagnostic testing because of availability and cost. GEP confirms BL as unique among lymphomas and supports the prognostic significance of a diagnosis of BL related to the requirement of intensive chemotherapy for overall survival [43]. BL variants of endemic and immune deficiency associated subtypes have similar genes but show consistent minor differences with sporadic BL [44]. The value of GEP to diagnosis is the prospect of identifying new immunohistochemical tests that improve the separation of BL from other Myc positive lymphomas and other confounders.

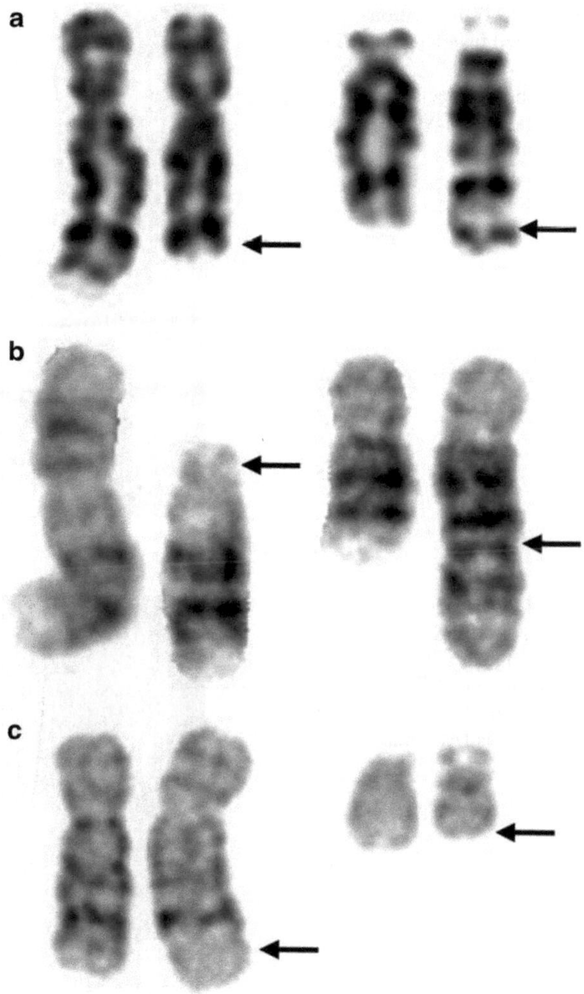

Fig. 2.6 Burkitt lymphoma Myc chromosome translocations at (**a**) t(8;14)(q24;q32), (**b**) t (2;8)(p12;q24) and (**c**) t(8;22)(q24;q11) (Karyotypes courtesy of Dr. Nyla Heerema)

Confounders

Lymphoblastic lymphoma is confused with BL as both occur in children and in immune-deficient adults [32]. Vacuoles in cytoplasm of medium-sized blastic cells on smears or imprints can mislead rather than be diagnostic for BL. Cells of acute lymphoblastic lymphoma/leukemia (LBL) can be intermediate in size and have a few prominent clear vacuoles in the cytoplasm. Nuclei in LBL are more varied in shape, less round; some are convoluted and have a thin rim of basophilic cytoplasm. The blastic nuclei resemble BL nuclei as they do not have prominent nucleoli. LBL has more intermixed lymphocytes than BL but can present the same tissue “starry sky” pattern associated with BL, can be CD44 negative and CD10 positive, can be

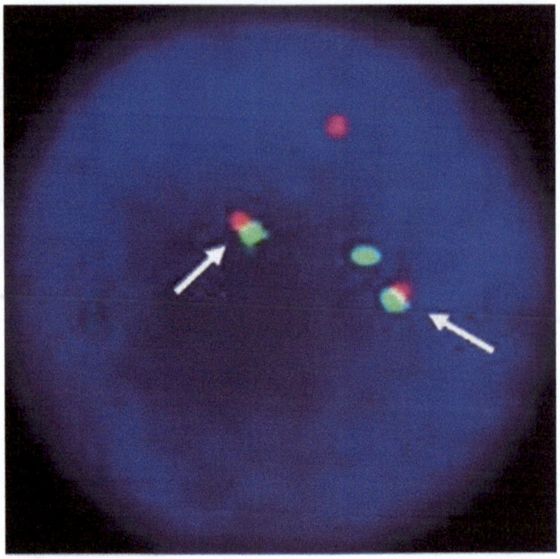

Fig. 2.7 Translocation generated fusion signal (FSH IgH-Myc dual fusion probe by Abbott Molecular, courtesy of Dr. Nyla Heerema)

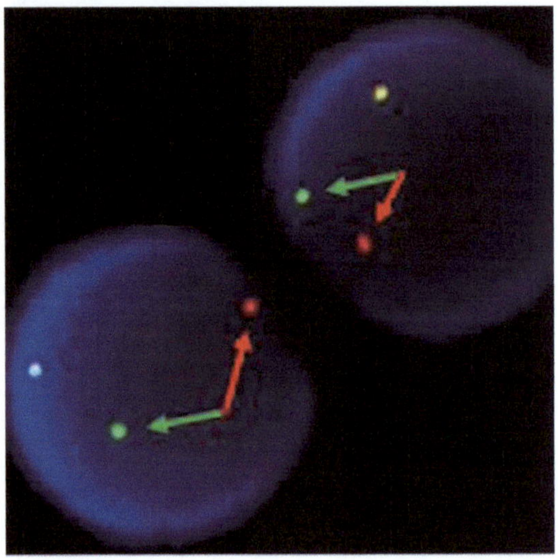

Fig. 2.8 Translocation generated split red–green probe signals (FISH c-Myc dual color break-apart probe by Abbott Molecular courtesy of Dr. Nyla Heerema)

EBV positive [45] but departs from BL by being TdT positive. If leukemic cells are present in the peripheral blood, acute lymphoblastic leukemia/lymphoma, a significantly more common leukemia, must be excluded before proceeding with a BL clinical diagnosis.

DLBCL of the germinal center type is CD44 negative, can have a similar BL immunophenotype with positive CD20, CD10, BCL6 and a high proliferation index in aggressive forms. Tissue areas may be *burkittoid* with cell clustering and phagocytic macrophages. Myc translocation will usually be negative. However, there are

DLBCL with similar BL appearance but with a positive Myc as well as a BCL2 or BCL6 translocations, called *double and triple hit* lymphomas. These DLBCL variants are high grade such as those that arise as relapse from lower grade lymphomas or arise *de novo* and may have a proliferation index >90%. In the activated B-cell DLBCL, the MUM1 positive feature, a positive BCL6 and high proliferation index may be confused with a MUM1-positive BL with a negative CD10, a positive BCL6 and a high proliferation index. EBV-positive DLBCL may also add to the confounding. Accuracy of separation of classic endemic BL from classic DLBCL when both are characteristic is good but clear separation throughout the spectrum of BL from gray zone BL/DLBCL or what has been called *B-cell lymphoma, unclassifiable, with features intermediate between BL and DLBCL* (WHO 2008) remains problematic [46]. The poor clinical response observed with some of the gray zone BL/DLBCL could occur because some of these tumors are genetic BL and require intensive chemotherapy for improved survival or because these tumors are simply very aggressive on their own.

So-called plasmacytoid BL creates a likely confounding with EMP that are EBER positive or negative, have immunoglobulin in their cytoplasm and characteristically have multinucleate and binucleate cells [47]. PBL has similar amphophilic, intermediate-sized cells but with prominent central nucleoli (immunoblastic) in tissue, are usually EBER positive and present prominent "starry sky" morphology. Confounding should be anticipated with smear or tissue morphologic interpretation (Fig. 2.9). The immunophenotypes and cytogenetics of these tumors differ significantly. CD45 and CD20 are always positive in BL, may be positive or negative in EMP while PBL is negative for both. All can be MUM-1 positive but CD138 is negative in BL, negative or weak for PBL and strongly positive for EMP. Myc is positive for both BL and many PBL but PBL has a complex karyotype and EMP is Myc negative. BL may uncommonly have a complex karyotype. It is possible that these plasma cell tumors were reported as BL in past literature using morphology alone, Myc alone or limited biomarkers to constitute a BL study set. As with other confounders, there is less difficulty between endemic BL and the confounders than with the BL variants and their confounders providing there is adequate experience, well-prepared smears and tissue and immunophenotyping and cytogenetics.

Summary

Treatment of BL is urgent due to the late stage of presentation and very short tumor doubling time. Patients risk the onset of tumor lysis syndrome even before the initiation of chemotherapy. An accurate diagnosis of BL requires integration of clinical, morphologic, immunophenotypic and genetic findings, all time consuming and medical laboratory resource intensive. A presumptive diagnosis for purposes of eminent treatment is commonly based on a typical clinical presentation in an at-risk patient. Because most cases of BL occur in resource constrained medical settings in equatorial Africa, clinicians may choose to proceed directly to treatment based on

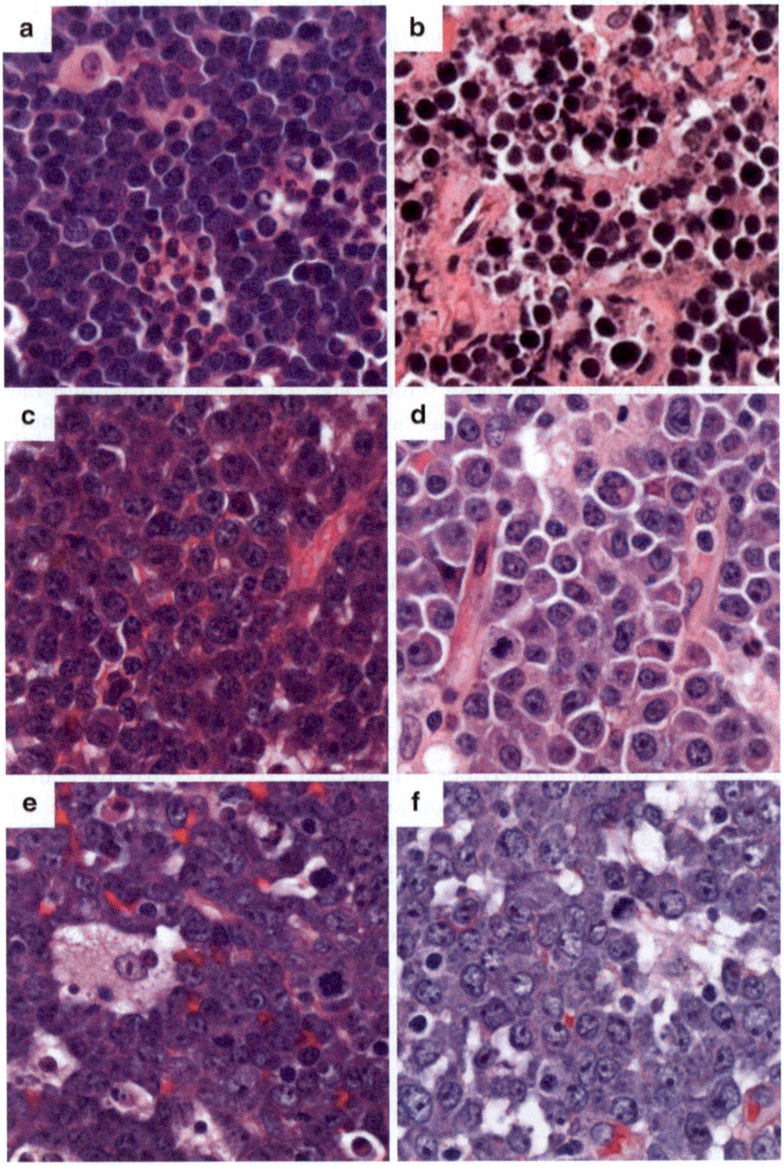

Fig. 2.9 Burkitt lymphoma (*BL*) confounders with diffuse growth of amphophillic, medium-sized cells and differential features: (**a**) BL cells with "squared off" feature, indistinct nucleoli, focal necrosis and (**b**) degenerated infiltrating cells with lost of features; (**c**) extramedullary plasmacytoma with amphophillic, medium-sized cells with indistinct nucleoli and (**d**) another area of this tumor showing plasma cell morphology including binucleate cells with nonspecific "squared off" appearance and central nucleoli; (**e**) plasmablastic lymphoma with diffuse pattern of amphophillic cells and prominent macrophages associated with "starry-sky" along with (**f**) cells showing the prominent PBL central nucleoli

clinical presumption of BL. Retrospective study of clinical presumption in northern Uganda, for example, demonstrated that BL presumption was correct at best in 80% of presumed cases, at worse in 40% of cases [18]. What clearly emerged is the presence in pediatric populations worldwide, including sub-Saharan Africa, of other malignancies that confound the clinical diagnosis of BL in children. Some are non-hematologic malignancies such as Ewing's Complex, undifferentiated neuroblastoma, rhabdomyosarcoma (alveolar, embryonal), synovial cell sarcoma, and renal rhabdoid tumors. Others are critical hematologic malignancies such acute myelogenous leukemia, (pre-T, pre-B) lymphoblastic lymphoma/leukemia, other NHL and Hodgkin's lymphoma that have treatment approaches different from BL. Where tissue was obtained and sent for pathology review, usually not relevant to initial treatment because of the time delay, there was relatively little overall improvement in BL diagnosis based on pathologist evaluation using morphology alone.

Where needle aspiration or biopsy tissue imprint showing characteristic BL cytomorphology is available especially when paired with immunophenotyping results from FC, there is opportunity for improved diagnosis without delay in appropriate treatment [48]. To the extent available, a presumptive clinical diagnosis of BL should be supported by FC of tumor cells for immunophenotype or examination of tissue for histomorphology and immunophenotype along with demonstration of Myc translocation by cytogenetics or FISH break-apart assay. Such full bodied confirmation of BL is usually available in well-resourced medical settings. If timely confirmatory tests are not available for the presumptive BL diagnosis, there should minimally be clinical confirmation of a positive treatment response to intensive chemotherapy within 24 h of initiation. If there is no clinical response within 24 h, then serious review to exclude BL confounders should be initiated.

References

1. Tumwine L, Campidelli C, Righi S, Neda S, Byarugaba W, Pileri S (2008) B-cell non-Hodgkin lymphomas in Uganda: an immunohistochemical appraisal on tissue microarray. Hum Pathol 39(6):817–823
2. Abayomi EA, Somers A, Grewal R, Sissolak G, Bassa F, Maartens D, Jacobs P, Stefan C, Ayers LW (2011) Impact of the HIV epidemic and Anti-Retroviral Treatment policy on lymphoma incidence and subtypes seen in the Western Cape of South Africa, 2002–2009: preliminary findings of the Tygerberg Lymphoma Study Group. Transfus Apher Sci 44(2):161–166
3. Wright D (1999) What is Burkitt's lymphoma and when is it endemic? Blood 93(2):758
4. Yustein JT, Dang CV (2007) Biology and treatment of Burkitt's lymphoma. Curr Opin Hematol. 2007 Jul;14(4):375–81. Review. PMID:17534164
5. Patuto N, Strebel B, Schmitt A, Tutuian R (2010) A gastric moonscape: lymph node penetration from subsequent Burkitt lymphoma after treatment of Hodgkin's lymphoma. Gastrointest Endosc 71(6):1089–1090
6. Wang SM, Huang FC, KO SF, Lee SY, Hsaio CC (2010) Ileocecal Burkitt's lymphoma presenting as ileocolic intussusceptions with appendiceal invagination and acute appendicitis. J Formosan Med Assoc 109(6):476–479
7. Kesik V, Safali M, Citak E, Kismet E, Koseoglu V (2010) Primary gastric Burkitt lymphoma: a rare cause of intraabdominal mass in childhood. Pediatr Surg Int 26(9):927–929

8. Millot F, Barboteau M, Loyer-Lecestre M, Brizard F, Levillain P, Guilhot F (2010) Endoscopic diagnosis of childhood Burkitt's lymphoma of the colon. J Clin Oncol 28(22):e374–e375
9. Amodio J, Brodsky J (2010) Pediatric Burkitt lymphoma presenting as acute pancreatitis: MRI characteristics. Pediatr Radiol 40(5):770–772
10. Aftandilian C, Friedmann A (2010) Burkitt lymphoma with pancreatic involvement. J Pediatr Hematol Oncol 32(8):e338–e340
11. Picarsic J, Jaffe R, Mazariegos G, Webber S, Ellis D, Green M, Reyes-Múgica M (2011) Post-transplant Burkitt lymphoma is a more aggressive and distinct form of post-transplant lymphoproliferative disorder. Cancer 117(19):4540–4550. doi:10.1002/cncr.26001
12. Camera A, Magri F, Fonte R, Villani L, Della Porta MG, Fregoni V, Manna LL, Chiovato L (2010) Burkitt-like lymphoma infiltrating a hyperfunctioning thyroid adenoma and presenting as a hot nodule. Thyroid 20(9):1033–1036
13. Fujiwara H, Odawara J, Hayama B, Takanashi Y, Iwama K, Yamakura M, Takeuchi M, Matsue K (2010) Gross hematopyuria presenting as a first symptom due to the bladder infiltration of extra nodal Burkitt's lymphoma. J Clin Oncol 28(16):e252–e253
14. Ageitos A, Bruno J, Vázquez A, López I, Freire A (2010) [Bilateral primary renal Burkitt lymphoma presenting with acute renal failure]. An Pediatr (Barc) 73(4):199–201 [Article in Spanish]
15. Calbi V, Mawanda M, Ogwang M (2010) Burkitt lymphoma with cutaneous involvement in Uganda. InCTR Network 9(4):21–22
16. Cyriac S, Srinivas L, Mahajan V, Sundersingh S, Sagar T (2010) Primary Burkitt's lymphoma of the ovary. Afr J Paediatr Surg 7(2):120–121
17. Minerbrook M, Schulman P, Budman DR, Teichberg S, Vinciguerra V, Kardon N, Degnan TJ (1982) Burkitt's leukemia. A re-evaluation. Cancer 49:1444–1448
18. Ogwang M, Zhao W, Ayers L, Mbulaiteye S (2011) Accuracy of Burkitt lymphoma diagnosis in constrained pathology settings: importance to epidemiology. Arch Pathol Lab Med 135(4): 445–450
19. Jeffers M, Milton J, Herriot R, McKean M (1998) Fine needle aspiration cytology in the investigation of non Hodgkin's lymphoma. J Clin Pathol 51:189–196
20. Magrath I (1973) Fine needle aspiration in the diagnosis of childhood malignant disease in Uganda. Br J Cancer 28(6):477–487
21. Wright C, Pienaar J, Marais B (2008) Fine needle aspiration biopsy: diagnostic utility in resource-limited settings. Ann Trop Paediatr 28:65–70
22. Van Noorden S, Lampert I, Xue S, Lykidis D, Phillips JA, Molyneux E, Griffin B (2011) Burkitt's lymphoma: maximising the use of fine needle aspirates by long-term preservation for diagnosis and research. Trans R Soc Trop Med Hyg 105(2):86–94
23. McPake B, Mensah K (2008) Task shifting in health care in resource-poor countries. Lancet 372(9642):870–871
24. Dong H, Harris N, Preffer F, Pitman M (2001) Fine-needle aspiration biopsy in the diagnosis and classification of primary and recurrent lymphoma: a retrospective analysis of the utility of cytomorphology and flow cytometry. Mod Pathol 14(5):472–481
25. Mayall F, Darlington A, Harrison B (2003) Fine needle aspiration cytology in the diagnosis of uncommon types of lymphoma. J Clin Pathol 56:821–825
26. Troxell M, Bangs C, Cherry A, Natkunam Y, Kong C (2005) Cytologic diagnosis of Burkitt lymphoma. Cancer 105(5):310–318
27. Swerdlow S, Campo E et al (2008) WHO classification of tumors of haematopoietic and lymphoid tissue. IARC, Lyon
28. Wakely PE Jr. (2010) The diagnosis of non-Hodgkin lymphoma using fine-needle aspiration cytopathology: a work in progress. Cancer Cytopathol. 2010 Oct 25;118(5):238–243. No abstract available. PMID:20737440
29. Howell L (2001) Challenging role of fine needle aspiration in the evaluation of paediatric masses. Diagn Cytopathol 24:65–70
30. Schniederjan S, Li S, Saxe D, Lechowicz M, Lee K, Terry P, Mann K (2010) A novel flow cytometric antibody panel for distinguishing Burkitt lymphoma from CD10+ diffuse large B-cell lymphoma. Am J Clin Pathol 133(5):718–726

31. Savage E, Vanderheyden A, Bell A, Syrbu S, Jensen C (2011) Independent diagnostic accuracy of flow cytometry obtained from fine-needle aspirates: a 10-year experience with 451 cases. Am J Clin Pathol 135(2):304–309
32. Mwanda W, Orem J, Fu P, Banura C, Kakembo J, Onyango C, Ness A, Reynolds S, Johnson J, Subbiah V, Bako J, Wabinga H, Abdallah F, Meyerson H, Whalen C, Lederman M, Black J, Ayers LW, Katongole-Mbidde E, Remick S (2009) Dose-modified oral chemotherapy in the treatment of AIDS-related non-Hodgkin's lymphoma in East Africa. J Clin Oncol 27(21):3480–3488
33. Mochen C, Giardini R, Costa A, Silvestrini R (1997) MIB-1 and S-phase cell fraction predict survival in non-Hodgkin's lymphomas. Cell Prolif 30(1):37–47
34. Ali AE, Morgen EK, Geddie WR, Boerner SL, Massey C, Bailey DJ, da Cunha Santos G. (2010) Classifying B-cell non-Hodgkin lymphoma by using MIB-1 proliferative index in fine-needle aspirates. Cancer Cytopathol. 2010 Jun 25;118(3):166–72. PMID:20544708
35. Kelly GL, Rickinson AB (2007) Burkitt lymphoma: revisting the pathogenesis of a virus-associated malignancy. Hematology Am Soc Hematol Educ Program:277–284
36. Montes-Moreno S, Roncador G, Maestre L, Martínez N, Sanchez-Verde L, Camacho F, Cannata J, Martinez-Torrecuadrada J, Shen Y, Chan W, Piris M (2008) Gcet1 (centerin), a highly restricted marker for a subset of germinal center-derived lymphomas. Blood 111(1): 351–358
37. Attarbaschi A, Mann G, Schumich A, König M, Pickl W, Haas O, Gadner H, Dworzak M (2007) CD44 deficiency is a consistent finding in childhood Burkitt's lymphoma and leukemia. Leukemia 21(5):1110–1113
38. Naresh K, Raphael M, Ayers L, Hurwitz N, Calbi V, Rogena E, Sayed S, Sherman O, Ibrahim H, Lazzi S, Mourmouras V, Rince P, Githanga J, Byakika B, Moshi E, Durosinmi M, Olasode B, Oluwasola OA, Akang E, Akenòva Y, Adde M, Magrath I, Leoncini L (2011) Lymphomas in sub-Saharan Africa - what can we learn and how can we help in improving diagnosis, managing patients and fostering translational research? Br J Haematol. doi:10.1111/j.1365-2141.2011.08772.x
39. Naresh K, Ibrahim H, Lazzi S, Rince P, Onorati M, Ambrosio M, Bilhou-Nabera C, Amen F, Reid A, Mawanda M, Calbi V, Ogwang M, Rogena E, Byakika B, Sayed S, Moshi E, Mwakigonja A, Raphael M, Magrath I, Leoncini L (2011) Diagnosis of Burkitt lymphoma using an algorithmic approach - applicable in both resource-poor and resource-rich countries. Br J Haematol. doi:10.1111/j.1365-2141.2011.08771.x
40. Leucci E, Cocco M, Onnis A, De Falco G, van Cleef P, Bellan C, van Rijk A, Nyagol J, Byakika B, Lazzi S, Tosi P, van Krieken H, Leoncini L (2008) MYC translocation-negative classical Burkitt lymphoma cases: an alternative pathogenetic mechanism involving miRNA deregulation. J Pathol 216(4):440–450
41. Sevilla DW, Gong JZ, Goodman BK, Buckley PJ, Rosoff P, Gockerman JP, Lagoo AS (2007) Clinicopathologic findings in high-grade B-cell lymphomas with typical Burkitt morphologic features but lacking the MYC translocation. Am J Clin Pathol 128(6):981–991
42. Hasserjian R, Ott G, Elenitoba-Johnson K, Balague-Ponz O, de Jong D, de Leval L (2009) Commentary on the WHO classification of tumors of lymphoid tissues (2008): "Gray zone" lymphomas overlapping with Burkitt lymphoma or classical Hodgkin lymphoma. J Hematop 2:89–95. doi:10.1007/s12308-009-0039-7
43. Dave S, Fu K, Wright G, Lam L, Kluin P, Boerma E, Greiner T, Weisenburger D, Rosenwald A, Ott G, Müller-Hermelink H, Gascoyne R, Delabie J, Rimsza L, Braziel R, Grogan T, Campo E, Jaffe E, Dave B, Sanger W, Bast M, Vose J, Armitage J, Connors J, Smeland E, Kvaloy S, Holte H, Fisher R, Miller T, Montserrat E, Wilson W, Bahl M, Zhao H, Yang L, Powell J, Simon R, Chan W, Staudt L (2006) Molecular diagnosis of Burkitt's lymphoma. N Engl J Med 354(23):2431–2442
44. Piccaluga P, De Falco G, Kustagi M, Gazzola A, Agostinelli C, Tripodo C, Leucci E, Onnis A, Astolfi A, Sapienza M, Bellan C, Lazzi S, Tumwine L, Mawanda M, Ogwang M, Calbi V, Formica S, Califano A, Pileri S, Leoncini L (2011) Gene expression analysis uncovers similarity and differences among Burkitt lymphoma subtypes. Blood 117(13):3596–3608

45. Sehgal S, Mujtaba S, Gupta D, Aggarwal R, Marwaha R (2010) High incidence of Epstein Barr virus infection in childhood acute lymphocytic leukemia: a preliminary study. Indian J Pathol Microbiol 53(1):63–67
46. Salaverria I, Siebert R. (2011) The gray zone between Burkitt's lymphoma and diffuse large B-cell lymphoma from a genetics perspective. J Clin Oncol. 2011 May 10;29(14):1835–1843. Epub 2011 Apr 11. Review. PMID:21482997
47. Yan B, Tan SY, Yau EX, Ng SB, Petersson F (2011) EBV-positive plasmacytoma of the submandibular gland-Report of a rare case with molecular genetic characterization. Head Neck Pathol 5(4):389–394
48. Tumwine L, Agostinelli C, Campidelli C, Othieno E, Wabinga H, Righi S, Falini B, Piccaluga P, Byarugaba W, Pileri S (2009) Immunohistochemical and other prognostic factors in B cell non Hodgkin lymphoma patients, Kampala, Uganda. BMC Clin Pathol 16(9):11

Chapter 3
Burkitt's Lymphoma: A View from the Bedside

Esther Lehman Kawira and Sam M. Mbulaiteye

Introduction

Burkitt's lymphoma clinical presentation is dramatic and always leaves an indelible memory. Typically, it presents as rapidly growing masses on the head or face—usually on the lower or upper jaw or around the eye. These growths may or may not be associated with other rapidly growing masses involving abdominal organs. Head or face and abdominal growths can erupt separately or simultaneously. Untreated, patients die. It was this dramatic presentation, and indelible memories it imparted, that compelled Dr. Denis Burkitt, after seeing several children when working at a rural hospital in the then Lango District of Uganda, to review clinical and autopsy records at Mulago Hospital, the largest hospital in Uganda, for all cases bearing similar symptoms and signs for clues about the nature of disease. He discovered that tumors, which hitherto were considered different because they erupted at different anatomic sites, shared the same characteristic of rapid progression, and concluded that they represented the same disease occurring at different sites—the disease now bearing his name—Burkitt's lymphoma [1]. Histological examination of tumor tissues revealed the disease to be a B-cell lymphoma and confirmed Burkitt's single-disease hypothesis.

In follow-up studies, Burkitt conducted a letter survey of doctors working at different hospitals in different regions of Africa—asking them whether they recalled treating children with rapidly growing facial tumors. His results established the geographic and climatic range of the lymphoma and became the basis for

E.L. Kawira
Shirati Health Education and Development (SHED) Foundation and EMBLEM Study,
P.O. Box 39, Shirati, Tanzania
e-mail: elkawira@gmail.com

S.M. Mbulaiteye (✉)
Division of Cancer Epidemiology and Genetics, 6120 Executive Blvd, Executive Plaza South,
Rm. 7080, Rockville Md, 20852
e-mail: mbulaits@mail.nih.gov

E.S. Robertson (ed.), *Burkitt's Lymphoma*, Current Cancer Research,
DOI 10.1007/978-1-4614-4313-1_3, © Springer Science+Business Media New York 2013

proposing by Haddow, an entomologist working at the East African Virus Research Institute in Entebbe, Uganda, the hypothesis that malaria, whose distribution tracked that of Burkitt's lymphoma, may be etiologically causal. Burkitt's lymphoma is not a new disease to Africa: a review of medical records at Mengo Hospital revealed a score of cases bearing the typical presentation recorded by Albert Cook, a pioneering missionary doctor in Uganda. Wood carvings depicting huge jaw tumors on the face, seen in far places such as Maputo in Mozambique or Lagos in Nigeria, have confirmed this view that Burkitt's lymphoma has afflicted Africans for long and left indelible memories in different cultures.

Today, when so much more is known about Burkitt's lymphoma [2–4], the view from the bedside is still largely an African view, as the great majority of cases occur there. While careful study of Burkitt's lymphoma, relying on its dramatic impression on clinicians and communities, gave a broadly informative picture of the disease, this picture is not complete and not very accurate. We believe clinical impressions have a role to play in the education and care of patients with Burkitt's lymphoma. In this chapter, we will share views from different perspectives, including the doctor, the parent, child, and nurse that span the Burkitt's lymphoma experience. We believe that these bedside views, rarely emphasized in modern teaching, are relevant to the understanding and wholesome treatment of Burkitt's lymphoma in the current modern era as they were in bygone days.

A Doctor's View

In the African setting, Burkitt's lymphoma involving the face, head, and abdomen is relatively easy to suspect and diagnose. With medical experience and a high index of suspicion, a clinical diagnosis can be presumed and the child referred to centers where cytology can be done and treatment given [5].

When I see, for the first time, a patient newly diagnosed with Burkitt's lymphoma, I see that here is a child I can treat and cure in a relatively straightforward manner. The face, though hugely distorted by tumor, will return to normal. The teeth loosened by tumor will become solid. The blind eye will see again. The abdomen distended by tumor masses and fluid will reduce to normal. The gait disturbance or paralysis of lower limbs will disappear, and the child will walk again. I can actually start feeling a kinship with the Almighty, as doctors are often accused of doing.

Burkitt's lymphoma is curable, but in Africa, the tumor frequently is fatal because of lack of effective treatment [6, 7]. In a child, the cure of an otherwise fatal illness saves many life years compared to cure of illness in elderly patients. That is true no matter what the illness. The life of a child is often not counted for much in Africa, especially in settings where child death from various causes is not that unusual. The acute illnesses of malaria, pneumonia, and diarrhea account for many more deaths than Burkitt's lymphoma, just because they are so much more frequent, and they are cheaper to treat. Not surprisingly, when resources are scarce, they will be devoted to these other illnesses and not for Burkitt's lymphoma, even if it is curable [6–9]. People don't think in terms of life years saved or lost. But as a doctor, even so, treating and curing a child with Burkitt's lymphoma is especially gratifying and, I know, restores many life-years to that child. It also helps to increase the confidence of the whole family and clan in modern medical treatment, reduce the belief in witchcraft and spells as the causes of terrible diseases (Fig. 3.1).

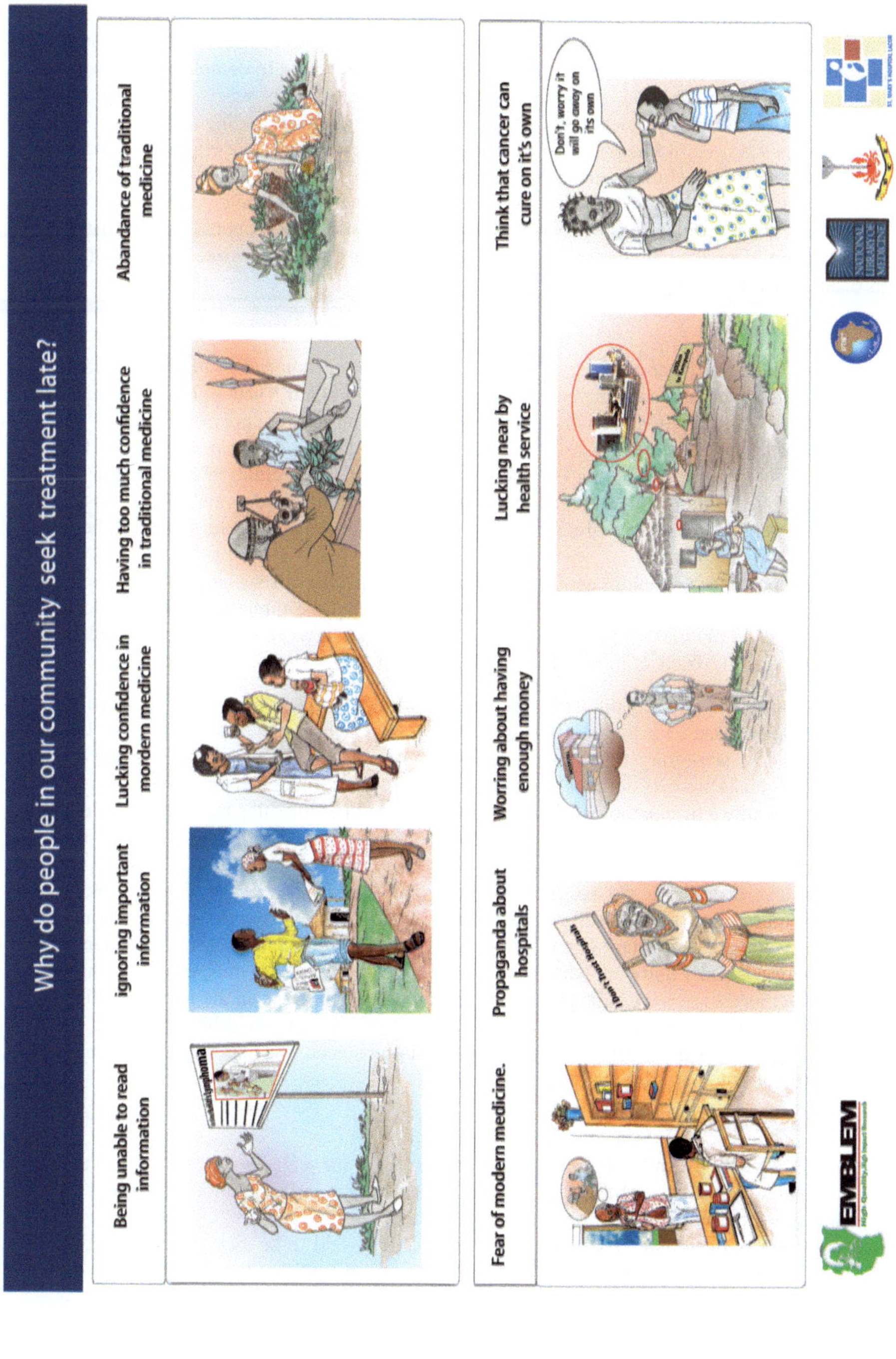

Fig. 3.1 A collection of drawings developed to assist nurses and doctors explain to patients the misconceptions about Burkitt's lymphoma in East Africa

Burkitt's lymphoma responds quickly and, usually, completely to chemotherapy alone. Radiation is not required. Surgery is usually indicated for diagnosis only. Usually, the child appears essentially well after the first round of chemotherapy. Ironically, this quick response often reduces compliance with the full course of chemotherapy. It is human nature to fail to remember final antibiotic or malarial doses when one is feeling well. Therefore, a parent of a child with Burkitt's lymphoma may decide not to bring the child to complete for chemotherapy doses when the child looks well, especially when the family survives only hand to mouth. Completion of treatment requires careful and continued counseling (Fig. 3.2).

Families whose child responds to treatment are understandably grateful to the doctor who treated them. The child's condition would have led them to assume that the child will die; their expectations of this terrible outcome would have been averted. Child death is still very common, from common illnesses such as malaria. With Burkitt's lymphoma, and its distortion of the child's body with tumor, and its relentless increase over a few weeks, expectation of death is that much higher.

Zebras in Indiana?

One year when I [EK] was working as a family physician in my home town in Indiana, USA, parents from the rural farming community nearby brought their 8 year old boy to see me. The boy had been having increasing difficulty in walking over the previous 3 days.

Except for the leg weakness, I found nothing remarkable on general examination. The symptoms being serious, I quickly referred the boy to the state children's hospital in the capital. Later, I found out that scanning had revealed a spinal cord tumor. The neurosurgeons opened him up for a biopsy, and the histopathology diagnosis turned out to be... Burkitt's lymphoma!

Of all the doctors who could have happened to see him initially, it was me, who had seen many children with Burkitt's lymphoma in Africa...and the thought of this diagnosis never crossed my mind. The old axiom is correct that when you hear hoof beats, think of zebras, yes, in Africa, but not in Indiana!"

As a doctor and an academician, I know that Burkitt's lymphoma is part of a heterogeneous group of diseases called non-Hodgkin lymphomas, which can be sub-classified into subtypes in the laboratory using methods beyond routine histology available in Africa. Clinical diagnosis alone is not ideal, or even sufficient, for optimal care and research studies, which require a firm pathologic diagnosis to be made [4]. Obtaining tissue for histology is invasive for the patient, sometimes complex for the doctor, so it is often dispensed with.

But even as a doctor concerned for the sensibilities of the child patient, I can support more invasive diagnostics if I see the potential good, for instance, if we were be able to detect subtypes that would actually need different chemotherapy from the start. Currently, we end up with some resistant or early relapse cases that we refer for second line chemotherapy without really knowing why this tumor relapsed compared to most others. Perhaps a different, more aggressive subtype was the reason. For the present, in the African setting, the chemotherapy drugs used are the same for all Burkitt's lymphoma, differing only in the number of cycles given for early (the minority) versus advanced (the majority) cases, which is a clinical decision at present [7, 8].

A tumor tolerant to delay

This tiny underweight child of age 3 years was brought to me with a swollen abdomen and a palpable left kidney. The child had been treated a year earlier at another hospital for Burkitt's lymphoma, but the parents had defaulted.

The family was in trouble. The child's mother was also said to be sick, and admitted at another facility. The father and the older brother promised that they would bring the child faithfully for chemotherapy treatments, but could not leave him at my facility as there was no family member who could stay with him.

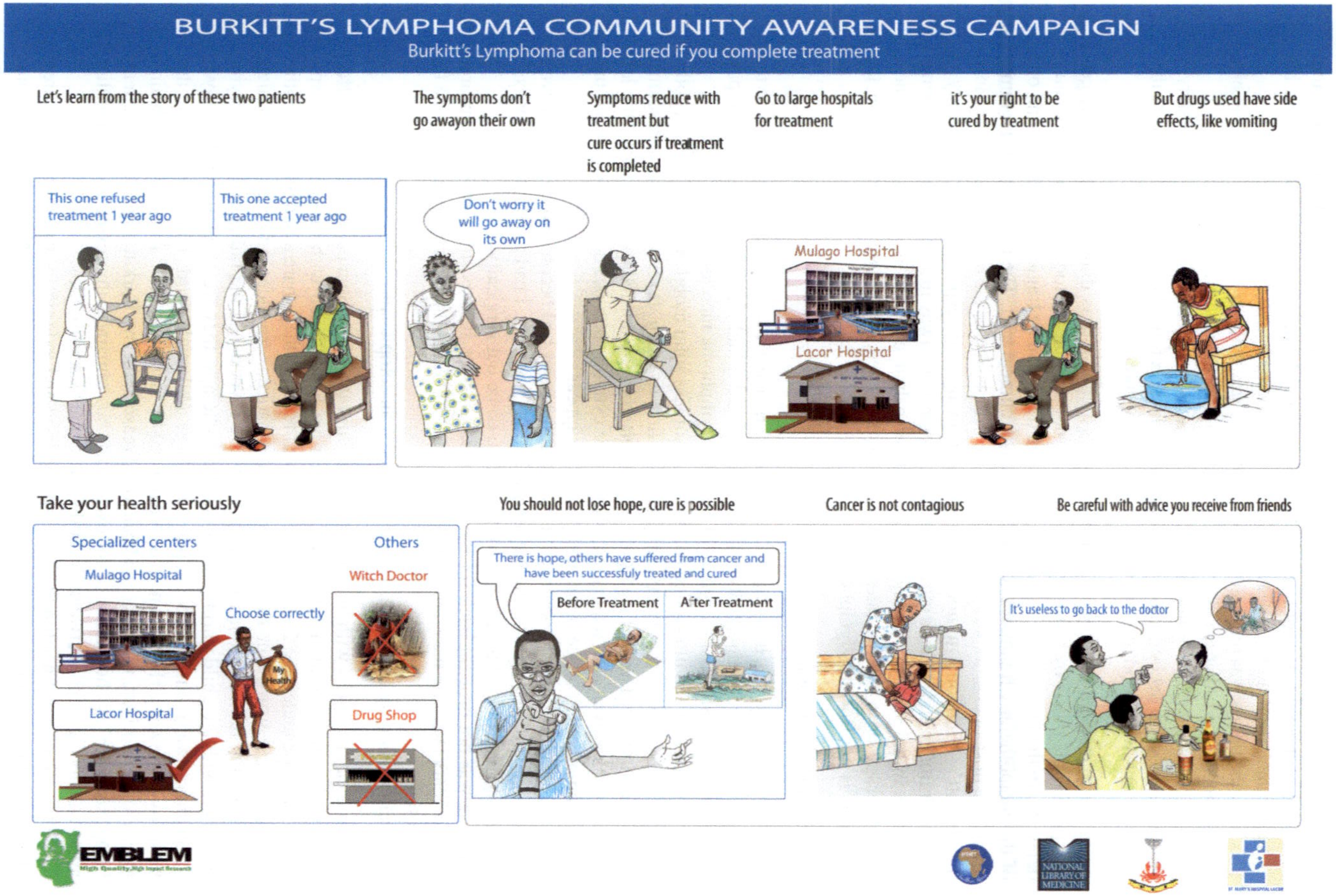

Fig. 3.2 A collection of drawings developed to assist nurses and doctors in East Africa to explain the process of treating Burkitt's lymphoma to patients

I gave round one of chemotherapy, and the child was taken away. He was not brought back, and since his condition had been so poor, I assumed he must have died.

A year later I was astonished when the child was brought to me again- to get his next round of chemotherapy! The one dose of chemotherapy I had given him had reduced his abdominal swelling for a year, but it had finally come back.

This time, the family was prepared to have the mother stay with her child for the full 12 weeks. He finished the full chemotherapy course, and all the palpable tumor went away.

A few months later, his tumor recurred, and he was brought back to me immediately. I referred him for second line chemotherapy at a large referral hospital. He completed that treatment, with good response, and is apparently cured.

In many medical settings in Africa, Burkitt's lymphoma is diagnosed clinically; getting precise diagnosis by histology is frequently not possible, or too costly, or would cause delay [5]. In the face of such rapid tumor growth, delay can be tragic. Therefore, round one of the chemotherapy treatment is often given as a clinical trial. The response of the tumor to this one dose of chemotherapy strengthens the impression of the clinical diagnosis. Since the Burkitt's lymphoma tumor is so rapidly growing, the response to chemotherapy is equally dramatic and appears miraculous. The tumor melts away in a few days, and, depending on its initial size, there may be no visible or palpable tumor by the time of the next chemotherapy dose a week later. If this does not happen, the doctor may reconsider the diagnosis is not Burkitt's lymphoma.

Is it Burkitt's lymphoma?

This 7 year old boy was brought by his mother, who gave a vague history of a mass in the abdomen since age three. However, when she said it had gotten a lot larger in the past 2 months, my index of suspicion of Burkitt's lymphoma increased.

My physical exam and ultrasound confirmed a painless solid mobile mass in the mid abdomen of about 10 × 15 cm size. The mass felt firm to touch. It reminded me of a splenecule, and in fact I wasn't sure there was a spleen in the normal location, above the left kidney. However, after a questionably positive cytology report, I decided to give a round of chemotherapy to see if the mass would disappear.

After the chemotherapy, I convinced myself that the mass had become smaller, and gave a second and third round of chemotherapy. Finally, however, I had to admit that it wasn't really going away. I decided it would need to come out surgically.

The boy was not brought back for the scheduled time for surgery. Instead, he reappeared two years later, the mass still present and a bit larger, but the patient none the worse for waiting.

Surgical excision by a visiting surgeon revealed…an ectopic spleen!

There can be issues with hospitalization of Burkitt's lymphoma patients that are different than for other children. Most sick children are hospitalized with their mothers, especially for those under age 2 and still being breast fed, and they share a bed with the mother in the pediatric ward. But Burkitt's lymphoma patients are older, and are often brought initially by the father. In one rural hospital where I worked, if the father ended up staying overnight with the child during the initial chemotherapy, they were not allowed to stay in the pediatric ward, but were being put in the large adult male ward. Thus it turned out that both boy and even girl children were surrounded by sick adult men. I managed to obtain a private or semiprivate room for medical/social reasons for my Burkitt's lymphoma patients being cared for by the father, at no extra cost, but remained impressed by the conflict, almost always ignored, between the child's and carer's sensibilities.

When we do have a setup that can provide food and lodging for the child and a parent during the three months, it is a great way to build trust with them. Normally they would never have seen a doctor before, much less have a close relationship over time. In the village, the doctor's role would be filled by the neighbors and the local traditional healer.

And naturally, those familiar and trusted and nearby would have been consulted first about this illness, sometimes causing harmful or fatal delay.

Waiting Too Long

This seven year old boy was carried into my clinic by several adult men. Seeing them approaching, we steered them directly to a bed. The boy was very ill and in a poor condition. He had been unable to walk for two months, I was told, and the family had been seeking treatment at a dispensary and also using local herbs.

Now he had severe pressure sores over sacrum and trochanters. He was thin, but had edema of the face and upper body from superior vena cava syndrome. In the abdomen, I could palpate hugely enlarged kidneys. One testis was also enlarged.

With such severe and neglected Burkitt's lymphoma, we really had no chance.

I cleaned the sores, cautiously hydrated, gave antibiotics, and gave round one of chemotherapy. I was gratified that the edema reduced and the kidney enlargement reduced. However, probably overwhelmed by sepsis and biochemical complications from very advanced disease, he died after about two weeks.

The best I could hope for this patient was that the parents would see our love and concern for their child, but the odds were stacked against us, and that there was indeed response to our drugs. Perhaps next time another child from that village will be brought to me sooner.

This case also illustrates the need for specialized pediatric oncology centers [6]. Such centers would have specialized staff and equipment to care for some of the sickest children. The complications of advanced cancer, especially in an African child, are myriad. In addition to sepsis, malnutrition, and common infections, like malaria, there is increased danger of tumor lysis syndrome when initially treating children who, like this patient, have delayed coming to medical attention and therefore have a large tumor burden.

If the treatment goes well, in a facility based setting, then I think there could be good opportunity to enrich the child's life, not to mention the parents, since most of the time the child is feeling well after the initial chemotherapy. If we could have videos, television, books, games, play materials available, this would be ideal. But so far, we are doing well if we manage to treat the illness well, and that of course has first priority. I do see children inventing their own games and amusements when, as usual, left to their own devices.

A Parent's View

"This illness, Burkitt's lymphoma, is VERY different from any other disease I have known to occur in my children. I am familiar with malaria, cold, pneumonia, and diarrhea. Those illnesses I expect to occur, even frequently, in all children. With the right treatment, the child gets better within a week or less.

Then, along came something else entirely. It caused disfigurement of my child's face that even the neighbors could see from a distance. It did not go away by itself, like a cold does, but continued and got worse", (Fig. 3.1).

"We went with her to a drug shop, and they said she had a tooth problem. In fact her teeth were loose in the swelling area, and one had fallen out just like that. They gave us treatment, but it didn't help." (*note - for Burkitt's lymphoma in the mouth, often there has been delay because the problem is suspected to be a dental infection. With chemotherapy, the teeth firm up, and do not need extraction, though unfortunately they are often extracted prior to presentation to the doctor*).

"We then suspected witchcraft could be responsible (Fig. 3.1). We took our child to a traditional healer to find out who was causing this illness. But our child just got worse, and we got no answers." (*note - for illness that is severe or persistent, the thought of witchcraft is normally somewhere in the parent's mind*).

Finally we heard that this illness is treated in a place farther away (Fig. 3.1). It took us some time to collect enough money to make the journey. By that time our child was really very sick, and we were losing hope.

A scourge for the poor?

In front of a group of visiting medical students from the U.S., a child was brought into the exam room who had the most distorted face I [EK] had ever seen. This is saying a lot, as I have seen and treated Burkitt's lymphoma for years.

The mother's tale was one of delay due to being a poor widow and the lack of travel money. Being from across the nearby border with Kenya, she had been advised to take the child to a major western Kenyan city, but did not have the money. Finally, someone advised her to come to my clinic, a shorter journey for her, and she had managed to scrape together the funds. Meanwhile, however, the tumor had grown frighteningly large. I was sure the child could no longer eat normally, or even breathe comfortably.

The child sat placidly and posed for photos, and agreed for smiley face stickers to be stuck onto her forehead and forearms. I cautioned the students not to show her the photos of how she looked. The mother, a good looking woman herself, sighed as she looked at Jacinta and said, "She used to be beautiful".

"She will be beautiful again", I told the mother.

The medical students, except for one, left the next day. The one who stayed longer documented for the others, by daily photos, the return of Jacinta's face to normal over the following week.

"Finally our child was seen by a doctor; we were told she has a cancer. The doctor told us the cancer was not just in her face, but in her abdomen. We had only seen the swelling in her face. We didn't think her abdomen was any bigger than usual in children." (*note - abdominal tumors can grow large unrecognized, as the natural lordosis plus worms or, in some areas, schistosomiasis, with hepatosplenomegaly, cause many village children to have protuberant abdomens*).

We were dismayed when we were told that the treatment takes three months. (*This is not as long as treatment for TB, that takes six months, but most of them have never known a child on TB treatment, much less one on HIV treatment for life….so dealing with this long treatment is a new experience and a significant burden.*)

We were told that the treatment would make our child have nausea, maybe vomit much (Fig. 3.2), for a few days. But what we saw- the swollen face went away-was like magic! Our child was able to eat again, and even started getting up, walking around, playing, being interested in life.

Difficult choices

By the time this child was brought to me, she had been to several other western and traditional medicine facilities without help. She had become thin, with stick limbs and a wizened face, but with a hugely swollen abdomen. She was also very pale from severe anemia. My exam revealed the palpably enlarged kidneys, most likely due to Burkitt's lymphoma.

She responded well to chemotherapy, and became a happy playful child around the hostel where she stayed with her mother.

Later the mother revealed to us, "We thought she would die".

"It looked like our child was well, and yet they said more treatment was needed. It was hard to see why, when our child now looked okay. We were supposed to bring the child every fortnight for treatment, but it wasn't easy to travel so much. It was costly, and we were barely feeding our other children. We wanted to do what the doctors said, but many times we just couldn't manage. Once we missed a treatment because one of our older children died and we had to bury him. We told the doctors why we missed, but they said we should have found someone to bring our child anyway." (*note - treating an apparently well child with toxic drugs is counter – intuitive to the parents, and needs careful explanation before and during chemotherapy, to encourage and support parents*).

"Once our child got fever at home between the chemotherapy treatments, so we took her to the local dispensary and they treated her for malaria. But when we told her cancer doctors later, they said we should have been brought her to them. They said her fever could be more serious than for other children without cancer, because her drugs for Burkitt's lymphoma weaken her immune system. But to us she looks just the same, and it looked like the usual malaria our other children get." (*note - understanding of suppressed immunity during chemotherapy is also counter-intuitive, and parents can delay returning when a Burkitt's lymphoma child becomes sick at home if being treated as an outpatient. Children who survive Burkitt's lymphoma remain at risk of death from malaria*).

"One good thing is that we don't have to pay for the treatment drugs, even though we still have to find money for all that travel back and forth. We were told that the drugs are very expensive, I don't know how expensive." (*note - in some settings the cost of drugs is supported by donors. The actual cost would often be more than a village family's annual income several times over, if they had to pay it.*)

"We usually get help from our clan when something like this comes along. The clan is used to contributing money when someone dies, or when someone wants to get married. But for illness in a child, they don't usually help out. And the doctors said we needed the treatment right away. We couldn't wait to collect money from people. So far, we are managing to take her for most of the treatments. We remember how sick she was, and how she got better so quickly, so we want to do what the doctors say, even if to us it doesn't always make sense and it is hard for us".

A (Child) Patient's View

"I don't feel like playing or going to school. I just want to stay in bed. It is hard to walk around. And I don't want to eat because my mouth hurts when I try." (*note - when parents bring a sick child to the doctor they often carry them but don't mention the fact. The doctor, if seeing the child in a bed, may not realize that the child is unable to walk. A child may actually have stopped walking due to being paralyzed from tumor, rather than just being unable or unwilling to walk around due to general debilitation and wasting. I always ask if the child can walk normally.*)

Life is not fun any more!

A concerned father brought his 10 year old daughter to my clinic. Though they happened to live very close by, he said he had carried her on the back of his bicycle. She was too weak to walk for the past few days, he said. There had been a heated family discussion about whether to take her to the traditional healer or bring her to me (Fig. 3.1), but fortunately they decided on me.

My exam revealed that the child could stand unsteadily, and was able to walk slowly, with a wide based stagger, for very short distance. There was no other definite finding, except that a dipstick showed blood in the urine.

Further diagnostics not being possible, and suspecting Burkitt's lymphoma in our setting, I started chemotherapy on her. Within a week she was walking normally again, and the blood disappeared from her urine. She completed the twelve week chemotherapy course without any further problems.

"I heard my parents saying that I used to be beautiful, but now I'm ugly. I feel like I have let them down, but I don't know why." (*note - children are often oblivious to facial disfigurement, even gross disfigurement, because there are no mirrors in the village, but of course they are exquisitely aware of comments*).

"People think maybe I can't see any more, but I can still see ok." (*note - child, and often parents, are oblivious of loss of eyesight in one eye, or don't consider it an emergency, since the child can still see from the unaffected eye*).

Light disappeared from my life!

A tall, dignified older woman walked into my consultation room and announced, "My grandson can't see for the past three days".

Looking up, I saw, trailing behind her and groping the walls for guidance, a boy of about six years of age. Further history revealed that he had a swelling abdomen for about two months, plus early swelling in one eye.

On physical exam I noted large fungating tumors on both sides of the palate, and a large abdominal mass. I suspected Burkitt's lymphoma and made a clinical diagnosis. I also thought the loss of sight was related to Burkitt's lymphoma. To save this child's eyesight, I prepared the child for chemotherapy and begun administering it within 24 hours.

After one day, the grandmother remarked, "He can see a little bit".

After two days the grandmother told me, "He can see a lot now".

After three days, the grandmother informed me, "He can see normally again"!

I wondered later what would have happened if this young boy had had Burkitt's lymphoma in only one eye, instead of both, and hadn't gone totally blind. Likely there would have been a much longer delay in bringing him for treatment.

A few months later, when he had finished his course of chemotherapy and was doing well, and seeing well, his father presented me with a chicken as a gift. I don't always eat gift chickens myself, but I made an exception of this one.

"I don't feel THAT bad. Not like malaria, when my head hurts and my body hurts and I feel hot. And I'm not coughing or having diarrhea. I just don't feel ok." (*note - this sub-acute nature of the illness also contributes to lag time until presentation*).

"I haven't gone to school for a while. I might go next year if I get better." (*with a persistent illness like Burkitt's lymphoma, most children by the time of presentation have left school. This is not a big issue to parents or children, and they simply resume the following year, repeating the missed year. Children get delayed or interrupted schooling for many reasons other than Burkitt's lymphoma, so it is not the issue that it would usually be in western countries, where schooling is even carried on in inpatient wards when the child is able*).

"I heard my parents saying they think I might die." (*note again - children overhear comments*).

I was scared when my parents took me on a long journey to the hospital. I never rode in a bus before, but that was fun. We went fast. I had only been carried on a bicycle before. At the hospital I saw a white person, and I got really afraid. My friend at home told me that white people will eat you. When they tried to make me lie down on a table, I fought as hard as I could. Even my dad tried to hold me down. They finally decided to let me go. I'm glad I fought so hard. I was afraid all the rest of the day, and I stayed as far away from that white person as I could.

I was Happy

I had just diagnosed this 6 year old child as having Burkitt's lymphoma. I had recently moved to my own clinic, so I was still giving intrathecal methotrexate myself, not having yet taught my nurse how to do it.

Happy was NOT happy, when we tried to position her for the intrathecal injection. In fact, she started screaming and writhing. When even her father jumped into the fray and tried to help hold her down without success, I soon saw that it was a losing battle.

"Back off", I told everyone. "We aren't going to do it this way".
"She is scared of white people", my nurse reluctantly revealed to me.
I decided then that instead of terrorizing Happy, I would have my nurse give her ketamine and have her soundly asleep before I ever entered the room.
It worked like a dream. Happy was still and relaxed. She could be positioned properly so that I could get the needle in the right place easily. And best of all, I was far away by the time she woke up.
Over time, Happy got accustomed to my face, and no longer feared me. I continue to use ketamine for many of the younger patients, for whom chemotherapy is therefore just a dreamlike experience.

"Lots of things in the hospital I never saw before. You flip a switch and a light comes on. I started flipping it on and off, on and off, till the nurse made me stop. And you turn a handle and water comes out. At home my mom has to walk a long way and bring back a bucket of water on her head. And here in the hospital, I take a bath in a special room, even short call or long call you have to do in a special room with a shiny hole in the floor. At home, we have to go outside to a latrine, even at night when it is scary." (*the hospital environment is often very different than home for the patients, even before considering the white coats, needle sticks, and aroma of alcohol*).

A Nurse's View

"Families who bring children with Burkitt's lymphoma need a lot of counseling. They are confused and bewildered by the disease. Many have heard of cancer and assume it means death. To be told that their child has cancer is a big blow, and I have to spend enough time reassuring them that this cancer is treatable and curable. They really want to trust what I say. But the thing that makes them really trust me is when they see the response to the first chemotherapy treatment.

I like that I can go ahead and treat this serious illness by myself, once the doctor has calculated the dosages of the drugs. Starting an intravenous line, giving intravenous fluids and drugs, observing for need of drugs for nausea- these are all routine nursing procedures, and they aren't very scary for the child or the parents. The thing that seems scarier, though, is giving the intrathecal drug. If I see that a child is very intimidated even by starting an intravenous, then I alert the doctor and we give the intrathecal drug under ketamine anesthetic. But if I see that a child is old enough, and mature enough, to cooperate well, then we just give intrathecal without anesthesia. Most children are younger, however, and do better when they don't know or remember what happened. They just wake up a bit later like after a nap, and get up and go to play as before.

The doctor taught me how to give the intrathecal injection, and it didn't take long to learn. Now I just give it myself. We just need to make sure that the child doesn't eat or drink anything if they need the anesthetic first".

They are children, again

These two Burkitt's lymphoma patients presented about the same time, and were undergoing chemotherapy together. They also got into mischief together. One was the 6 year old boy who came blind in both eyes, and now was able to see who was the ringleader and a 5 year old boy David, who was the devoted follower.
One day we noticed that the middle of David's back was covered with a patch of blistered and rashy skin.
I finally figured out that the two boys had been playing doctor. One boy, the "doctor", had "washed" the other's back in preparation for intrathecal injection.

It appeared they had used some kind of irritating poison ivy type of leaf that caused his skin to break out. This causes us to delay the intrathecal chemotherapy for the "patient" boy by a few weeks while it healed.

Giving the three iv drugs, iv fluids, plus the intrathecal drug takes several hours of time, but we only need to do it all once every two weeks. On alternate weeks they just get the intrathecal drug, and that doesn't take long. They don't need iv fluid for that. So we just make out a schedule and plan to set aside the needed time, and that makes it go smoothly. Even if we have more than one patient on treatment, we can treat them all the same day of the week for the follow-up treatments.

We do warn the family about side effects of the drugs, especially nausea (Fig. 3.2). For that, we routinely give an antiemetic drug along with the chemotherapy drugs to try to prevent that symptom. Once in a while a child gets sores in the mouth, and we just give them liquid pain medication and wait it out. Rarely severe and fatal complications can occur.

Even in sickness, they teach us

This five year old child presented with classic Burkitt's lymphoma swelling of the right orbit and left mandible. She responded well to chemotherapy, and had already finished five of the six courses. Her mother, aunt, and older sibling had been taking turns staying with her.

Suddenly, over the course of a few days, she developed blistering of small areas, then large sheets, of skin. A visiting nursing student who had worked in a burn unit in the US told us it looked like TENS (toxic epidermal necrolysis syndrome). I had to look it up in my books, as I had never seen such a condition before.

I am sure that was the right diagnosis, and it could have been related to the chemotherapy or to the underlying tumor, out of the many possible causes listed.

Sadly, she died within three days, in spite of our attempts to treat what in the US would have been intensive care, referral burn unit level treatment with a guarded prognosis.

Of course children usually lose their hair, but that is not a big deal here. So many younger children have their heads routinely shaved anyway, that people are used to seeing all or most children bald. But it does bother some of the older girl patients. Sometimes they do have hair to start with, and then they see it falling out. Usually they just ask me to shave off the rest, and they are happy when I assure them that it will grow back later. Most of the patients are still primary school age, and primary schools require girl students to have short hair anyway, I guess so they don't waste a lot of time braiding each other's hair instead of studying.

I am usually the one who needs to help the family discuss things related to the treatment support. The first major issue is who can be available to stay with the child. Sometimes they try to leave an older child as the companion, but we don't usually allow that, especially when that child ought to be in school. For mothers, the issue is usually that they have other children at home to care for. But with our extended family system being the norm, sometimes the mother can be able to stay during treatment with her Burkitt's lymphoma child if a co-wife or sister- in- law or grandmother is there at home to take care of her other children. If a younger child is still breast-feeding, we sometimes find that the mother has brought it to the ward to stay with her and the Burkitt's lymphoma child patient (Fig. 3.3). We try to discourage that also, because of increased risk of childhood infections being passed around…on the other had we do support prolonged breast feeding…so sometimes we just let them all stay, if there is no other better way.

The main thing that makes Burkitt's lymphoma patients special for me as a nurse is that I really get to know the patient and the family well, because we are together for such a long time. I get to know their family problems and relationship issues. They really need emotional support more than other families, because of the long treatment required. I have to encourage them to stick with it, to get a good outcome. They really thank me, later. And if they have grown to like and trust me and the other staff, they are happier to make the effort to come for the follow-up visits even if the child is doing fine.

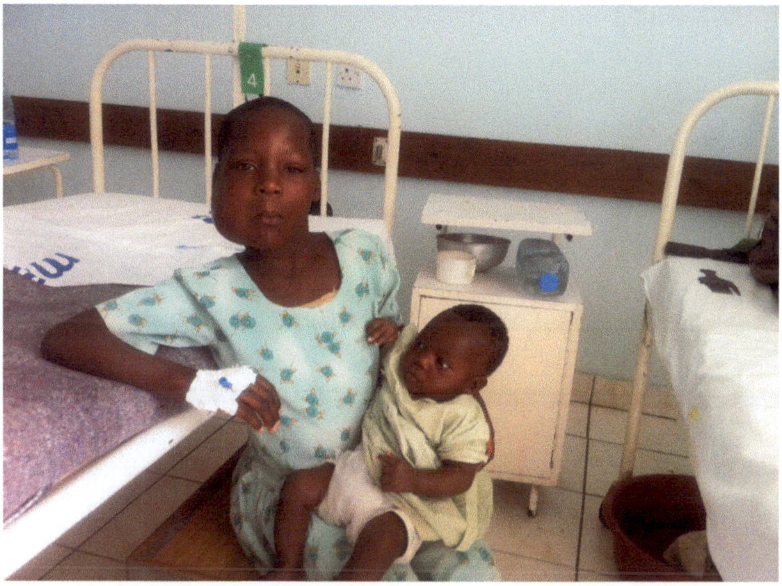

Fig. 3.3 A child with Burkitt's lymphoma helping to care for her younger sibling. Please note familial Burkitt's lymphoma can occur, but it is rare (Photo taken by SMM)

References

1. Burkitt D (1958) A sarcoma involving the jaws in African children. Br J Surg 46:218–223
2. Ziegler JL (1981) Burkitt's lymphoma. N Engl J Med 305:735–745
3. van den Bosch CA (2004) Is endemic Burkitt's lymphoma an alliance between three infections and a tumour promoter? Lancet Oncol 5:738–746
4. Ogwang MD, Bhatia K, Biggar RJ, Mbulaiteye SM (2008) Incidence and geographic distribution of endemic Burkitt lymphoma in northern Uganda revisited. Int J Cancer 123:2658–2663
5. Ogwang MD, Zhao W, Ayers LW, Mbulaiteye SM (2011) Accuracy of burkitt lymphoma diagnosis in constrained pathology settings: importance to epidemiology. Arch Pathol Lab Med 135:445–450
6. Mbulaiteye SM, Talisuna AO, Ogwang MD, McKenzie FE, Ziegler JL, Parkin DM (2010) African Burkitt's lymphoma could collaboration with HIV-1 and malaria programmes reduce the high mortality rate. Lancet 375:1661–1663
7. Molyneux E (2003) Post-conference thoughts from Malawi. Lancet 362:2117
8. Israels T, Chirambo C, Caron H, de Kraker J, Molyneux E, Reis R (2008) The guardians' perspective on paediatric cancer treatment in Malawi and factors affecting adherence. Pediatr Blood Cancer 51:639–642
9. Hesseling PB, Broadhead R, Molyneux E et al (2003) Malawi pilot study of Burkitt lymphoma treatment. Med Pediatr Oncol 41:532–540

Chapter 4
Clinical Implications of Burkitt Lymphoma

Jakub Svoboda and Stephen J. Schuster

Introduction

Patients with Burkitt lymphoma present a unique challenge to clinicians because of the highly aggressive nature of this neoplasm. Three variants of Burkitt lymphoma are recognized: endemic, sporadic, and immunodeficiency-related [1]. While the epidemiology and some clinical characteristics differ among subtypes, the unifying features are rapid tumor cell growth and a propensity to involve extranodal sites. This chapter will focus on the clinical consequences of these biologic features, which frequently present as oncologic emergencies. These aspects of Burkitt lymphoma need to be readily recognized by physicians caring for these patients since delays in providing optimal therapy can result in poor outcome and early mortality.

Tumor Lysis Syndrome

Tumor lysis syndrome (TLS) can cause significant morbidity and mortality at presentation, during therapy, and at relapse in patients with Burkitt lymphoma. This clinical syndrome results from massive tumor cell lysis, followed by release of intracellular potassium, phosphate, and nucleic acids into the circulation [2–4]. Hyperphosphatemia from release of intracellular phosphate also causes secondary hypocalcemia due to precipitation of serum calcium into calcium phosphate crystals.

While TLS in most malignancies occurs after initiating cytotoxic therapy, TLS can develop spontaneously prior to any therapy in patients with Burkitt lymphoma [4–6].

J. Svoboda (✉) • S.J. Schuster
Lymphoma Program, Abramson Cancer Center, University of Pennsylvania,
3400 Civic Center Blvd., Philadelphia, PA 19104, USA
e-mail: Stephen.Schuster@uphs.upenn.edu; Jakub.Svoboda@uphs.upenn.edu

E.S. Robertson (ed.), *Burkitt's Lymphoma*, Current Cancer Research,
DOI 10.1007/978-1-4614-4313-1_4, © Springer Science+Business Media New York 2013

Table 4.1 Cairo–Bishop definition of tumor lysis syndrome (TLS).

A. Laboratory TLS: any two or more serum values of uric acid, potassium, phosphate, and calcium within 3 days before or 7 days after the initiation of chemotherapy.	
Uric Acid	≥ 8 mg/dL or 25 % increase from baseline
Potassium	≥ 6 mmol/l or 25 % increase from baseline
Phosphate	≥ 6.5 mg/dL (children) or ≥ 4.5 mg/dL (adults) or 25 % increase from baseline in either age group
Calcium	≤ 7 or 25 % decrease from baseline
B. Clinical TLS: laboratory evidence of TLS and presence of any one or more of the criteria.	
Creatinine ≥ 1.5 upper limit of normal	
Cardiac arrhythmia/sudden death	
Seizure	

From: Cairo, M. S., & Bishop, M. (2004). Tumour lysis syndrome: New therapeutic strategies and classification. *British Journal of Haematology, 127*(1), 3-11.

The etiology of spontaneous TLS in Burkitt lymphoma is unclear. Some hypothetical causes for TLS include increased production of endogenous stress-related glucocorticoids and fever causing hyperthermic toxicity in the rapidly dividing, highly metabolic tumor cells [7, 8]. Kinetic studies have revealed that the potential doubling time of Burkitt lymphoma cells is about 24 h with a cell-loss rate of 70% of the cell-renewal rate, making Burkitt lymphoma the fastest growing human tumor [9].

The electrolyte and metabolic abnormalities caused by TLS affect various organs and result in several symptoms and clinical signs. Patients with TLS may present with malaise, altered mental status, and/or oliguria due to renal failure. The mechanism of renal failure is multifactorial, involving both injury from intrarenal precipitation of calcium phosphate, uric acid, and xanthine crystals, as well as crystal-independent mechanisms such as vasoconstriction, hypoperfusion, and inflammation [10–12].

Hyperkalemia arises from release of intracellular potassium and may be exacerbated by concurrent renal failure. It may cause cardiac arrhythmias which can manifest as subjective palpitations, heart failure, hypotension, or even sudden death. Hypocalcemia may cause neuromuscular issues including seizures or muscular irritability. Calcium phosphate crystals can also precipitate outside of the kidneys and may involve the cardiac conduction system, further increasing the possibility of cardiac arrhythmias [3]. Tumor lysis may also stimulate cytokine release and induce the systemic inflammatory response syndrome [13, 14]. Ultimately, TLS may evolve into multi-organ failure and death.

Several groups have defined TLS in objective terms [15, 16]. The commonly used Cairo-Bishop definition provides specific criteria for TLS at presentation and within 7 days of treatment (see Table 4.1) [15]. These criteria use laboratory and clinical findings to objectively define TLS. The laboratory criteria include uric acid ≥8 mg/dL or 25% increase from baseline, potassium ≥6.0 mmol/L or 25% increase from baseline, serum phosphate ≥6.5 mg/dL in children or ≥4.5 mg/dL in adults or a 25% increase from baseline in either age group, serum calcium ≤7 mg/dL or 25% decrease from baseline [15]. *Laboratory TLS* is defined by abnormality in two or more of these laboratory studies, occurring within 3 days before or 7 days after chemotherapy. *Clinical TLS* is defined as laboratory TLS with at least one of the following clinical findings: cardiac arrhythmia, hypotension, heart failure, neuromuscular irritability, seizure, renal insufficiency documented by increased creatinine level, or oligouria. Not all patients with laboratory TLS develop clinical TLS. Sudden death in a patient with laboratory TLS also defines clinical TLS.

There are limited data on the incidence of TLS in patients with Burkitt lymphoma, especially in adult patients. Most studies combine patients with B-cell acute lymphoblastic leukemia (ALL) and Burkitt lymphoma together for the purpose of reporting TLS. Moreover, the incidence is affected by management at the time of presentation. It has been estimated that prior to the availability of urate oxidase agents, about 15–25% of pediatric patients with Burkitt lymphoma developed clinical TLS [17–20]. Data from B-cell ALL and Burkitt lymphoma pediatric patients who were treated on a multicenter international trial in both Europe and the USA were analyzed for the need of hemodialysis due to TLS [18]. Patients in Europe had significantly lower need for dialysis when compared to the USA. This was thought to be due to the availability of urate oxidase agents approved for prevention and management of TLS in Europe which were not approved in the USA at that time [18]. Comparison of outcomes between periods before and after the introduction of urate oxidase agents shows that these agents can reduce incidence of TLS and anuria [20].

Management of TLS can be divided into two parts: prophylactic measures in patients at risk of developing TLS and treatment of established TLS. The scope of this chapter does not allow for providing detailed management algorithms, but we will review the main concepts and interventions.

The major goal for Burkitt lymphoma patients at risk for TLS or with established TLS (spontaneous or therapy-induced) is preservation of renal function since the kidneys are essential for excretion of potassium, uric acid and phosphate. Aggressive hydration with intravenous fluid, maintenance of adequate urine output, and use of agents to reduce the level of uric acid are effective interventions for prevention and treatment of TLS. Urinary alkalinization remains controversial in the management of patients at high risk for TLS. This treatment may offer benefit for patients with metabolic acidosis by increasing the solubility of uric acid and reducing urate nephropathy [21]. However, urinary alkalization is not recommended for patients with hyperphosphatemia since it decreases calcium phosphate solubility.

Traditionally, allopurinol has been used to reduce the level of uric acid. It is usually administered orally, but an intravenous formulation is now available. Allopurinol inhibits xanthine oxidase, the enzyme responsible for the conversion of hypoxanthine to xanthine as well as xanthine to uric acid (Fig. 4.1) [22]. Allopurinol is metabolized to oxypurinol which is also an inhibitor of xanthine oxidase. While it prevents formation of new uric acid, existing uric acid must still be excreted by the kidneys.

Rasburicase is an intravenous recombinant urate oxidase enzyme, which has been approved for the treatment of hyperuricemia associated with TLS in the USA since 2009. A nonrecombinant form has been used in Europe for many years. Rasburicase converts uric acid to allantoin, an inactive, soluble metabolite [23].

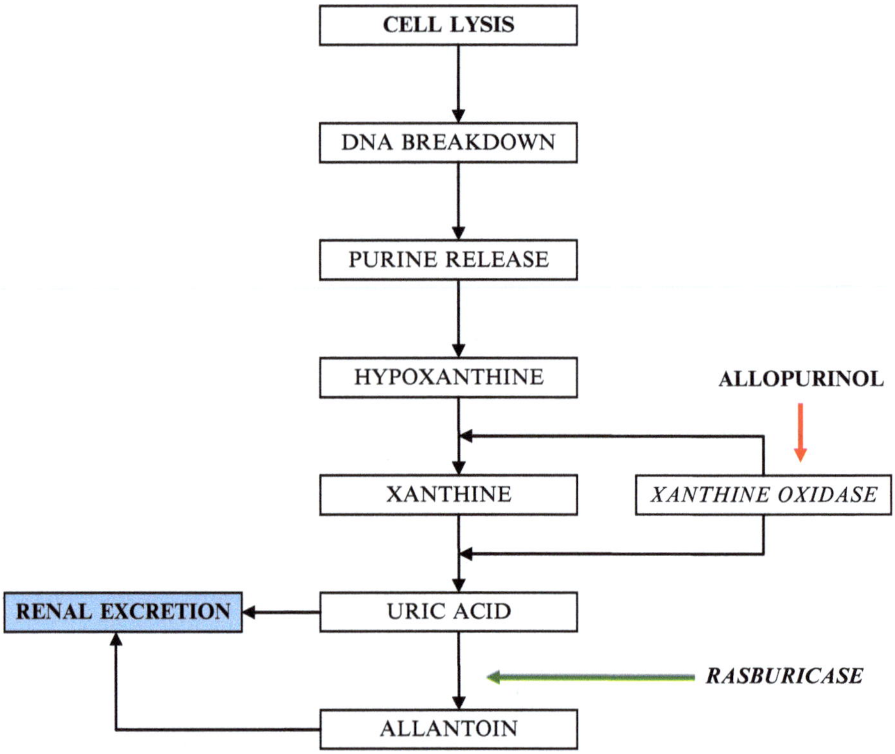

Fig. 4.1 Purine metabolism. Different mechanisms of action by allopurinol versus rasburicase in reducing uric acid levels. Allopurinol acts by inhibiting the endogenous enzyme xanthine oxidase, thereby preventing formation of new uric acid. Rasburicase is a recombinant form of urate oxidase and promotes conversion of uric acid to allantoin which is then excreted by kidneys. Adapted from Goldman SC et al. [30]

Rasburicase is highly effective in reducing serum uric acid; levels usually decrease within 4 h of initial administration [23]. While the Food and Drug Administration recommends dosing rasburicase at 0.2 mg/kg once daily for up to 5 days, several other alternative dosing schedules have been suggested, including a single dose of 3–7.5 mg [24–28]. Of note, rasburicase causes degradation of uric acid in vitro if blood samples are left at room temperature before performing the assay. Therefore, care must be taken to place blood samples on ice to avoid spuriously low serum uric acid concentrations and missing hyperuricemia in the setting of TLS.

A phase III trial comparing rasburicase versus allopurinol in 280 adults with hematological malignancies included patients with Burkitt lymphoma or B-cell ALL [29]. The patients were randomized into three treatment groups: allopurinol alone; combination rasburicase and allopurinol; and rasburicase alone. In patients with hyperuricemia or at high risk for TLS, rasburicase provided more rapid control of plasma uric acid than allopurinol (4 h for rasburicase alone or rasburicase with allopurinol versus 27 h for allopurinol alone). Rasburicase was well tolerated as a single agent and in sequential combination with allopurinol [29]. A randomized trial in 56 children with hematological malignancies also demonstrated more rapid control and lower levels of plasma uric acid in patients at high risk for tumor lysis who received rasburicase compared to allopurinol [30].

Patients from populations in which glucose-6-phosphate dehydrogenase (G6PD) deficiency is common should undergo screening for this condition before treatment with rasburicase [31]. G6PD deficiency is most common in patients of Mediterranean and African descent [32]. In patients with a prior history of G6PD deficiency or those who test positive, rasburicase is contraindicated and allopurinol should be utilized instead. The reason for this contraindication is that hydrogen peroxide liberated from the breakdown of urate to allantoin may induce severe hemolytic anemia and methemoglobinemia in G6PD-deficient patients [33].

There have been efforts to develop management guidelines to reduce the incidence of TLS in patients with aggressive hematological malignancies such as Burkitt lymphoma. The most recent model categorizes patients with hematological malignancies into low, intermediate, and high-risk TLS groups and provides TLS prophylaxis recommendations for each group [34]. Patients with advanced Burkitt lymphoma and those with early stage disease with elevated lactate dehydrogenase (LDH) are considered to be in the high risk group for development of TLS [34]. Patients with early stage Burkitt lymphoma and normal LDH are considered at intermediate risk unless they have renal dysfunction, renal involvement by Burkitt lymphoma, or if their serum uric acid, serum phosphate or serum potassium levels are elevated [34].

These guidelines recommend that patients at high risk for TLS undergo frequent monitoring of electrolytes, aggressive intravenous hydration (at 3 L/m^2 daily with the goal urine output of at least 80–100 mL/m^2 per hour), and prophylactic treatment with rasburicase (at 0.1–0.2 mg/kg as a single dose). Repeated doses of rasburicase should be administered only if clinically necessary [34]. The guidelines defer management of hyperkalemia and hyperphosphatemia to institutional norms or previous TLS treatment guidelines from 2008 [21]. Patients initially classified as low or intermediate risk who develop laboratory features of TLS should also receive rasburicase according to the most recent guidelines. The rare Burkitt lymphoma patients who are considered only intermediate risk of developing TLS (early stage, no significant LDH elevation or laboratory TLS) should be monitored for electrolyte abnormalities, receive intravenous hydration at 3 L/m^2 per day, and be started on allopurinol (100–300 mg orally every 8 h daily) without urinary alkalization [34].

For those Burkitt lymphoma patients who develop TLS spontaneously or who are found to have TLS during induction therapy despite appropriate preventive measures, management focuses on preserving renal function, reversing electrolyte abnormalities, and closely monitoring for impending arrhythmias or neurological complications.

Hyperkalemia is the most serious acute issue and potassium levels should be closely monitored (about every 4–6 h). High potassium foods should be avoided in this setting (e.g., bananas, beans, beets). In patients with mildly elevated potassium levels, the use of oral sodium polystyrene sulfonate resin can be effective. This agent removes potassium by exchanging sodium ions for potassium ions in the intestine before the resin is passed from the body. However, in patients who have GI involvement by Burkitt lymphoma with associated symptoms such as constipation or impending obstruction sodium polystyrene sulfonate must be used with caution. This agent has been associated with intestinal necrosis in patients with intestinal disease or recent surgery, especially when administered in sorbitol [35]. Transient decrease in the serum potassium level can also be rapidly achieved by administration of insulin (with concurrent glucose) which promotes potassium uptake into skeletal muscle by stimulating the activity of the Na+-K+ pump [36, 37]. Beta-2 adrenergic agonists can also drive potassium into cells and may be effective in the management of hyperkalemia [36, 38]. Calcium salts (gluconate or chloride) can be used to temporarily antagonize the effect of hyperkalemia on the myocardium, but this effect is short-lived [39].

Ultimately, hemodialysis may be necessary in patients with active TLS failing more conservative measures, although the need for hemodialysis decreased significantly since the introduction of rasburicase. While there are no specific guidelines or cutoff values, clinical experience suggests that oligouria and symptomatic hypocalcemia may be appropriate triggers for initiating hemodialysis. Hemodialysis removes excess serum potassium and phosphate, which in turn improves serum calcium levels. Correcting hypocalcemia with supplemental calcium is limited by calcium-phosphate crystallization while phosphate levels are high. Persistent or progressive electrolyte abnormalities may also be an indication for dialysis. Continuous hemofiltration has also been used in this setting and might have potential benefits in reducing phosphate when compared to intermittent hemodialysis [40].

TLS remains a major concern when managing patients with Burkitt lymphoma. Current guidelines consider any patient with advanced Burkitt lymphoma to be at high risk for development of TLS [34]. Aggressive prevention and early recognition of TLS are essential for successful outcomes for patients with Burkitt lymphoma.

Obstruction, Compression, and Other Anatomic Complications

Patients with Burkitt lymphoma may develop emergent issues due to mechanical obstruction or compression of vital structures by rapidly enlarging lymph nodes or extranodal masses of malignant lymphocytes. Frequent obstructive and compressive complications of Burkitt lymphoma are discussed below.

Superior Vena Cava Syndrome

Superior vena cava (SVC) syndrome occurs in Burkitt lymphoma patients due to extrinsic compression of the SVC by a large tumor or obstruction of the SVC by thrombosis [41]. Most patients with SVC syndrome present with edema of the face, neck, and upper extremities which can be associated with superficial venous dilation in these areas. Some patients may also develop hoarseness and dysphagia [42, 43]. At times, syncope, headache, or mental status change can also occur [43]. A large mass in the superior mediastinum may compress the airway and cause pulmonary symptoms such as cough and dyspnea. This is more common in pediatric patients, since their airway is smaller and the cartilaginous rings of the trachea are more compliant [42].

The diagnosis of SVC syndrome is usually confirmed by radiologic imaging, most often CT scan, revealing a large mediastinal mass with associated anatomic complications. Additional studies, such as ultrasound, may be helpful in detecting associated venous thrombosis. Management of SVC syndrome in patients with Burkitt lymphoma depends on the clinical scenario and whether a diagnostic tissue biopsy has been obtained. In the most severe cases, patients may require emergent interventions prior to obtaining tissue for diagnosis. However, emergent treatment of a symptomatic mediastinal mass prior to tissue biopsy may result in lower diagnostic yield. In a group of 19 patients emergently irradiated for a symptomatic mediastinal mass, only 11 patients were able to have a pathological diagnosis established by later biopsy [44]. Steroids can also reduce compression of vital structures by the mass, but may cause tumor necrosis and thus interfere with the quality of the biopsy specimen.

Supportive measures, such as supplemental oxygen and optimal positioning to limit compression of mediastinal structures by the mass, can be effective. If venous thrombosis is detected, anticoagulation is usually started unless there is a contraindication, such as concurrent GI bleeding. Endovascular stenting of SVC has been shown to be an effective way to treat SVC syndrome in epithelial malignancies, such as lung cancer [45]. However, stenting is not usually necessary in Burkitt lymphoma since most patients usually respond to steroids, radiation, or systemic chemotherapy,

Abdominal Emergencies

Patients with Burkitt lymphoma have high likelihood of gastrointestinal (GI) involvement and may present with acute abdominal symptoms due to bowel obstruction, perforation, GI bleeding, or intussusception (Fig. 4.2). In pediatric patients with Burkitt lymphoma, intussusception is a common presenting feature of the disease [46]. Intestinal obstruction can also occur secondary to extrinsic compression of bowel or intrinsic involvement of intestine by tumor causing mechanical obstruction or intussusception. Malignant lymphocytes infiltrating the bowel wall may also cause GI bleeding and perforation at presentation. Bleeding or perforation can also follow chemotherapy when the responding tumor necrotizes causing thinning of the bowel wall. Other causes of abdominal emergencies that occur include infection (typhilitis) or direct mucosal ulceration during neutropenia following chemotherapy. Patients with Burkitt lymphoma may also develop severe

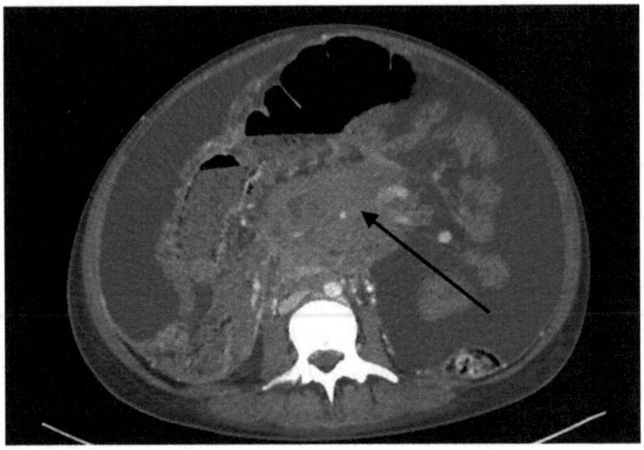

Fig. 4.2 Abdominal presentation of sporadic Burkitt lymphoma. Computed tomography (CT) image from a 24 year old patient who developed progressive abdominal distention, emesis, and pain. Her CT scan revealed a large, necrotic retroperitoneal soft tissue mass (see arrow) encasing the aorta and major branches with extension to the root of the mesentery and small bowel. Cytology from the peritoneal fluid was consistent with involvement by Burkitt lymphoma

ileus from vinca alkaloid chemotherapy such as vincristine, or from opioids used for pain, as well as pseudo-obstruction related to metabolic derangements.

The diagnosis of an acute abdomen is based on clinical and radiographic findings. The clinical features of obstruction include abdominal pain, distention, and emesis. Imaging usually identifies air-fluid levels or free air when perforation is present. Barium enemas, which are often used for diagnosis and treatment of intussusception in children without lymphoma, should be avoided in patients receiving chemotherapy due to the increased risk of rupturing thinned gut mucosa.

Management of abdominal emergencies in Burkitt lymphoma patients is generally coordinated with the surgical team. Surgery may be indicated for complete bowel obstruction, but partial small bowel obstruction may be managed conservatively using decompression with nasogastric suction and bowel rest. Bowel perforation and hemorrhage usually require emergent surgical repair. Severe constipation due to decreased gut motility in Burkitt lymphoma patients with GI involvement may require adjustment of treatment strategies, e.g., eliminating or reducing vinca alkaloids from the treatment.

Renal and Urologic Emergencies

While the most common cause of renal failure in Burkitt lymphoma is TLS, urinary tract obstruction and/or mechanical compression of renal vascular structures by bulky lymph nodes can also result in renal emergencies [47]. In some cases, direct tumor infiltration of kidneys without obstruction may also affect renal function [48, 49].

Obstructive nephropathy is diagnosed by imaging studies that reveal hydronephrosis in a patient with decreased urinary output and elevated serum creatinine. The goal of management should be decompression and urinary drainage since prolonged obstruction may lead to irreversible renal injury and renal insufficiency due to obstruction may promote TLS. Percutaneous nephrostomy tubes or ureteral stenting prior to chemotherapy may occasionally be necessary to decompress the urinary tract and avoid dialysis.

Malignant Effusions (Pleural and Pericardial)

Patients with Burkitt lymphoma may develop pleural or pericardial effusions that can cause cardiopulmonary emergencies. At diagnosis, effusions in patients with Burkitt lymphoma are usually the result of involvement of serosal surfaces by lymphoma; during therapy, secondary processes such as infection or volume overload may present as effusions. Patients usually present with respiratory distress or cough. The diagnosis is based on imaging such as chest X-ray or CT scan. Echocardiography is used to assess pericardial effusion. Cardiac tamponade may occur in Burkitt lymphoma patients who have severe compression of cardiac chambers by pericardial effusion resulting in significant decrease in cardiac output [50]. Symptomatic patients are usually managed by pericardiocentesis or thoracentesis which may be both therapeutic and diagnostic [51].

Neurological Emergencies

Patients with Burkitt lymphoma may develop neurological complications due to the direct involvement of the central nervous system (CNS) by lymphoma or from secondary effects of electrolyte imbalance and hematologic derangements. There have also been several cases of primary CNS Burkitt lymphoma reported in the literature [52, 53]. Immunosuppression may be associated with higher risk of meningeal infections in these patients [54].

Symptoms that should alert clinicians to involvement of the CNS by Burkitt lymphoma may range from subtle mental status change, vomiting, or headache to obvious cranial nerve deficits, seizures, or, in extreme cases, coma. Diagnosis of CNS involvement by Burkitt lymphoma is based on imaging, such as contrast-enhanced magnetic resonance imaging (MRI) and analysis of cerebrospinal fluid (CSF) obtained by lumbar puncture. Brain biopsy may rarely be necessary for diagnosis. Occasionally, one must accept the presence of cranial nerve palsy with negative imaging and CSF examination in a patient with known Burkitt lymphoma as evidence of CNS involvement. Of note, all patients with Burkitt lymphoma, even those without clinical suspicion for CNS involvement, should undergo lumbar puncture at diagnosis to obtain CSF for cytology and receive prophylactic chemotherapy aimed at the CNS as part of initial therapy.

The management of CNS complications in Burkitt lymphoma patients depends on the underlying process. Lymphomatous involvement of CNS can be treated with systemic agents that penetrate the blood–brain barrier, such as high-dose methotrexate, or by delivering chemotherapy directly into the spinal fluid by lumbar puncture or use of an Ommaya reservoir [55, 56]. Radiation may be employed for treatment of parenchymal CNS lesions [57]. An important part of the treatment of Burkitt lymphoma in patients without evidence of CNS involvement is the use of intrathecal chemotherapy for prophylaxis. Prior to the use of prophylaxis, the CNS was a common site of relapse, occurring in about 50% patients with highly aggressive lymphomas and leukemias including Burkitt lymphoma [56].

Spinal cord compression is another neurological complication that may occur in Burkitt lymphoma. Patients with spinal cord compression may present with back pain and/or neurological deficits such as paraplegia or anal/bladder sphincter dysfunction [58]. These symptoms are caused by compression of the spinal cord by adjacent tumor growth and associated vasogenic edema. Diagnosis is usually made by MRI, which should be considered emergently in any patient with Burkitt lymphoma and concerning symptoms. Acute management includes high-dose steroids and may involve neurosurgical decompression, radiation therapy, chemotherapy, or a combination of these approaches.

Metabolic Abnormalities Other Than TLS

While TLS causes hypocalcemia in Burkitt lymphoma, high levels of calcitriol and osteolytic lesions may cause hypercalcemia in some patients [59, 60]. Symptoms associated with hypercalcemia depend on the severity of the abnormality. Mild hypercalcemia is usually asymptomatic, but patients with moderate and severe elevation of calcium levels can develop polyuria, constipation, confusion, and lethargy. Cardiac arrhythmias may also be associated with severe hypercalcemia. Hypercalcemia in Burkitt lymphoma patients is usually managed acutely with aggressive hydration, steroids, and bisphosphonates; ultimately, treatment of the lymphoma will correct this metabolic complication.

Hyponatremia due to the syndrome of inappropriate secretion of antidiuretic hormone (SIADH) can also cause a spectrum of symptoms depending on the degree of the abnormality and the acuteness of change in the serum sodium level. Patients may present with subtle symptoms, such as malaise and nausea; severe hyponatremia may cause seizures or coma. Any CNS process including involvement by Burkitt lymphoma, infection, or hemorrhage can cause enhanced production of the antidiuretic hormone (ADH). Pulmonary disease due to lymphoma or infection can also result in SIADH. Some of the drugs used for treatment of Burkitt lymphoma, such as vincristine and cyclophosphamide, have been associated with SIADH and may rarely complicate Burkitt lymphoma therapy [61].

The management of SIADH depends on etiology; free water restriction and treatment of the underlying cause remain the mainstays of therapy. The use of salt tablets, ADH antagonists, and diuretics can also be effective in certain clinical settings [62].

Hematological Complications

Patients with Burkitt lymphoma may experience medical emergencies related to severe cytopenias from bone marrow infiltration by malignant lymphocytes or from myelotoxic chemotherapy. Patients with low white blood cell counts are at high risk for infection and may develop sepsis or atypical infections. Anemia may result in a variety of symptoms ranging from fatigue to heart failure, depending on severity. Thrombocytopenia may result in coagulopathy and spontaneous bleeding.

Conclusion

Burkitt lymphoma is a highly aggressive lymphoma characterized by rapid tumor growth and frequent extranodal involvement. These biologic features result in unique clinical complications, including tumor lysis syndrome, CNS and GI emergencies, and major renal, electrolyte, and metabolic disturbances (Table 4.2). An understanding of the biology of Burkitt lymphoma, as well as its clinical complications and response to therapy, has resulted in successful treatment outcomes for most patients with Burkitt lymphoma.

Table 4.2 Common medical emergencies in Burkitt lymphoma patients.

1. **Tumor lysis syndrome**
2. **Obstruction, compression, and other anatomic complications**
Superior vena cava syndrome
Gastrointestinal emergencies
Bowel obstruction
Perforation
Gastrointestinal bleeding
Intussusception
Urologic emergencies
Obstructive nephropathy and hydronephrosis
Direct tumor infiltration by lymphoma
Vascular compromise to kidneys
Malignant effusions
Pleural
Pericardial (cardiac tamponade)
Ascites
3. **Neurological emergencies**
Direct involvement of central nervous system
Spinal cord compression
4. **Metabolic abnormalities other than TLS**
Syndrome of inappropriate secretion of antidiuretic hormone
Hypercalcemia
5. **Hematological complications**
Cytopenias
Coagulopathy

Acknowledgements The authors thank Amanda Gordon, MSN and Elise Chong, MSIII for assistance in preparation of this manuscript.

References

1. Swerdlow SH, Campo E, Harris NL, Jaffe ES, Pileri SA, et al (2008) WHO classification of tumours of haematopoietic and lymphoid tissues, fourth edition. International Agency for Reserach on Cancer, 150 cours Albert Thomas, 69372 Lyon Cedex 08, France in 2008
2. Gertz MA (2010) Managing tumor lysis syndrome in 2010. Leuk Lymphoma 51(2):179–180
3. Howard SC, Jones DP, Pui CH (2011) The tumor lysis syndrome. N Engl J Med 364(19): 1844–1854
4. Magrath IT, Semawere C, Nkwocha J (1974) Causes of death in patients with Burkitt's lymphoma–the role of supportive care in overall management. East Afr Med J 51(9):623–632
5. Agha-Razii M, Amyot SL, Pichette V, Cardinal J, Ouimet D, Leblanc M (2000) Continuous veno-venous hemodiafiltration for the treatment of spontaneous tumor lysis syndrome complicated by acute renal failure and severe hyperuricemia. Clin Nephrol 54(1):59–63
6. Jasek AM, Day HJ (1994) Acute spontaneous tumor lysis syndrome. Am J Hematol 47(2):129–131
7. Levin M, Cho S (1996) Acute tumor lysis syndrome in high grade lymphoblastic lymphoma after a prolonged episode of fever. Med Pediatr Oncol 26(6):417–418
8. Riccio B, Mato A, Olson EM, Berns JS, Luger S (2006) Spontaneous tumor lysis syndrome in acute myeloid leukemia: two cases and a review of the literature. Cancer Biol Ther 5(12):1614–1617
9. Iversen OH, Iversen U, Ziegler JL, Bluming AZ (1974) Cell kinetics in Burkitt lymphoma. Eur J Cancer 10(3):155–163
10. Ejaz AA, Mu W, Kang DH, Roncal C, Sautin YY, Henderson G et al (2007) Could uric acid have a role in acute renal failure? Clin J Am Soc Nephrol 2(1):16–21
11. LaRosa C, McMullen L, Bakdash S, Ellis D, Krishnamurti L, Wu HY et al (2007) Acute renal failure from xanthine nephropathy during management of acute leukemia. Pediatr Nephrol (Berlin, Germany) 22(1):132–135
12. Shimada M, Johnson RJ, May WS Jr, Lingegowda V, Sood P, Nakagawa T et al (2009) A novel role for uric acid in acute kidney injury associated with tumour lysis syndrome. Nephrol Dial Transplant 24(10):2960–2964
13. Hijiya N, Metzger ML, Pounds S, Schmidt JE, Razzouk BI, Rubnitz JE et al (2005) Severe cardiopulmonary complications consistent with systemic inflammatory response syndrome caused by leukemia cell lysis in childhood acute myelomonocytic or monocytic leukemia. Pediatr Blood Cancer 44(1):63–69
14. Soares M, Feres GA, Salluh JI (2009) Systemic inflammatory response syndrome and multiple organ dysfunction in patients with acute tumor lysis syndrome. Clinics (Sao Paulo, Brazil) 64(5):479–481
15. Cairo MS, Bishop M (2004) Tumour lysis syndrome: new therapeutic strategies and classification. Br J Haematol 127(1):3–11
16. Hande KR, Garrow GC (1993) Acute tumor lysis syndrome in patients with high-grade non-Hodgkin's lymphoma. Am J Med 94(2):133–139
17. Bowman WP, Shuster JJ, Cook B, Griffin T, Behm F, Pullen J et al (1996) Improved survival for children with B-cell acute lymphoblastic leukemia and stage IV small noncleaved-cell lymphoma: a pediatric oncology group study. J Clin Oncol 14(4):1252–1261
18. Cairo MS, Gerrard M, Sposto R, Auperin A, Pinkerton CR, Michon J et al (2007) Results of a randomized international study of high-risk central nervous system B non-Hodgkin lymphoma and B acute lymphoblastic leukemia in children and adolescents. Blood 109(7):2736–2743

19. Stapleton FB, Strother DR, Roy S 3rd, Wyatt RJ, McKay CP, Murphy SB (1988) Acute renal failure at onset of therapy for advanced stage Burkitt lymphoma and B cell acute lymphoblastic lymphoma. Pediatrics 82(6):863–869
20. Wossmann W, Schrappe M, Meyer U, Zimmermann M, Reiter A (2003) Incidence of tumor lysis syndrome in children with advanced stage Burkitt's lymphoma/leukemia before and after introduction of prophylactic use of urate oxidase. Ann Hematol 82(3):160–165
21. Coiffier B, Altman A, Pui CH, Younes A, Cairo MS (2008) Guidelines for the management of pediatric and adult tumor lysis syndrome: an evidence-based review. J Clin Oncol 26(16):2767–2778
22. Murrell GA, Rapeport WG (1986) Clinical pharmacokinetics of allopurinol. Clin Pharmacokinet 11(5):343–353
23. Coiffier B, Mounier N, Bologna S, Ferme C, Tilly H, Sonet A et al (2003) Efficacy and safety of rasburicase (recombinant urate oxidase) for the prevention and treatment of hyperuricemia during induction chemotherapy of aggressive non-Hodgkin's lymphoma: results of the GRAAL1 (groupe d'etude des lymphomes de l'adulte trial on rasburicase activity in adult lymphoma) study. J Clin Oncol 21(23):4402–4406
24. Campara M, Shord SS, Haaf CM (2009) Single-dose rasburicase for tumour lysis syndrome in adults: weight-based approach. J Clin Pharm Ther 34(2):207–213
25. Giraldez M, Puto K (2010) A single, fixed dose of rasburicase (6 mg maximum) for treatment of tumor lysis syndrome in adults. Eur J Haematol 85(2):177–179
26. Liu CY, Sims-McCallum RP, Schiffer CA (2005) A single dose of rasburicase is sufficient for the treatment of hyperuricemia in patients receiving chemotherapy. Leuk Res 29(4):463–465
27. McDonnell AM, Lenz KL, Frei-Lahr DA, Hayslip J, Hall PD (2006) Single-dose rasburicase 6 mg in the management of tumor lysis syndrome in adults. Pharmacotherapy 26(6):806–812
28. Reeves DJ, Bestul DJ (2008) Evaluation of a single fixed dose of rasburicase 7.5 mg for the treatment of hyperuricemia in adults with cancer. Pharmacotherapy 28(6):685–690
29. Cortes J, Moore JO, Maziarz RT, Wetzler M, Craig M, Matous J et al (2010) Control of plasma uric acid in adults at risk for tumor lysis syndrome: efficacy and safety of rasburicase alone and rasburicase followed by allopurinol compared with allopurinol alone–results of a multicenter phase III study. J Clin Oncol 28(27):4207–4213
30. Goldman SC, Holcenberg JS, Finklestein JZ, Hutchinson R, Kreissman S, Johnson FL et al (2001) A randomized comparison between rasburicase and allopurinol in children with lymphoma or leukemia at high risk for tumor lysis. Blood 97(10):2998–3003
31. Elitek (rasburicase) prescribing information. www.PDR.net (Revised 2010)
32. Beutler E (1991) Glucose-6-phosphate dehydrogenase deficiency. N Engl J Med 324(3):169–174
33. Browning LA, Kruse JA (2005) Hemolysis and methemoglobinemia secondary to rasburicase administration. Ann Pharmacother 39(11):1932–1935
34. Cairo MS, Coiffier B, Reiter A, Younes A, TLS Expert Panel (2010) Recommendations for the evaluation of risk and prophylaxis of tumour lysis syndrome (TLS) in adults and children with malignant diseases: an expert TLS panel consensus. Br J Haematol 149(4):578–586
35. McGowan CE, Saha S, Chu G, Resnick MB, Moss SF (2009) Intestinal necrosis due to sodium polystyrene sulfonate (kayexalate) in sorbitol. South Med J 102(5):493–497
36. Allon M, Copkney C (1990) Albuterol and insulin for treatment of hyperkalemia in hemodialysis patients. Kidney Int 38(5):869–872
37. Ferrannini E, Taddei S, Santoro D, Natali A, Boni C, Del Chiaro D et al (1988) Independent stimulation of glucose metabolism and na+-K+exchange by insulin in the human forearm. Am J Physiol 255(6 Pt 1):E953–E958
38. Brenner BM (ed) (2008) Brenner and rector's the kidney, 8th edn. W.B. Saunders Co, Philadelphia
39. Sood MM, Sood AR, Richardson R (2007) Emergency management and commonly encountered outpatient scenarios in patients with hyperkalemia. Mayo Clin Proc 82(12):1553–1561
40. Tan HK, Bellomo R, M'Pis DA, Ronco C (2001) Phosphatemic control during acute renal failure: intermittent hemodialysis versus continuous hemodiafiltration. Int J Artif Organs 24(4):186–191

41. Juimo AG, Temdemno AM, Tapko JB, Yomi J, Teyang A, Tagny G et al (1997) Superior vena cava tumoral thrombosis revealing a Burkitt's lymphoma and a lymphoblastic non-Hodgkin's lymphoma. A case report. Angiology 48(3):263–268
42. Ingram L, Rivera GK, Shapiro DN (1990) Superior vena cava syndrome associated with childhood malignancy: analysis of 24 cases. Med Pediatr Oncol 18(6):476–481
43. Parish JM, Marschke RF Jr, Dines DE, Lee RE (1981) Etiologic considerations in superior vena cava syndrome. Mayo Clin Proc 56(7):407–413
44. Loeffler JS, Leopold KA, Recht A, Weinstein HJ, Tarbell NJ (1986) Emergency prebiopsy radiation for mediastinal masses: impact on subsequent pathologic diagnosis and outcome. J Clin Oncol 4(5):716–721
45. Lanciego C, Pangua C, Chacon JI, Velasco J, Boy RC, Viana A et al (2009) Endovascular stenting as the first step in the overall management of malignant superior vena cava syndrome. AJR Am J Roentgenol 193(2):549–558
46. Gupta H, Davidoff AM, Pui CH, Shochat SJ, Sandlund JT (2007) Clinical implications and surgical management of intussusception in pediatric patients with Burkitt lymphoma. J Pediatr Surg 42(6):998–1001, discussion 1001
47. Mantadakis E, Aquino VM, Strand WR, Quigley R (1999) Acute renal failure due to obstruction in Burkitt lymphoma. Pediatr Nephrol (Berlin, Germany) 13(3):237–240
48. Castellano I, Hernandez MT, Gomez-Martino JR, Covarsi A, Bergua J, Gonzalez MA (2000) Acute renal failure as presentation of a Burkitt's lymphoma. Am J Kidney Dis 36(6):E32
49. Siegel MB, Alexander EA, Weintraub L, Idelson BA (1977) Renal failure in Burkitt's lymphoma. Clin Nephrol 7(6):279–283
50. Kaul P, Javangula K (2007) Burkitt lymphoma masquerading as cardiac tamponade. J Cardiothorac Surg 2:30
51. McLean TW, Farber RS, Lewis ZT, Wofford MM, Pettenati MJ, Pranikoff T et al (2007) Diagnosis of Burkitt lymphoma in pediatric patients by thoracentesis. Pediatr Blood Cancer 49(1):90–92
52. Gu Y, Hou YY, Zhang XB, Hu F (2010) Primary central nervous system burkitt lymphoma as concomitant lesions in the third and the left ventricles: a case study and literature review. J Neurooncol 99(2):277–281
53. Valsamis MP, Levine PH, Rapin I, Santorineou M, Shulman K (1976) Primary intracranial Burkitt's lymphoma in an infant. Cancer 37(3):1500–1507
54. Balkundi DR, Murray DL, Patterson MJ, Gera R, Scott-Emuakpor A, Kulkarni R (1997) Penicillin-resistant streptococcus mitis as a cause of septicemia with meningitis in febrile neutropenic children. J Pediatr Hematol Oncol 19(1):82–85
55. Gokbuget N, Hartog CM, Bassan R, Derigs HG, Dombret H, Greil R et al (2011) Liposomal cytarabine is effective and tolerable in the treatment of central nervous system relapse of acute lymphoblastic leukemia and very aggressive lymphoma. Haematologica 96(2):238–244
56. Pui CH, Thiel E (2009) Central nervous system disease in hematologic malignancies: historical perspective and practical applications. Semin Oncol 36(4 Suppl 2):S2–S16
57. Norin T (1977) Radiation therapy in Burkitt's lymphoma of the central nervous system. Acta Radiol Ther Phys Biol 16(1):73–80
58. Dechambenoit G, Piquemal M, Giordano C, Cournil C, Ba Zeze V, Santini JJ (1996) Spinal cord compression resulting from burkitt's lymphoma in children. Childs Nerv Syst 12(4):210–214
59. Seymour JF, Gagel RF (1993) Calcitriol: the major humoral mediator of hypercalcemia in Hodgkin's disease and non-Hodgkin's lymphomas. Blood 82(5):1383–1394
60. Spiegel A, Greene M, Magrath I, Balow J, Marx S, Aurbach GD (1978) Hypercalcemia with suppressed parathyroid hormone in Burkitt's lymphoma. Am J Med 64(4):691–695
61. Hammond IW, Ferguson JA, Kwong K, Muniz E, Delisle F (2002) Hyponatremia and syndrome of inappropriate anti-diuretic hormone reported with the use of vincristine: an over-representation of Asians? Pharmacoepidemiol Drug Saf 11(3):229–234
62. Esposito P, Piotti G, Bianzina S, Malul Y, Dal Canton A (2011) The syndrome of inappropriate antidiuresis: pathophysiology, clinical management and new therapeutic options. Nephron Clin Pract 119(1):c62–c73; discussion c73

Chapter 5
Definition of Burkitt Lymphoma

Lorenzo Leoncini and Harald Stein

Definition

Burkitt lymphoma (BL) is defined by the World Health Organization (WHO) as a highly aggressive lymphoma often presenting at extranodal sites [1], or as an acute leukemia [2], composed of monomorphic medium-sized B-cells with basophilic cytoplasm and numerous mitotic figures [3, 4]. Chromosomal translocation involving *MYC* is the most frequent genetic feature [4–6]. Epstein–Barr Virus (EBV) is found in a variable proportion of cases. Three clinical variants of Burkitt lymphoma are recognized; these differ in geographic distribution, clinical presentation, as well as association with infectious agents and cell biology (Table 5.1).

Epidemiology and Clinical Features

Endemic BL (eBL) occurs in the malaria belt of equatorial Africa and in Papua New Guinea. In endemic regions there is a correlation between the geographical occurrence and some climatic factors (rainfall, altitude, etc.), which corresponds to the geographical distribution of endemic malaria, vectors of certain arboviruses such as Chikungunya Virus (CHIKV), and EBV-activating plants such as *Euphorbia tirucalli* [1, 7–9]. BL represents the most common childhood malignancy in these areas,

L. Leoncini
Department of Human Pathology and Oncology, Anatomic Pathology Section,
University of Siena, Via delleScotte 6, 53100 Siena, Italy
e-mail: leoncinil@unisi.it

H. Stein (✉)
Pathodiagnostik Berlin, Komturstr. 58-62, 12099 Berlin, Germany
e-mail: harald.stein@charite.de; info@pathodiagnostik.de; h.stein@pathodiagnostik.de

E.S. Robertson (ed.), *Burkitt's Lymphoma*, Current Cancer Research,
DOI 10.1007/978-1-4614-4313-1_5,

Table 5.1 Characteristic features of BL subtypes

	Endemic Burkitt's lymphoma	Sporadic Burkitt's lymphoma	AIDS-related BL
Geographical distribution	Equatorial Africa	Worldwide	Worldwide
Incidence	Children	Children and adults	Adults
Sites	Jaws, facial bones, kidneys, liver, gonads, breast	Ileocecal region, Waldeyer's ring, gonads, breast	Nodal, central nervous system (CNS)
EBV infection	100%	5–30%	25–40%
Enviromental factor	Malaria, arbovirus, euphorbia	–	–
Myc breakpoint in t(8;14)(q24;32)	Far 5′ (centromeric) of MYC (class III)	Exon and intron 1 (class I) and 5′ (centromeric) of MYC (class II)	Exon and intron 1 (class I)
Predominant IGH breakpoint in t(8;14)(q24;32)	VDJ region	Switch region	Switch region
Somatic IGH mutation	Yes	Yes	Yes

with a peak in incidence between 4 and 7 years and a male-to-female ratio of 2 to 1. Endemic BL is associated with EBV infection in almost 100% of cases. In endemic BL, the jaws and other facial bones (orbit) are the sites of presentation in about 50% of cases [1, 4]. The distal ileum, cecum and/or omentum, gonads, kidneys, long bones, thyroid, salivary glands, and breast may also be involved. Breast involvement, often bilateral and massive, has been associated with onset during puberty, pregnancy or lactation. Retro-peritoneal masses may result in spinal cord compression with paraplegia. Involvement of the lungs, mediastinum, and spleen is relatively rare. Although localization may sometimes occur in the bone marrow, no manifestation of leukemia in the peripheral blood has been reported [1, 4].

Sporadic BL (sBL) is seen throughout the world, and shows age-specific incidence peak occurring near 10 and 70 years [6, 10, 11]. The incidence is low, representing 1–2% of all lymphomas in Western Europe and the USA. However, sporadic BL accounts for approximately 30–50% of all childhood lymphomas. The male-to-female ratio is about 2 or 3 to 1, and is even higher in children [12]. EBV is seen in less than 30% of cases, and in most Western countries it is found in 10–20%. In some parts of the world, e.g. in South America and North Africa, the incidence is intermediate between true sporadic and endemic variants [9]. Low socioeconomic status and early EBV infection are associated with a higher prevalence of EBV-positive BL. Sporadic BL can also occur in people leaving in endemic regions and may account for some cases of atypical presentation and a lack of association with infectious agents [13]. In sporadic BL, jaw tumors are very rare, while the majority of cases present with abdominal masses ([6, 10]) and the ileocecal region represents the most frequent site of involvement [14]. Similar to endemic BL, the ovaries, kidneys, and breasts are also frequently involved. Lymph node presentation is seen more commonly in adults than in children. Waldeyer's ring and mediastinal involvement are rare. A leukemic phase can be observed in patients with bulky disease, but only rare cases present purely as acute leukemia [1], with bone marrow involvement and circulating B-blasts resembling Burkitt cells [10, 15].

Immunodeficiency-associated BL (ID-BL) is primarily seen in association with human immunodeficiency virus (HIV) infection, often occurring as the initial manifestation of acquired immunodeficiency syndrome (AIDS) [16]. EBV is identified in 25–40% of cases [16]. In some cases, tumors may arise in immunocompetent patients, when the CD4 count is still high, thus suggesting that HIV itself may have an oncogenic role [17].

BL is seen less often in other immunodeficiency states. In immunodeficiency-associated BL, nodal localization is frequent, as is bone marrow involvement [16, 18].

Morphology

The prototype of BL is observed in endemic BL and in a high percentage of sporadic BL cases, particularly in children [19]. The tumor cells of BL are medium-sized and show a diffuse monomorphous and cohesive pattern of growth. Rare cases with a follicular pattern may be seen, but is not possible to distinguish a true follicular growth pattern from colonization of residual benign lymphoid follicles in the majority of cases [20]. The nuclei are round with clumped chromatin and relatively clear parachromatin, and contain multiple basophilic, medium sized, centrally situated nucleoli. The cytoplasm is deeply basophilic and usually contains lipid vacuoles. Such cellular details are better seen in imprint preparations or fine needle aspiration cytology (FNAC) (Fig. 5.1). The tumor has an extremely high proliferation rate (Ki-67-index >95%) as well as a high rate of spontaneous cell death (apoptosis). A "starry sky" pattern is usually present, due to numerous benign macrophages that have ingested apoptotic tumor cells (Fig. 5.2). The nuclei of the tumor cells approximate

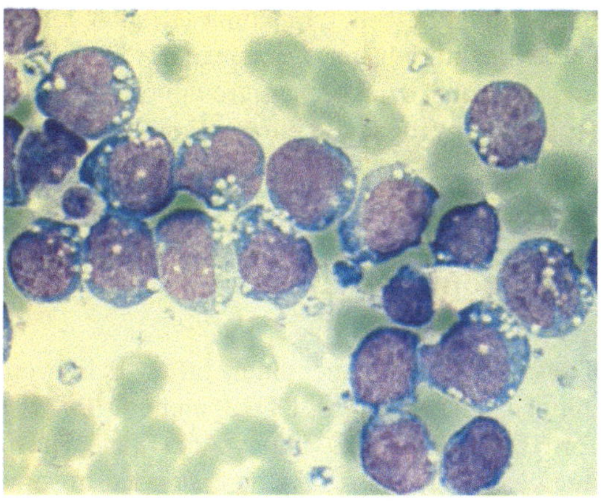

Fig. 5.1 The neoplastic cells show basophilic cytoplasm and contain lipid vacuoles on FNAC

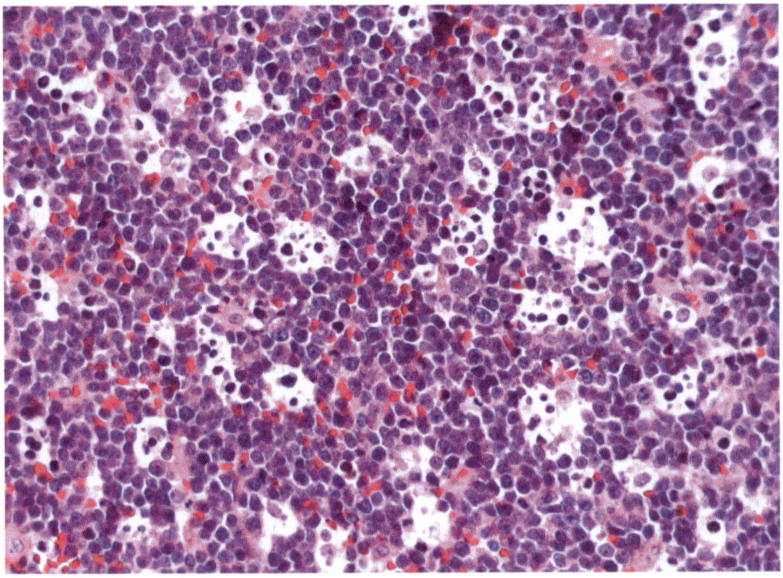

Fig. 5.2 A starry-sky pattern is present, due to numerous benign macrophages [Hematoxylin and Eosin, Original Magnification (O.M.): 20×]

in size those of the admixed starry-sky histiocytes. However, some cases of BL may show greater nuclear pleomorphism, despite clinical, immunophenotypical, and molecular characteristics all pointing to typical BL. In these cases the nucleoli may be more prominent and fewer in number. In other cases, the tumor cells exhibit plasmocytoid differentiation with eccentric basophilic cytoplasm and often a single central nucleolus. Such cases can be observed in children but are more common in immunodeficiency states [16]. These morphological features are in line with gene expression profile studies suggesting that the morphological spectrum of BL is broader than previously expected [21]. Undoubtedly, borderline cases between BL, diffuse large B-cell lymphoma (DLBCL), and "double-hit" lymphoma do exist. These might be better designated as "high-grade B cell lymphoma, unclassifiable" and additional data, such as growth fraction and molecular abnormalities, should be reported for prognostic information and to facilitate the choice of treatment.

Immunophenotype

Tumor cells express membrane IgM with light chain restriction and B-cell-associated antigens CD19, CD20, CD22, and CD79a [19]. The neoplastic cells are negative for CD23, CD44, CD138, cyclinD1, and TdT [22, 23]. BCL2 is characteristically negative, although it may be expressed in some cases and its expression does not exclude the diagnosis of BL [19]. It should be considered, however, that phenotypic heterogeneity is more common in sporadic BL, while endemic BL shows a more homogenous immunoprofile.

The expression of CD10, BCL6, and CD38 point towards a germinal center origin for the tumor cells. CD21, the receptor for C3d, can be expressed in the endemic form, but sporadic cases are usually negative [15]. A very high growth fraction is observed: nearly 100% of the cells are positive for Ki-67 [19]. Tumor-infiltrating T cells are few in number. Blasts of BL presenting with leukemia have a mature B-cell phenotype, in contrast to the blasts of precursor B-cell acute lymphoblastic leukemia (B-ALL). The blasts of BL are CD34 negative and TdT negative. They express membrane light chain restricted Ig and usually are positive for CD19, CD20, CD22, and CD79a.

Genetics

BL was the first lymphoma for which a recurrent chromosomal aberration was detected. The molecular hallmark of BL is, in fact, a translocation of *MYC* at band q24, from chromosome 8 to the Immunoglobulin (Ig) heavy chain region on chromosome 14 [t(8;14)] at band q32 or, less commonly, to light chain loci on 2p12 [t(2;8)] or 22q11[t(8;22)]. The molecular breakpoint within the *MYC* locus at 8q24 depends on the translocation partners and shows considerable inter-individual variation. In the case of classic t(8;14), the breakpoints in 8q24 typically lie within the centromeric (5′) part of the *MYC* locus. These have been classified according to the position of the chromosomal breakpoints in relation to the *MYC* gene translocations, with breakpoints in the first (5′) exon or intron of *MYC* being designated as class I, those with breakpoints immediately upstream of the gene designated as class II, and those with distant breakpoints as class III. In sporadic and immunodeficiency-associated BL, class I (and II) translocations are predominant, whereas in endemic African cases, class III translocations with breakpoints dispersed over several hundred kilo bases upstream of the gene are most frequent. The t(8;14) leads to activation of *MYC* on the der(14) chromosome, containing the intact coding region of the gene. The deregulation of *MYC* plays a decisive role in lymphomagenesis, by driving the cells through the cell cycle [24, 25]. The breakpoints in the *IGH* locus at 14q32 usually occur 5′ of the intron enhancer in a joining (J) or diversity (D) segment in endemic BL and 3′ of the intron enhancer in the switch mu region in sporadic and HIV-associated BL, suggesting that these translocations occur during an aberrant VDJ or class switch recombination process, respectively. There is also evidence that Burkitt translocation might be the result of a misdirected somatic mutation. Somatic and, in part, ongoing VH mutations have been observed in several cases of BL [26]. Similarly, mutations of the *MYC* gene are very frequent, presumably owing to somatic hypermutation driven by the immunoglobulin sequences juxtaposed to the *MYC* locus on the derivative chromosome 14. Mutations in *MYC* may further enhance its tumorigenicity and some of these mutations lead to decreased expression of *BIM*, which binds and inactivates BCL-2 [27]. Enigmatically, in normal cells *MYC* activation leads to two counteracting effects, i.e. induction of proliferation and apoptosis, but genetic and epigenetic alterations other than *MYC* have been reported in BL. These include *P53* point mutation and *P16INK4a* gene silencing by promoter methylation [28]. Other genetic alterations occurring in a subset of BL, including *P73*, *BAX*, *RBL2*, *BCL6*, and *A20* may promote cell growth and/or antagonize apoptosis [13, 29, 30]. In recent years, global genetic analyses, including conventional karyotyping, comparative genomic hybridization, and array-based comparative genomic hybridization, have described secondary genomic alterations in BL. One of the larger studies using CGH described gains of 12q, 22q, Xq, and losses of 13q as the most frequent alterations in BL. Moreover, abnormalities in 1q and 7q were associated with an inferior outcome [31].

Gene Expression Profile

Gene expression profiling (GEP) analysis by microarray has become an important part of biomedical and clinical research. The resulting data may provide important information regarding pathogenesis and may be extrapolated for the diagnosis and prognosis of non-Hodgkin lymphomas (NHLs) [32]. In particular, this technology has revealed that the existing diagnostic categories of NHLs are comprised of multiple molecularly and clinically distinct diseases. In addition, GEP studies may lead to the identification of novel targets for the development of new therapeutic agents for NHL.

Great progress in understanding the molecular features of BL was made by two gene expression profile studies, which differ in many important ways, but both reach the same conclusion: the gene-expression profiling of cases classified as Burkitt lymphoma identifies a characteristic genetic signature that clearly distinguishes this tumor from cases of DLBCL [21, 33]. In particular, the signature NF-κB target genes and MHC class I genes were expressed at very low levels in BL, whereas, due to the very nature of BL pathogenesis, the MYC and target gene signatures were increased. Germinal center B cell-associated genes showed a heterogeneous picture. In addition, these studies identified a new provisional category with morphologic features that are intermediate between those of Burkitt lymphoma and those of diffuse large B-cell lymphoma, which has been termed B-cell lymphoma, unclassifiable, with features intermediate between DLBCL and BL (DLBCL/BL) [34]. Despite the existence of some cases with an ambiguous gene expression signature, the studies by Dave et al. [33] and Hummel et al. [21] clearly show that categories which are homogeneous according to gene expression patterns overlap only partially with categories which are homogeneous according to the traditional criteria of morphology and immunophenotype, and two additional criteria should be applied: correlation with cytogenetic abnormalities and with clinical features. Both these studies were mainly performed on sporadic BL cases. We have more recently performed GEP including endemic and HIV-related BL cases [35].

This study demonstrated that, although BL is relatively homogeneous, differences among BL subtypes exist. In particular, a differential expression profile was observed between eBL and sBL, clustering HIV-BL with eBL and mainly involving genes controlling the cell cycle, proliferation, transcription, and nucleic acid metabolism. In particular, gene set enrichment revealed an enhancement of the B-cell receptor (BCR) signaling pathway in eBL, thus suggesting an active role for chronic antigenic stimulation and infectious agents in these cases and pointing to a possible different pathogenetic mechanism. Because the terms sporadic and endemic are mainly based on epidemiology, a better classification should take into account the causative pathogenetic mechanisms.

Another important finding that emerged from these molecular studies was the identification of BL cases that cluster as molecular Burkitt lymphomas, but do not carry *MYC* translocation. Interestingly, these cases express *MYC* at comparable levels to translocated ones. This prompts the question whether *MYC* translocation should still be considered the gold standard for defining BL [36]. We can conclude that *MYC* rearrangement alone is not sufficient for a diagnosis of BL and that *MYC*-negative cases may have a different pathogenetic mechanism. This issue will be discussed at length in the next paragraph.

More recently, dysregulation of small noncoding RNAs, known as microRNAs (miRNAs), has been proposed as a cofactor for Burkitt lymphomagenesis. MicroRNAs are a class of small (~22nt) noncoding RNAs that are able to regulate gene expression by miRNA cleavage or translational inhibition [37]. They are usually expressed in a tissue-specific manner and play important roles in apoptosis, differentiation, and cell proliferation [38]. Several experimental studies have reported miRNA involvement in cancer and their association with fragile sites in the genome [39–41], suggesting that these molecules could act as tumor suppressors or oncogenes [42]. Even though an increasing amount of evidence highlights their possible role in malignant transformation, little is known about their expression and deregulation in malignant lymphomas. A recent study compared BL with DLBCL to determine whether miRNA profiles reflect the molecular differences between BL and DLBCL revealed by mRNA profiling. The miRNA profiling confirmed that BL and DLBCL represent distinct lymphoma categories, thus endorsing the GEP data [43]. Interestingly, a few BL cases were included in the miRNA DLBCL category, thus identifying a subgroup reminiscent of the cases intermediate between BL and DLBCL, as detected by mRNA expression profiling. In addition, a comparison of sBL and eBL revealed only a few differentially expressed miRNAs and demonstrated that the three BL variants are representative of the same biological entity, with only marginal differences in miRNA expression between eBL and sBL.

MYC-Translocation Negative BL Cases

Two pivotal studies, aimed at unraveling the differences between various lymphoma entities, have revealed the existence of BL cases with comparable GEP to the classical profiles, but lacking the typical translocation [21, 33]. These cases were negative for *MYC* translocation by FISH analysis using both split and fusion probes for t(8;14), as well as using IgH and IgL split probes. There is increasing evidence that about 10% of classical BL cases lack an identifiable *MYC* rearrangement. The current WHO classification states that the diagnosis of this subset of BL must be confirmed by typical morphology, immunophenotyping and clinical features. In other words, these cases must be typical in all other aspects for a diagnosis of BL to be made. Although none of the techniques currently used to diagnose genetic changes can unambiguously rule out all *MYC* translocations [44], it can be postulated that alternative molecular mechanisms, possibly resulting in *MYC* deregulation, also exist.

Quantitative Reverse Transcriptase-Polymerase Chain Reaction (qRT-PCR) has been used to identify two miRNAs, hsa-miR-34b and hsa-miR-9*, which are differentially expressed between *MYC* translocation-positive and negative BL cases [45, 46]. In particular, a strong down-regulation of both miRNAs was only reported in *MYC*-translocation-negative BLs, due to epigenetic events. This finding suggests that a dysregulated expression of miRNAs may represent one of the mechanisms leading to *MYC* over-expression in BL cases lacking a *MYC* translocation, through either a direct or indirect mechanism. In addition, it may be argued that *MYC* itself also induces a specific miRNA pattern that, in turn, might be responsible for differential gene expression, and for functional alterations in tumor cells. A miRNA microarray strategy has recently been developed in order to gain an overview of the differences between the miRNA expression profile of *MYC* translocation-positive and negative BL cases [46]. Using this approach, a clear-cut microRNA signature has been identified, which distinguishes between *MYC* translocation-positive and negative BLs. Of note, these miRNAs control relevant biological processes, such as angiogenesis, apoptosis, and cell proliferation, according to Gene Ontology categories. Furthermore, the impact of miRNA deregulation on the gene expression pattern identified genes, which are more likely to be regulated by the selected miRNA.

The identification of miRNAs, which are specifically altered in BL cases lacking *MYC* translocation, may represent a model for understanding the *MYC* regulatory network not only in BL but also in other human cancers. In fact, their deregulation may represent a valid alternative molecular mechanism leading to MYC over-expression in the absence of genetic alteration.

A Practical Approach to the Diagnosis of Burkitt Lymphoma

For therapeutic and prognostic purposes, BL needs to be distinguished from the subset of lymphomas that compose the newly identified borderline category DLBCL/BL. Moreover, it should be remembered that a proportion of cases of DLBCL may also have some of the individual characteristics of BL. In children, Burkitt and non-Burkitt types seem not to differ clinically, whereas in adults, most cases classified as non-Burkitt lymphoma are similar to diffuse large B-cell lymphoma [19].

RNA extraction and microarray analysis are laborious and expensive and therefore not ready for real-time diagnosis, but other tools currently available to pathologists can be used to identify some of the distinguishing features of cases with the molecular signature of BL [36]. IGH, IGL, MYC, BCL2, and BCL6 rearrangement can be detected by FISH in paraffin sections, while down-regulation of class I HLA and CD44 and up-regulation of germinal center markers can be detected by immunohistochemistry [36]. In conclusion, no single parameter, such as morphology, genetic analysis, or immunophenotyping, can be used as a gold standard for the diagnosis of BL, but a combination of diagnostic techniques is necessary. The combined application of genomics and immunophenotyping, in conjunction with consensus reviewed histology and clinical features, appear to constitute a reliable approach that enables a reproducible and clinically meaning full characterization of BL [19].

Most endemic BL and a large portion of other BL occur in locations in which the necessary infrastructures and technical expertise are not currently available, and may not be available in the near future. This aspect makes it pertinent to construct a diagnostic algorithm that would facilitate reliable diagnosis of BL using less resources. Such a systematic approach is also relevant in the setting of developed countries, as none of the parameters currently used in diagnostic evaluation can clearly distinguish between BL, DLBCL/BL, and DLBCL on an individual basis.

A feasible scoring system has recently been proposed for the differential diagnosis between BL and non-BL. This scoring system [20] was applied to 252 cases and was based on morphology, immunohistochemistry, and fluorescent in situ hybridization (FISH), employed in three phases: phase 1 (morphology with CD10 and BCL2 immunostainings), phase 2 (CD38, CD44, and Ki-67 immunostainings) and phase 3 (FISH on paraffin sections for *MYC*, *BCL2*, *BCL6*, and immunoglobulin family genes). Using this algorithm, a specific diagnosis of BL or non-BL was determined in 82, 92, and 95% cases in phase 1, 2, and 3, respectively (Fig. 5.3).

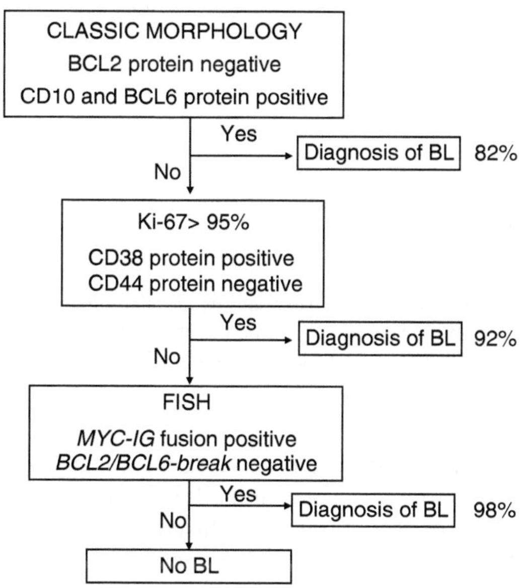

Fig. 5.3 Using the algorithm proposed by Naresh et al. [20] a specific diagnosis of BL or non-BL was determined in 82, 92, and 95% cases in phase 1, 2, and 3

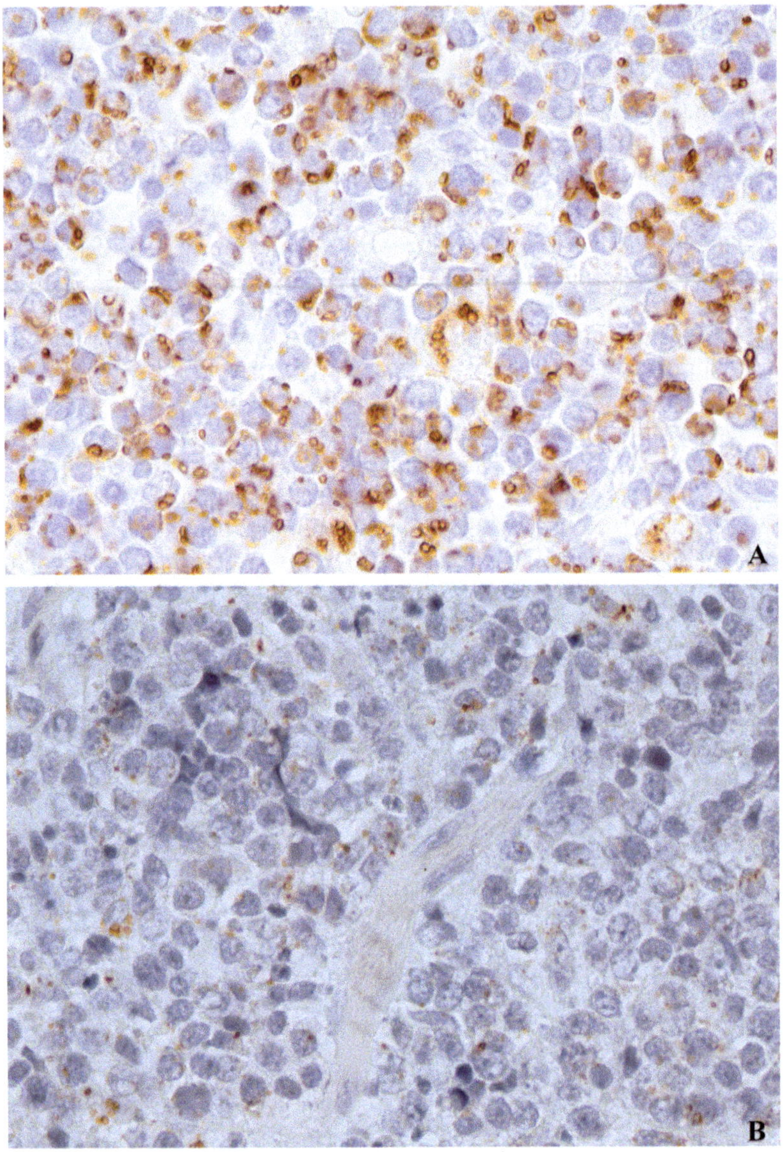

Fig. 5.4 A monoclonal antibody against the adipophilin is able to specifically recognize cytoplasmic vacuoles in typical BL (**a**); on the other hand, in non-BL adipophilin shows a weak positivity in few cells (**b**) (**a–b**: Adipophilin stain, OM: 10×)

With FNAC, diagnosis of BL is facilitated by the identification of the characteristic cytoplasmic vacuoles in the lymphoid cells [48]. However, these lipid-containing vacuoles cannot be seen on histological preparations. A recently performed GEP of BL cases found a marked up-regulation of some genes (*ADPF, SCD5, FASN, USF1*) involved in lipid metabolism in BL. One of these genes (*ADPF*) encodes for a protein, known as adipophilin (adipocyte differentiation-related protein), which is a member of the PAT (perilipin, adipophilin, and TIP47) family of proteins and is mainly involved in fatty acid transport and in preserving the cellular content of triacylglycerols. A monoclonal antibody against the adipophilin is able to specifically recognize the cytoplasmic vacuoles of BL by immunohistochemistry and was tested on a large series of aggressive B-cell lymphomas (Fig. 5.4). The preliminary results suggest adipophilin as a novel marker that maybe useful for the diagnosis of BL in histological sections, especially in challenging cases, such as DLBCL/BL [49].

Acknowledgement The authors would like to thank Maria Raffaella Ambrosio, Cristiana Bellan, Giulia De Falco, Stefano Lazzi and Anna Onnis, Department of Human Pathology and Oncology, University of Siena, for their contribution.

References

1. Burkitt DP (1958) A sarcoma involving the jaws in African children. Br J Surg 46:218
2. Soussain C, Patte C, Ostronoff M et al (1995) Small noncleaved cell lymphoma and leukemia in adults. A retrospective study of 65 adults treated with the LMB pediatric protocols. Blood 85:664–674
3. Harris NL, Jaffe ES, Stein H et al (1994) A revised European-American classification of lymphoid neoplasms: a proposal from the International Lymphoma Study Group. Blood 84:1361–1392
4. Wright DH (1971) Burkitt's lymphoma: a review of the pathology, immunology and possible aetiological factors. Pathol Annu 6:337–363
5. Pelicci PG, Knowles DM, Magrath I et al (1986) Chromosomal breakpoints and structural alterations of the c-myc locus differ in endemic and sporadic forms of Burkitt lymphoma. Proc Natl Acad Sci USA 83:2984–2988
6. Wright DH (1997) What is Burkitt's lymphoma? J Pathol 182:125–127
7. Mannucci S, Luzzi A, Carugi A et al (2012) EBV reactivation and chromosome polysomies: Euphorbia tirucalli as a possible cofactor in Endemic Burkitt lymphoma. Adv Hematol 2012:149780
8. Rochford R, Cannon MJ, Moormann AM (2005) Endemic Burkitt lymphoma: a polymicrobial disease? Nat Rev Microbiol 3(2):182–187
9. Van den Bosch C (2012) A role for RNA viruses in the pathogenesis of Burkitt lymphoma: the need for reappraisal. Adv Hematol 2012:494758
10. Magrath IT, Sariban E (1985) Clinical features of Burkitt's lymphoma in the USA. IARC Sci Publ 60:119–127
11. Mbulaiteye SM, Anderson WF, Ferlay J et al (2012) Pediatric, elderly, and emerging adult-onset peaks in Burkitt's lymphoma incidence diagnosed in four continents, excluding Africa. Am J Hematol. doi:10.1002/ajh.23187
12. Boerma EG, van Imhoff GW, Appel IM et al (2004) Gender and age-related differences in Burkitt lymphoma–epidemiological and clinical data from The Netherlands. Eur J Cancer 40:2781–2787
13. Bellan C, Lazzi S, De Falco G et al (2003) Burkitt's lymphoma: new insights into molecular pathogenesis. J Clin Pathol 56:188–192
14. Levine PH, Kamaraju LS, Connelly RR et al (1982) The American Burkitt's Lymphoma Registry: eight years' experience. Cancer 49:1016–1022
15. Magrath IT, Janus C, Edwards BK et al (1984) An effective therapy for both undifferentiated (including Burkitt's) lymphomas and lymphoblastic lymphomas in children and young adults. Blood 63:1102–1111

16. Raphael M, Gentilhomme O, Tulliez M et al (1991) Histopathologic features of high-grade non-Hodgkin's lymphomas in acquired immunodeficiency syndrome. The French Study Group of Pathology for Human Immunodeficiency Virus-Associated Tumors. Arch Pathol Lab Med 115:15–20
17. De Falco G, Bellan C, Lazzi S (2003) Interaction between HIV-1 Tat and pRb2/p130: a possible mechanism in the pathogenesis of AIDS-related neoplasms. Oncogene 22:6214–6219
18. Ziegler JL, Beckstead JA, Volberding PA et al (1984) Non-Hodgkin's lymphoma in 90 homosexual men. Relation to generalized lymphadenopathy and the acquired immunodeficiency syndrome. N Engl J Med 311:565–570
19. Leoncini L, Raphael M, Stein H et al (2008) Burkitt lymphoma. In: WHO classification of tumours of haematopoietic and lymphoid tissues. IARC Press, Lyon
20. Naresh KN, Ibrahim HA, Lazzi S et al (2011) Diagnosis of Burkitt lymphoma using an algorithmic approach - applicable in both resource-poor and resource-rich countries. Br J Haematol. doi:10.1111/j.1365-2141.2011.08771.x
21. Hummel M, Bentink S, Berger H et al (2006) Molecular Mechanisms in Malignant Lymphomas Network Project of the Deutsche Krebshilfe a biologic definition of Burkitt's lymphoma from transcriptional and genomic profiling. N Engl J Med 8:2419–2430
22. Braziel RM, Arber DA, Slovak ML et al (2001) The Burkitt-like lymphomas: a Southwest Oncology Group study delineating phenotypic, genotypic, and clinical features. Blood 15(97):3713–3720
23. McClure RF, Remstein ED, Macon WR et al (2005) Adult B-cell lymphomas with Burkitt-like morphology are phenotypically and genotypically heterogeneous with aggressive clinical behavior. Am J Surg Pathol 29:1652–1660
24. Gaidano G, Ballerini P, Gong JZ et al (1991) p53 Mutations in human lymphoid malignancies: association with Burkitt lymphoma and chronic lymphocytic leukemia. Proc Natl Acad Sci USA 88:5413–5417
25. Gutierrez MI, Bhatia K, Barriga F et al (1992) Molecular epidemiology of Burkitt's lymphoma from South America: differences in breakpoint location and Epstein-Barr virus association from tumors in other world regions. Blood 79:3261–3266
26. Bellan C, Lazzi S, Hummel M et al (2005) Immunoglobulin gene analysis reveals 2 distinct cells of origin for EBV-positive and EBV-negative Burkitt lymphomas. Blood 106:1031–1036
27. Hemann MT, Bric A, Teruya-Feldstein J et al (2005) Evasion of the p53 tumour surveillance network by tumour-derived MYC mutants. Nature 11(436):807–811
28. Sánchez-Beato M, Sáez AI, Navas IC et al (2001) Overall survival in aggressive B-cell lymphomas is dependent on the accumulation of alterations in p53, p16, and p27. Am J Pathol 159:205–213
29. De Falco G, Leucci E, Lenze D et al (2007) Gene expression analysis identifies novel RBL2/p130 target genes in endemic Burkitt's lymphoma cell lines and primary tumors. Blood 15(110):1301–1307
30. Lindstrom MS, Wiman KG (2002) Role of genetic and epigenetic changes in Burkitt lymphoma. Semin Cancer Biol 12:381–387
31. Salaverria I, Zettl A, Beà S et al (2008) Chromosomal alterations detected by comparative genomic hybridization in subgroups of gene expression-defined Burkitt's lymphoma. Haematologica 93:1327–1334
32. Staudt LM, Dave S (2005) The biology of human lymphoid malignancies revealed by gene expression profiling. Adv Immunol 87:163–208
33. Dave SS, Fu K, Wright GW et al (2006) Molecular diagnosis of Burkitt's lymphoma. N Engl J Med 354:2431–2442
34. Kluin P, Harris NL, Stein H et al (2008) B cell lymphoma, unclassifiable, with features intermediate between diffuse large B-cell lymphoma and BurkittlymphomaIn: WHO classification of tumours of haematopoietic and lymphoid tissues. IARC Press, Lyon
35. Piccaluga PP, De Falco G, Kustagi M et al (2011) Gene expression analysis uncovers similarity and differences among Burkitt lymphoma subtypes. Blood 117:3596–3608

36. Harris NL, Horning SJ (2006) Burkitt's lymphoma – the message from microarrays. N Engl J Med 354:2495–2498
37. He L, Hannon GJ (2004) MicroRNAs: small RNAs with a big role in gene regulation. Nat Rev Genet 5:522–531
38. Bartel DP (2004) MicroRNAs: genomics, biogenesis, mechanism, and function. Cell 116:281–297
39. Calin GA, Sevignani C, Dumitru CD et al (2004) Human microRNA genes are frequently located at fragile sites and genomic regions involved in cancers. Proc Natl Acad Sci USA 101:2999–3004
40. Cullen BR (2004) Transcription and processing of human microRNA precursors. Mol Cell 16:861–865
41. Lu J, Getz G, Miska EA et al (2005) MicroRNA expression profiles classify human cancers. Nature 435:834–838
42. Volinia S, Calin GA, Liu CG et al (2006) A microRNA expression signature of human solid tumors defines cancer gene targets. Proc Natl Acad Sci USA 103:2257–2261
43. Lenze D, Leoncini L, Hummel M et al (2011) The different epidemiologic subtypes of Burkitt lymphoma share a homogenous micro RNA profile distinct from diffuse large B-cell lymphoma. Leukemia 25:1869–1876
44. Jaffe ES, Harris NL, Vardiman JW et al (2011) Hematopathology. Elsevier, London
45. Leucci E, Cocco M, Onnis A et al (2008) MYC translocation-negative classical Burkitt lymphoma cases: an alternative pathogenetic mechanism involving miRNA deregulation. J Pathol 216:440–450
46. Onnis A, De Falco G, Antonicelli G et al (2010) Alteration of microRNAs regulated by c-Myc in Burkitt lymphoma. PLoS One 5(9). pii: e12960
47. Onnis A, Morettini F, Fuligni F et al (2012) MicroRNA expression profile identifies a distinct molecular signature between MYC translocation-positive and negative Burkitt lymphoma cases. Submitted to Blood
48. Swerdlow SH, Campo E, Harris NL et al (2008) WHO classification of tumours of haematological and lymphoid tissues. IARC Press, Lyon
49. Ambrosio MR, Piccaluga PP, Ponzoni M et al (2012) The alteration of lipid metabolism in Burkitt lymphoma identifies a novel marker: adipophilin. PLoS ONE 7(8): e44315

Chapter 6
Endemic Burkitt's Lymphoma

Elizabeth Molyneux, Trijn Israels, and Thomas Walwyn

Brief History

Doctors working in West, East and Central Africa at the turn of the nineteenth century described an unusual but fairly common jaw tumour in children [1–5].

It was in 1957 that Denis Burkitt, an Irish surgeon at Mulago Hospital in Uganda published a report of a series of children with rapidly growing jaw tumours that he thought were round cell sarcoma [1], but in 1960 O'Connor, a pathologist confirmed that the tumours were of lymphoma lineage [2]. In 1964 Epstein, Achong and Barr, three virologists, identified viral particles in the tumour cells; and the virus became known as the Epstein Barr virus (EBV) [3]. Burkitt and two physician colleagues from Uganda then toured the hospitals of Eastern and Central Africa to map the geographical extent of the tumour [4, 5]. They found hospital records of children with similar tumours from all the malarial areas of the countries that they visited and proposed that malaria and this tumour (now called Burkitt's tumour) were linked in some way.

E. Molyneux (✉)
Paediatric Department, College of Medicine, Queen Elizabeth Central Hospital, Box 360, Blantyre, Malawi, C.Africa
e-mail: emmolyneux@gmail.com

T. Israels
VU University Medical Center, Department of Pediatric Oncology, Amsterdam, The Netherlands
e-mail: trijnisraels@hotmail.com

T. Walwyn
Princess Margaret Hospital for Children, Perth, Western Australia
e-mail: tomwalwyn@hotmail.com

E.S. Robertson (ed.), *Burkitt's Lymphoma*, Current Cancer Research,
DOI 10.1007/978-1-4614-4313-1_6, © Springer Science+Business Media New York 2013

Epidemiology

Endemic BL (eBL) is found in areas of equatorial Africa, Brazil and Papua New Guinea where malaria is holo-endemic and EBV infections are acquired in early childhood [4–10]. In Africa this means that eBL is found in hot, wet areas of the continent, 15° on either side of the equator where the rainfall is >50 mm per annum [1]. This area is known as the Burkitt Belt and matches the epidemiological map of malaria (Fig. 6.1). The annual incidence of eBL in the high-risk areas of Africa is estimated at 40–50 per million children under 18 years of age per year [11]. It accounts for half of all the malignancies and 90% of the lymphomas diagnosed in children [11]. The disease is more common in boys than in girls, with various reports of being twice as common in rural boys but with less gender difference in urban areas such as Nairobi where the ratio of boys to girls with eBL was reported as 1.2:1 [12, 13]. This is in contrast to resource-rich settings where the gender disparity is more marked with about 80% of BL occurring in boys [14]. The peak age of presentation is at about 6 years [13, 15]. In Kenya over a 10-year period from 1988 to 1997, the age of presentation was around 3 years of age in 5.6%, 6 years in 19.5% and 17 years in 13.6% of cases. Four percent of the 1,005 cases of eBL were in adults [15]. There is a smaller peak in presentation in early adolescence when the sex difference is less marked and abdominal tumours predominate [16]. In Malawi the mean age at presentation was 7.1 ± 2.9 years, ranging from 1 to 17 years. The majority of children were boys (62.4% ± 2.2%) [12]. Almost all the children with eBL come from poor rural communities [11].

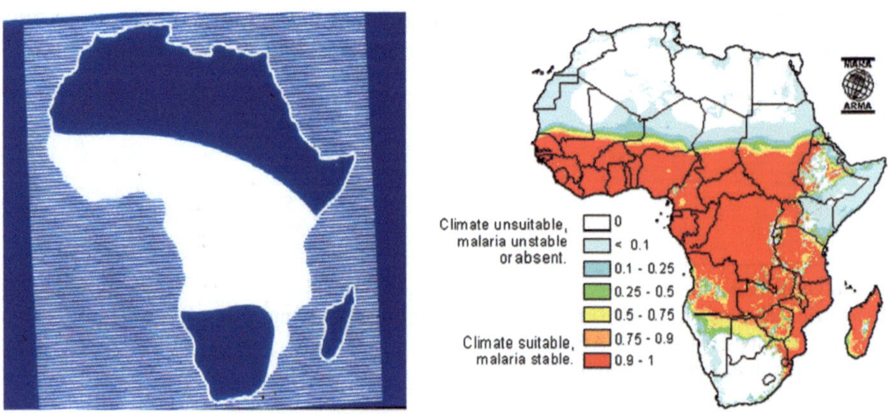

Burkitt belt of Africa

Malaria Transmission in Africa

Fig. 6.1 The (endemic) Burkitt lymphoma belt of Africa and the map of endemic malaria

Cofactors

The important interactions of malaria, EBV, and eBL are covered in chapters. Other cofactors have been raised as possible causative agents in the development of eBL. The impact of HIV infection on the development of eBL is unclear. HIV-infected children may present with eBL in less usual sites (e.g., bone, scalp) but initial reports from Uganda claiming that there was an association between HIV and eBL were not confirmed in Côte d'Ivoire, where none of the 78 HIV infected patients had eBL, [17–19] nor in Zambia where no increase in the number of eBL cases was seen after the HIV pandemic emerged [20].

Preliminary data from Malawi suggested an increased risk of BL but updated analyses found no significant association. Twenty of 263 (7%) children with eBL were HIV infected with an odds ratio (OR) for developing eBL of 2.2 [(95% CI 0.8–6.4); $p=0.13$] [21]. Few HIV-positive children with eBL have been reported, and so the role of HIV (if any) in the aetiology of eBL remains uncertain.

Arboviruses and schistosomiasis have both been suggested as causative cofactors of eBL, but the evidence is not convincing [10].

The plants *Euphorbia tirucalli* and *Jatropha caveas* are common in areas where eBL occurs. The dipterene esters found in their milky sap can activate latent EBV and induce rearrangements of chromosomes in about 10% of EBV-infected B cells exposed to them [22, 23]. Euphorbia sap is used in religious ceremonies, weddings and at some twin births in the Lake Victoria Basin. It is also used by children as a sticky "glue" when they make toys [22]. Fishermen, in the same area, use the sap as a fish poison [24].

Sickle cell trait protects against malaria and eBL [23]. Sickle cell disease is more common in West than East Africa that may account partially for the higher rates of eBL in the eastern part of the African continent.

Cytology

eBL is a highly aggressive B-cell non-Hodgkin's lymphoma (NHL). Its cells are monomorphic, medium in size and have a high proliferation rate. The cells contain coarse chromatin and prominent basophilic nucleoli though atypical variants may show more nuclear pleomorphism. In tissue sections the cells appear to be moulded and the cytoplasm is deeply basophilic with squared off cytoplasmic margins. A "starry sky" appearance is due to scattered tingible body-laden macrophages that contain apoptotic tumour cells.

Chromosomal Rearrangements

The chromosomal translocation, t(8;14)(q24;32), is the hallmark of eBL. It occurs in 70–80% of patients with the variant translocations, t(2;8)(p12;q24) and t(8;22)(q24;q11), accounting for 10–15% [23, 25, 26]. The molecular consequence of the three translocations is deregulated expression of the *MYC* oncogene, which plays an essential role in cell cycle control. It arises as a result of juxtaposition of *MYC* to the enhancer elements of one of the immunoglobulin genes (*IG*); the heavy chain (*IGH*) at 14q32, the kappa light chain (*IGK*) at 2p12 or the lambda light chain (*IGL*) at 22q11. There is overlap between disease types but usually endemic, sporadic and immunodeficiency-associated BL show different clustering of breakpoints of both chromosome partners. Usually eBL have breakpoints upstream of *MYC* and originate from aberrant somatic hypermutation within the *IG* loci, whereas sporadic Burkitt's lymphoma (sBL) breakpoints are closer to *MYC* and mostly involve the switch regions of the *IG* loci [25, 26]. The differences in *MYC* breakpoint are most likely due to the EBV-positive nature of eBL compared to the EBV-negative nature of sporadic BL [27].

Clinical Presentation

The classical and best known presentation of eBL is a rapidly growing jaw tumour. The history is therefore short—usually 3–4 weeks. In Malawi median duration of symptoms was 1 month ranging from 1 week to 36 months (personal communication EMM). In Ghana, Owuru et al. found 48% of children presented with facial tumour; in Kenya it was 52% and in Malawi 63% [12, 15, 16].

The mass is painless and inside the mouth, the gum is swollen and teeth are displaced at the site of the tumour. Facial tumours may affect the maxillary areas, mandibles or be retro-orbital, pushing the eye forward and causing proptosis (Figs. 6.2 and 6.3). Abdominal masses, often multiple, also are common (Fig. 6.3). In Kenya 25% of 1,005 children over the periods 1988–1992 and 1993–1997 presented with abdominal masses and 14% presented with both facial and abdominal tumours. The presentations in Ghana were similar; 23% were abdominal and 16% were of face and abdomen [15, 16]. Central nervous system (CNS) involvement occurs, even at diagnosis; in Malawi CNS involvement was found in 15% of cases, in Kenya BL cells were found in cerebro-spinal fluid (CSF) in 18% of 1,005 cases but the diagnosis was only suspected clinically in 6% [12, 28].

The Kenyan study also reported that CNS presentation tended to occur in older children (11–15 years) compared to jaw masses that peaked in presentation at 6 years of age [28]. Paraplegia may be caused by direct cord involvement or pressure from a tumour mass lying outside the dura. Figure 6.4 shows an MRI scan of a boy with paraplegia due to eBL. eBL is multifocal and so the tumours often present at several sites simultaneously. Table 6.1 shows the most common sites and Table 6.2

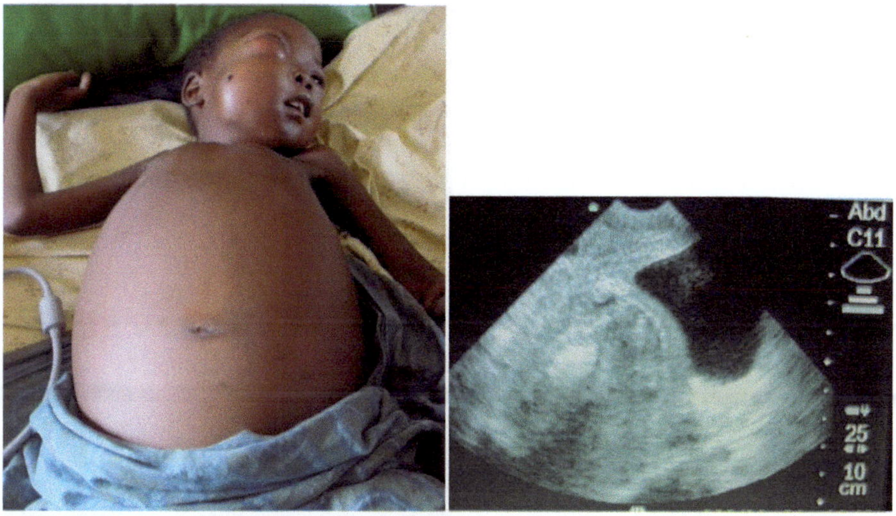

Fig. 6.2 Patient presenting with Burkitt lymphoma of the jaw, peri-orbital area and abdomen. Ultrasound scans of the abdominal masses

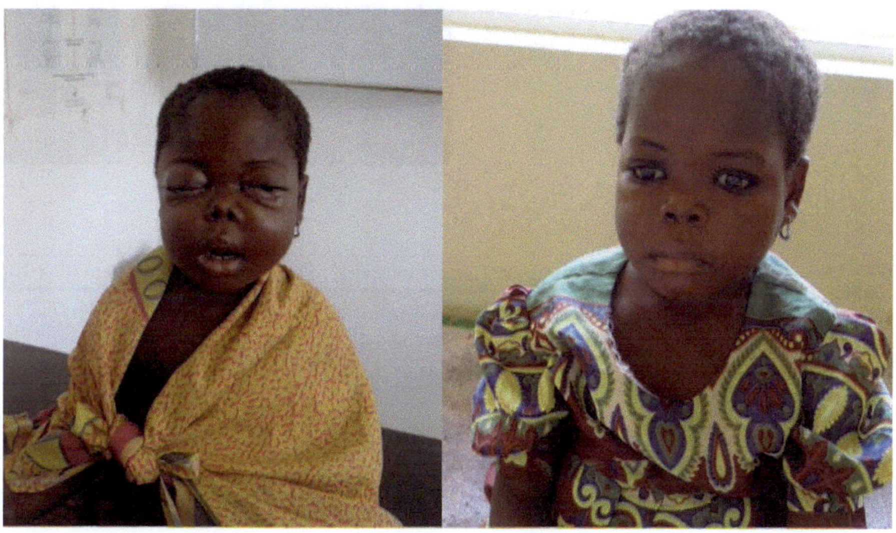

Fig. 6.3 Patient presenting with retro orbital Burkitt lymphoma

the presenting signs and symptoms in children with eBL in Blantyre Malawi. Other centres also report that most children present with advanced disease [12, 15, 16].

Often the children are malnourished and may have other co-infections [12, 29]. Many children in the communities where these children live are chronically undernourished. In sub-Saharan Africa 42% of all children less than 5 years of age are

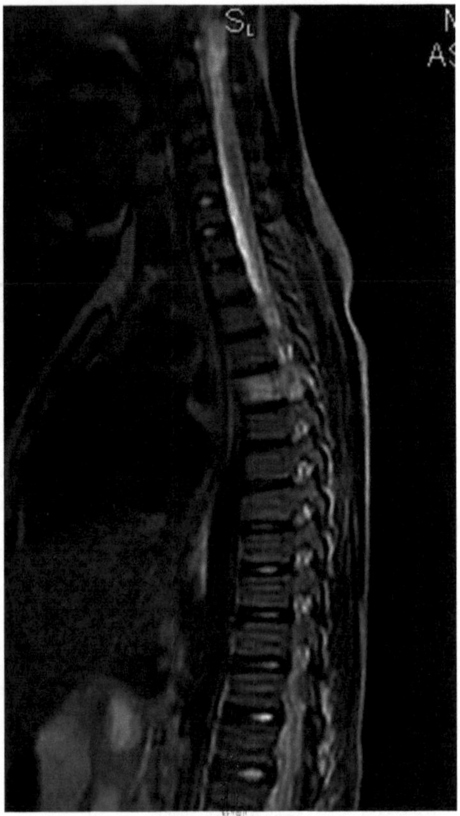

Fig. 6.4 MRI showing Burkitt lymphoma of the spine

Table 6.1 Location of tumour(s)[a] for endemic Burkitt's Lymphoma patients at QECH 2000–2009 (n=475)

Tumour location	Present [N, (%)]	Absent [N, (%)]
Face	306 (63.3)	177 (36.7)
Abdomen	303 (62.7)	180 (37.3)
Orbital	148 (30.6)	335 (69.4)
Limb	14 (2.9)	469 (97.1)
Bony	8 (1.7)	475 (98.3)

[a]Patients could have more than one tumour location

stunted (the result of chronic poor nutrition) and 9% are wasted [30] (Table 6.3). Many children with eBL have acute malnutrition adding to their underlying chronic under-nutrition. Israels et al. [29] found that 69% of children with eBL were acutely malnourished at admission. In a study reported by Hesseling et al. from Malawi a third of children had a co-infection of one or more of malaria, schistosomiasis or hookworm [12].

Table 6.2 Common presenting signs of endemic Burkitt's lymphoma in Malawi

Symptom	Present [N, (%)]	Absent [N, (%)]
CSF infiltrated	35 (10.3)	305 (89.7)
BM infiltrated	21 (6.3)	314 (93.7)
Lower limb weakness	19 (3.9)	463 (96.1)
Paraplegia	46 (9.5)	436 (90.5)
Urinary incontinence	36 (7.4)	446 (92.6)
Stool incontinence	31 (6.4)	451 (93.6)
Malnutrition	223 (46.3)	259 (53.7)
Lymphadenopathy	183 (37.9)	300 (62.1)
Hepatomegaly	113 (23.4)	369 (76.6)
Splenomegaly	209 (43.4)	273 (56.6)
Abdominal distension	151 (31.3)	331 (68.7)
Pedal oedema	81 (16.8)	401 (83.2)
Ascites	40 (8.3)	442 (91.7)
Weight loss	83 (17.2)	399 (82.8)

Symptoms at presentation in endemic Burkitt's Lymphoma patients at QECH, 2000–2009 (n=475)

Table 6.3 Some comparative demographic data of selected countries in sub-Saharan Africa, North Africa, and Latin America

	Malawi	Senegal	Tanzania	Ghana	S. Africa	Morocco	Brazil
Socioeconomic and demographic indicators							
Population (millions)[a]	13.6	12.1	39.5	23.0	48.3	30.9	189.3
Population < 15 years (millions)[a]	6.4	5.8	17.6	8.9	14.0	8.9	53.0
Gross national income per capita (US$)[b]	170	750	350	520	5,390	1,900	4,730
Total per capita expenditure on health (US$)[c]	64	72	N.A.	N.A.	869	N.A.	765
Per capita govt expenditure on health (US$)[c]	14	12	N.A.	N.A.	437	N.A.	164
Under 5 mortality rate (1990)[b]	221	149	161	120	60	89	57
Under 5 mortality rate/1,000 (2006)[b]	120	116	118	120	69	37	20
Under 5 mortality rank (2006)[b]	32	35	34	32	55	78	113
Life expectancy (years)[b]	47	53	52	59	50	71	72
Nutrition							
Children <5 years, % stunted[b]	46	16	38	22	25[1]	18	11[1]
Children <5 years, % wasted[b]	3	8	3	5	3[1]	9	2[1]
HIV							
HIV prevalence rate (age 15–40 year) (2005)[b]	14.1	0.9	6.5	2.3	18.8	0.1	0.5
No. of HIV-infected children (×1,000)[b]	91	5	110	25	240		
Health							
Access to clean water (%)[b]	73	76	62	75	88	81	90

[a]US Census Bureau, International Data Base. http://www.census.gov/ipc/www/idb/ [3]
[b]UNICEF, The State of the World's Children 2008: child survival. http://www.unicef.org/publications [2]
[c]World Health Organization. National Health Accounts. http://www.who.int/nha/en/ [4]

Differential Diagnosis

A careful history and examination will help in making the diagnosis of eBL especially with a classical jaw mass on presentation. Retro-orbital tumours could be, amongst others, rhabdomyosarcoma or non-Hodgkin's lymphoma (NHL). When the eye is already destroyed it is important to elicit where the mass started (in the eye as a white spot or outside the orbit) and the length of history. Retinoblastomas present usually at an earlier age than eBL but advanced retinoblastoma and peri-orbital eBL have been mistaken for each other. Abdominal masses are often very large and multiple. They may arise within any organ or from the retro-peritoneum. Renal involvement is not uncommon and must sometimes be differentiated from a Wilm's tumour. Bone infiltration with eBL does occur and can be mistaken radiologically for a primary bone cancer such as osteosarcoma or chronic osteomyelitis (Fig. 6.5).

Investigations

In many places where eBL is common the ability to undertake diagnostic tests is limited. It is important to confirm the diagnosis and fine needle aspiration (FNA) is easy to do and has a characteristic morphological appearance (Fig. 6.6). Of 475 cases of eBL that presented to QECH from January 2000 to August 2009, 83.8%

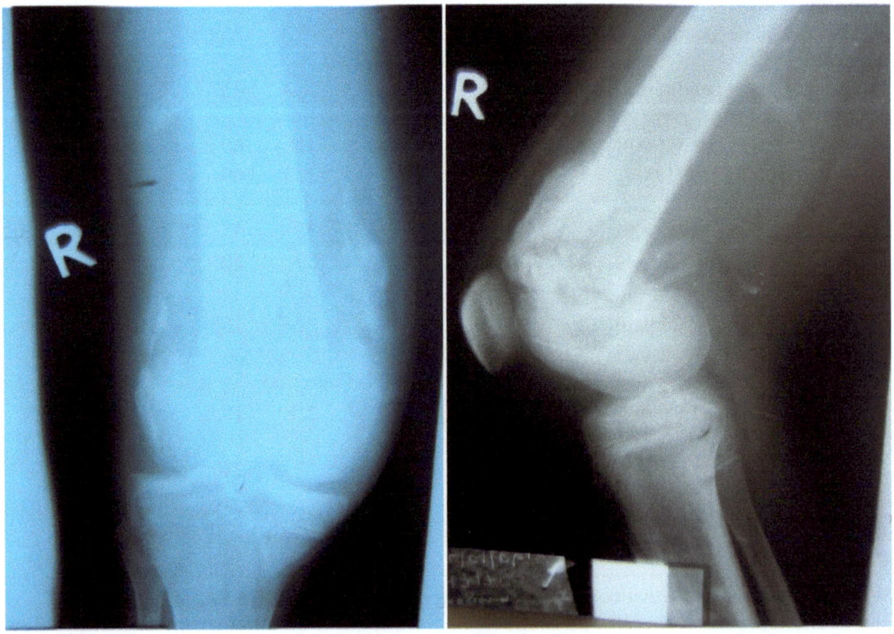

Fig. 6.5 X-ray of the femur of a patient with Burkitt lymphoma

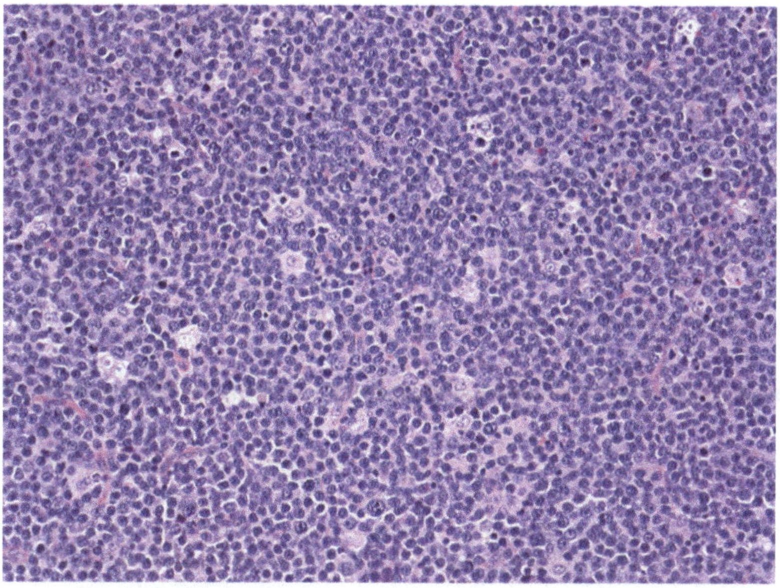

Classic Burkitt's lymphoma showing starry sky appearance

Fig. 6.6 Burkitt's lymphoma: H&E stain. Classic Burkitt's lymphoma showing starry sky appearance

were confirmed by FNA (Personal communication EMM). Sometimes it is difficult to differentiate other small round blue cell tumours from eBL but immunocytochemistry and cytogenetics are seldom available to confirm the diagnosis and clinical judgement must be deployed. If they are available it is helpful in the diagnosis of BL to demonstrate *MYC* deregulation and the presence of additional cytogenetic abnormalities, some of which have been shown to have prognostic significance [31]. The cells are always of B cell lineage (CD20 and CD79a positive); co-expression of CD10 and bcl-6 are often present, but the cells are usually negative for bcl-2. There is a paucity of T cells in the background [32].

EBV EBER may be identifiable by fluorescence in situ hybridization (FISH). It can be difficult to distinguish diffuse large B-cell lymphoma (DLBCL) with genetic and immunophenotypic features of BL from BL and some of these cases are now classified as "B-cell lymphoma—unclassifiable", as they have features between diffuse large B-cell lymphoma and BL. Distinct molecular changes in BL may provide a more reliable diagnosis.

Van Noorden et al. described the preservation of eBL cells for immunocytochemistry, in situ hybridisation and polymerase chain reaction in a buffered solution (PreserveCyt). These samples can be kept at room temperature and provide adequate cells for testing for many months. Though this does not help with immediate diagnosis it is a valuable tool for retrospective review, to confirm the diagnosis and as a tool to explore immunocytochemical markers for treatment failure [33].

It is also necessary to assess tumour spread. A thorough physical examination, ultrasound scan (USS) of the abdomen, chest X-ray, examination of bone marrow and cerebro-spinal fluid (CSF) will assist in evaluating the extent of the disease. Ideally lactic dehydrogenase, liver function tests, urea and electrolytes and full blood count should also be done.

One needs to know if it is safe to treat and a haemoglobin level, full blood count and differential, HIV test, stool and urine microscopy will identify any co-infections that require treatment or gross anaemia that needs correction prior to initiating treatment.

Staging

The St Jude/Murphy staging classification for Burkitt's lymphoma is the most common in current use (Table 6.4). Many children with eBL present in Africa with very advanced, stage III or IV disease. In three, combined studies of 208 consecutively recruited patients in Malawi, Cameroon and Ghana, 75% presented with Murphy stage III/IV disease, which is similar to the corresponding 79% who presented with stage III/IV disease in the Lymphome Malins de type B (LMB '89) study of 561 children [12, 34–36]. In the first publications investigating the treatment of eBL, the need to be able to classify tumours by their stage of advancement was apparent. Burkitt initially commented only on primary tumour size with a subjective categorisation as small, medium and large (stages A–C) [37, 38]. Others in the field soon felt that a description of disease stage was more useful [39]. John Ziegler and colleagues working in Kampala, Uganda in collaboration with the National Cancer Institute (NCI), of the USAA developed a staging system for eBL based on earlier work by Morrow et al. in Mulago Hospital, Uganda [40]. This gave four stages, from

Table 6.4 The St Jude Staging system for non-Hodgkin's lymphoma in children

Stage I	A single tumor (extranodal) or anatomic area (nodal) excluding the mediastinum or abdomen
Stage II	A single tumor (extranodal) with regional node involvement
	Two or more nodal areas on the same side of the diaphragm
	Two single (extranodal) tumors ± regional node involvement on the same side of the diaphragm
	A primary gastrointestinal tract tumor ± mesenteric lymph node involvement that is grossly completely resected
Stage III	Two single extranodal tumors on both sides of the diaphragm
	Two or more nodal areas on both sides of the diaphragm
	All primary intrathoracic tumors
	All extensive primary unresectable intra-abdominal disease
	All primary paraspinal or epidural tumors (CNS and CSF not involved)
Stage IV	Any of the above with initial CNS or bone marrow involvement

Note: Elective surgery for presumed abdominal BL is not recommended and abdominal tumours are classified as stage III disease

isolated facial tumours, through to multiple facial tumour masses and disseminated disease to CNS or bone marrow disease [41]. This system was modified further by Nkrumah et al. in Ghana, during work supported, again, by the NCI. They more clearly separated intra-abdominal disease from other non-facial sites [42]. Following additional clinical observations in which it was found that the resection of limited extent abdominal disease (of the ileo-caecal area) conferred a survival benefit, the NCI staging system in its full form was reached [43]. In 1980, Murphy proposed the staging system for non-Hodgkin Lymphoma that remains in use today [44]. Staging is different from the treatment group assignment used by LMB and Berlin-Frankfurt-Munster (BFM) protocols.

Treatment

In well-resourced centres BL is treated aggressively with remarkably good results [45, 46]. In resource-limited centres the intensity of treatment must be tempered by the level of locally available supportive therapy, staffing numbers, expertise, drug availability, patient's co-morbidity, and nutritional status.

The more intense the treatment, the better the long-term outcome. Each centre needs to decide what level of intensity their children can safely tolerate. Unacceptable high treatment-related morbidity and mortality due to unduly toxic regimens must be avoided. It must be decided how staff will monitor safety and progress, and what treatment is available for rescue therapy.

Chemotherapy

Burkitt's lymphoma (BL) was one of the first tumours to be found to be curable with chemotherapy alone [47]. At a time when BL and most other neoplasms were almost universally fatal, the prospect of long-term cure was tantalising and resulted in the testing of multiple single cytotoxic agents together with various combinations (Table 6.5) [13].

The agents that emerged at that time as being of particular use were cyclophosphamide (CPM), methotrexate (MTX) and vincristine (VCR). At the same time there was concern, in conjunction with the discovery of the link with Epstein–Barr Virus (EBV), that bolstering the host immune response could be an important avenue for therapy. The immune suppression induced by cytotoxic therapies was thought to be of concern for the same reason [38]. Approaches that were tested include scarification with the attenuated mycobacterium tuberculosis vaccination Bacille-Calmette-Guerin (BCG) [48]. Although various immunologically based avenues continue to attract research attention, their places in the treatment of eBL in resource-poor settings are minimal at present. The place of other non-chemotherapeutic modalities such as radiotherapy and surgery waxed and eventually waned over the following years. Of these, surgery alone has survived, though limited to

Table 6.5 History of the treatments with single cytotoxic agents for endemic Burkitt's lymphoma

Drug[a]	No. of patients	CR	CR+PR	% RR
Cyclophosphamide	163	43	132	81
Orthomerphalan	14	?	14	100
Chlorambucil	12	3	10	83
Nitrogen mustard	61	10	44	72
Melphalan	26	8	16	61
Procarbazine	6	0	0	0
BCNU	5	0	4	80
Vincristine	21	10	17	81
Vinblastine	2	0	0	0
Methotrexate	45	11	26	58
6-Mercaptopurine	3	0	0	0
Cystosine arabinoside	3	2	2	100
Epipodophyllotoxin	3	2	2	100
Actinomysin D	4	1	4	100

CR complete response; *PR* partial response; *RR* response rate; BCNU, carmustine
[a]Variety of doses and regimens were used [13].

resection of localised disease (e.g. nodal or ileo-caecal abdominal disease) or biopsy of more extensive disease. Radiotherapy has now been shown to have no place in the treatment of BL in resource-rich settings, but historically its use in resource-poor settings was limited by extremely poor access to radiotherapy facilities rather than by lack of inclination to use it [13, 49].

Although local intra-arterial administration of chemotherapy to the tumour mass was explored in the 1960s by Oettgen and Burkitt, the importance of *systemic* and *central nervous system* (CNS) coverage was quickly discovered [37, 50]. The propensity of BL to relapse in untreated sanctuary sites, particularly the CNS has proved to have important implications for the design of treatment regimens. BL is characterised by extremely rapid growth, and this is reflected in its chemo-sensitivity. In resource-rich settings the progressive refinement of treatment protocols has resulted in short, very intense and expensive multi-agent regimens that cure the majority of children even with advanced disease, but they require a considerable contribution in supportive care (Table 6.6). Over time the focus of research into potential treatments for BL, which was heavily concentrated in Africa and eBL during the 1960s and 1970s, has moved away. There was a notable paucity of research published from the resource-poor African settings during the 1980s and 1990s. During this period the research interest was concentrated on the treatment of sporadic BL (sBL) by single centres and large national and multinational cooperative groups. More recently there has been a resurgence in publications addressing eBL in non-resource-rich environments (Fig. 6.7). Sadly, the countries with the highest incidence of eBL have the least resources. The Burkitt Belt corresponds remarkably

Table 6.6 Cost of treatments for Burkitt's lymphoma in rich countries

Locale	Year	First author	*N*	Stage	%TRM	Outcome (%EFS)	Comments
Malawi	2009	Hesseling [12]	40	All	5	47	28 day CPM based protocol
North Africa	2008	Harif [54]	187	LMB Groups B & C	28	56	Reduced intensity LMB 89 protocol (GFA 2001)
Iraq	2011	Moletti [58]	239	All	29	53	Reduced intensity LMB 96 protocol. 12% abandonment included in events
Central America	2009	Peña [66]	114	All	6.1	83	Reduced intensity BFM protocol
Brazil	2009	Klumb [67]	85	All	1.2	80	Reduced intensity BFM 90 protocol
Argentina	2009	Chantada [68]	44	All	9	83	Reduced intensity BFM 95 protocol
France, etc.	2001	Patte [36]	561	All	1.4	91	LMB 89
Germany, etc.	2005	Woessmann [69]	362	All		89	BFM 95

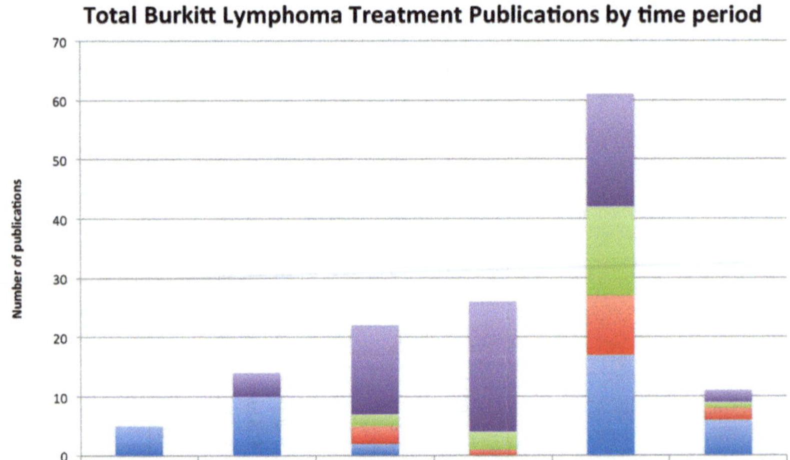

	1960-1969	1970-1979	1980-1989	1990-1999	2000-2009	2010 onwards
THEpC >1001 USD/year	0	4	15	22	19	2
THEpC 301<1000 USD/year	0	0	2	3	15	1
THEpC 51<300 USD/year	0	0	3	1	10	2
THEpC < 50 USD/year	5	10	2	0	17	6

Fig. 6.7 Total publications for eBL by time period

well to the countries where total health expenditure per capita is <USD 50 per year. This in turn leads to greater barriers to research. Only more recent multi-centre studies (e.g. ongoing work of the International Network for Cancer Treatment and Research, INCTR) have patient numbers comparable to those enrolled in the LMB or BFM trials.

At a basic level the chemotherapy for eBL in the most resource-poor settings has not changed significantly since the 1960s. In 1967 after his earlier papers had described disease responses, Denis Burkitt published a paper describing long-term remissions using one or two 30–40 mg/kg body weight doses of cyclophosphamide (CPM) [47]. In 1970 Ziegler published a study of 57 patients comparing a single 40 mg/kg dose of CPM given 6 times, every 2–3 weeks with an event-free survival (EFS) of 42% and 17% treatment-related mortality (TRM) in the 21 patients receiving the multi-dose regimen [41]. In 2009, Hesseling et al. published their 28-day regimen of four doses of CPM; the first dose given intravenously followed by oral dosing, combined with intrathecal methotrexate (MTX) and hydrocortisone as both CNS treatment and prophylaxis (Fig. 6.8) [12]. This prospective single-centre study of 40 patients achieved a projected 1 year EFS of 47% and TRM of 5% in conjunction with rigorous and pragmatic supportive care guidelines. Unfortunately this "basic minimum" approach does not treat stage IV disease adequately (13% EFS). Attempts to replicate these results in multi-centre settings have been carried out by the French–African Pediatric Oncology Group GFAOP). Traoré et al. performed an international multi-centre trial in Burkino Faso, Cameroon, Cote D'Ivoire, Mali, Madagascar and Senegal. Over a 3-year period (April 2005 to March 2008) there

"Malawi 2006" Protocol (Hesseling 2009)

Day	1	8	*18*	22	*28*	43	57
CPM 40mg/kg iv	↓						
CPM 60mg/kg iv/oral		↓	↓		↓		
IT MTX/HC 12.5mg each	↓	↓	↓		↓		

Fig. 6.8 Twenty-eight-day treatment schedule for eBL in Malawi

were 257 consecutive patients with eBL registered in the central trial database. After excluding patients with advanced disease (patients with CNS or bone marrow disease, equivalent to LMB Group C disease), HIV and poor clinical condition, they recruited 178 subjects. Their chemotherapy was stratified by St Jude stage at presentation and response at 21 days. Stage I/II patients received 3 weekly 1.2 g/m^2 CPM doses (equivalent to 40 mg/kg) with concomitant intrathecal MTX/hydrocortisone (HC), and Stage III/IV patients showing a complete response (CR) at 21 days were given a further three doses together with intrathecal MTX/HC. After this CR was observed in 83 of 176 evaluable patients (47%), and EFS was 33% at 18 months with a TRM of 7% for CPM monotherapy. The authors commented that in comparison with the Hesseling Malawi results their approach was hampered by advanced disease and a lower standard of supportive care [51].

There have been many studies performed to investigate the augmentation of a basic CPM backbone with other agents in the African setting. The most commonly used additional agents are vincristine (VCR) and methotrexate (MTX). The majority of the earlier studies were hampered by the inherent difficulties of conducting useful studies in situations where consistency of recruitment, treatment, supportive care and follow-up are very difficult. There are now a number of studies aimed at addressing this issue [52]. An example is a multicentre prospective study set in Cameroon, using a pragmatic response and stage-based regimen that builds on the backbone of the Hesseling et al. [12] Malawi 28-day first-line and subsequent relapse protocols (Fig. 6.9). In this approach, after the initial "core" courses of chemotherapy, children with known advanced disease (St Jude stage III or IV) or incomplete response on either clinical examination or abdominal ultrasound receive either additional CPM or additional agents (VCR and 1 G/m^2 MTX). In another multi-centre African study, INCTR are investigating a risk stratified 3 or 6 cycles of COM (cyclophosphamide, vincristine and methotrexate) as a first-line regimen with intrathecal cytotoxics followed by a secondline regimen of 4 cycles of ifosfamide, etoposide and cytosine arabinoside for children with incomplete responses or relapse within 3 months of completion of first-line therapy. The progression to integration of first-line and relapse strategies in a more seamless way is common to both

"Cameroon 2008 protocol" (Katayi 09, Hesseling 10)

<u>Risk group 1:</u> *St Jude stages I & II in CCR*

<u>Risk group 2:</u> *St Jude stage III or stage unconfirmed in CCR $\pm$ abdominal tumour! 30ml @ D29*

<u>Risk group 3:</u> *St Jude stage IV, all patients not in CCR or with abdominal tumour" 30 ml @ D29*

Induction (all stages)

Day	1	8	15	22	29
CPM 40mg/kg iv/po	!	!	!		
MTX/HC 12.5mg IT	!	!	!		

Consolidation (Risk group 1)

Day	29	36	43	57	65
CPM **60mg/kg** iv/po	!				

Consolidation (Risk group 2)

Day	29	36	43	57	65
CPM **60mg/kg** iv/po	!	!			

Consolidation (Risk group 3)

Day	29	36	43	57	65
CPM **60mg/kg** iv/po	!	!		!	
VCR 1.5mg/m^2 iv	!	!		!	
MTX 1.0g/m^2 iv	!				

Fig. 6.9 Cameroon protocol for endemic Burkitt's lymphoma

these studies and the French African Cooperative Group (GFAOP) work. The approach used in the Traoré et al. study was to proceed to second-line chemotherapy if there was not a complete response at 21 days (1 week earlier than in the Hesseling Cameroon study). This consisted of two courses of COPM (CPM 1.5 g/m^2 over 3 days, vincristine, prednisone and 3 G/m^2 HD MTX with intrathecal MTX/HC) followed by two courses of CYM (low-dose cytarabine arabinoside, 3 G/m^2 HD MTX and further intrathecal MTX/HC and cytarabine arabinoside). Including the initial CPM monotherapy, Traoré et al. were able to demonstrate an overall survival (OS) of 50.5% with a total TRM of 14%. In the context of countries where the total health expenditure per capita is under 30 US dollars per year, the average cost of treatment per patient, in this protocol, of 685 US dollars is problematic.

The alternative approach to building on to the most basic CPM-based regimen is to modify one of the "gold standard" protocols currently used in resource-rich settings. Again, there have been a number of studies where this approach has been investigated. Following the first African Continental Conference of the International Society of Paediatric Oncology (SIOP) in 1994, the regimen used in Malawi was based on Lymphome Malins de type B (LMB) '89 Group B therapy, with omission of doxorubicin and reduction in CPM and high-dose MTX doses. In 44 patients with St Jude stage I–III disease this achieved a 1-year projected EFS of 57%, but at the expense of 23% TRM [53]. Reduced-dose LMB/Berlin-Frankfurt-Munster (BFM) protocols have been more successful in less resource-poor settings, but the spectre of significant (>10%) TRM is ever present. The GFAOP has tested a variety of reduced-intensity LMB-based regimens. Harif et al. [54] describe two regimens in a total of 306 children after 37 children had been excluded (reasons being, among others, very limited stage disease, disease too advanced to be treated and parental refusal). The lower intensity regimen (GFA 2001) produced results not dissimilar to the initial Malawi experience with an EFS of 55.6% and TRM of 28.3%. The higher intensity regimen (MAT) used in the more experienced Moroccan units gave an EFS of 75.2%, but still with an undesirable TRM of 15.1%. Subsequent GFAOP studies have attempted to further modify the MAT regimen to minimise TRM [55]. Modified Berlin-Frankfurt-Munster (BFM) protocols used in central and south America now give somewhat better outcomes with EFS of above 80% and TRM <10%. These centres have made a greater number of iterations to achieve these results and are possibly better resourced (Table 6.6). In a retrospective analysis of the non-modified use of the French American British LMB 96 in Pakistan, Ahmad et al. demonstrate the hazards of not adapting to local circumstances. Over a 12-year period, they treated 122 consecutive children under 18 years of age with mature B-cell non-Hodgkin lymphoma (NHL), including 95 (78%) with BL. Despite unrestricted access to diagnostic facilities and antibiotics comparable with resource-rich settings, the EFS was 55% at 5 years with 30% TRM and 24% loss to follow-up. The authors attributed the difference between their results and those in the FAB/LMB '96 study to late presentation, poor nutritional state and delays in recognition of potential infection during treatment [56].

It might be thought that simply omitting or reducing the doses of drugs that have significant potential for morbidity and mortality without appropriate supportive care would be sufficient to design a protocol for middle-income countries. Cytotoxics that are commonly modified or omitted are high-dose methotrexate (HD MTX), high-dose cytosine arabinoside (HD Ara-C), etoposide (VP16), cyclophosphamide (CPM) and doxorubicin (Dox). HD MTX is a particular example of a cytotoxic drug that can be relatively well tolerated if there is good supportive care and the ability to measure blood levels in a timely and accurate manner. The potential for harm or death if mistakes are made with the doses commonly used for advanced disease in LMB (8 G/m^2) or BFM (5 G/m^2) schedules is large. Experience of relatively lower, but still "high", doses of MTX in settings where the measurement of blood levels to guide folinic acid (FA) rescue therapy can be done has shown that 3 G/m^2 or less may be used safely as long as a cautious fluid and FA regimen is adhered to strictly [57]. Other studies suggest that there are factors other than dose intensity alone to consider. The experience of the treating unit, together with factors discussed in the supportive care section of this chapter, and local patient factors such as malnutrition all play their part [58].

Supportive Care

Adequate and timely supportive care, even if not as intense as in high income countries, is essential. This should include measures to prevent and manage tumour lysis syndrome (hyper-hydration, allopurinol and rarely frusemide). It is essential to be able to manage malaria, fevers, oral candidiasis and herpetic ulceration. Anti-emetics, for example metoclopramide, are needed to prevent nausea. Blood must be available for transfusion and analgesia of varying strengths. A protocol for the rapid institution of antibiotics for fever is vital. A "fever guideline" needs to empower nurses to initiate therapy without having to wait for a clinician. The choice of antibiotics should be informed by local bacterial patterns of antimicrobial resistance.

Central lines are rarely used in sub-Saharan Africa. They are expensive, require operative placement and need meticulous, aseptic handling. This means that children have frequent venous sampling for full blood counts, and when febrile, for blood cultures. Finger pricks are carried out to make thick blood films to look for malarial parasitaemia. It is not surprising if children are traumatised by frequent blood sampling and intra-thecal injections. It is important to do these as frequently as necessary but not unnecessarily. The fact that central lines are not in place also means that the causative agents of bacteraemia tend to be similar to those found in other community-acquired infections and not the line-induced non-pathogens of well resourced settings.

Oral tumours can be ulcerated on presentation and may have superimposed secondary infections. The infection causes pain and an offensive smell. Liquid metronidazole (or powder from crushed metronidazole tablets) swilled around the mouth reduces the pain, controls the infection and as chemotherapy is given and the tumour regresses, the problem resolves.

Nutritional support can be a major need. Malnourished children have reduced immunity, increased risk of infection and increased risk of surgical complications and mortality [59]. Malnutrition is also associated with more severe chemotherapy-related neutropenia [29, 60] (Table 6.7). Hospital food is often inadequate and parents are far from home. Children may be anorexic because of the disease or the drugs and oral sores make swallowing painful. Many mothers fear naso-gastric tubes (as a sign of poor prognosis) and will not allow their children to have one inserted making it necessary to rely on high calorie oral foods. One such food is a peanut based, high density, ready-to-use therapeutic food (RUTF) with added micronutrients. It has a calorific value of 540 kcal per 100 g which means that a small quantity can provide good nutritional support, essential in the anorexic child. Furthermore it tastes good and children like it [61].

Table 6.7 The association of malnutrition and neutropaenia in Malawian patients with Burkitt's lymphoma

Neutropenia in Malnourished children with eBL		
Malnourished	Odds ratio	*p* value
Neutropenic episodes	1.4(0.5 to 3.7)	0.5
Profound neutropenia	12(1.5 to infinity)	0.01
Prolonged neutropenia	5.9 (0.7 to infinity)	0.1
Febrile neutropenia	3.0 (0.6 to 28)	0.2
Death	3.6 (0.4 to infinity)	0.3

Pain control is vital. The WHO ladder for pain management guides therapy [62]. Oral morphine is cheap and should be available to the children who need it. Unfortunately, availability of morphine in low-income countries is still often a problem, due to several reasons such as import regulations and inappropriate fear of addiction. Not all children will be cured and many will benefit from palliative care. Members of the palliative care team should be part of the core clinical team for cancer care. In our units we do ward rounds together and the palliative care team has the time to counsel families, to give pain control, to assist with transport home or communicate with distant relatives. They take part in the care of many of the children who will eventually do well, but at critical times in the hospital stay they may have needed, for example, extra time, pain control, mouth care or bladder training.

There is urgent need to treat retro-orbital masses as increasing pressure on and distortion of the retinal vessels may lead to blindness, orbital ischaemia and loss of the eye.

Monitoring Treatment

Children require high fluid intake immediately prior to and during the time they receive chemotherapy. This is especially important when there is a large tumour load. Careful monitoring of fluid input and urine output is required. Body temperature should be checked at least twice a day.

Full blood counts and differentials need to be done regularly. At a minimum they should be done before each cycle of treatment and the absolute neutrophil count should be greater than 500 cells $\times 10^6/\text{mm}^3$ for chemotherapy to be given. The haemoglobin level, neutrophil count and platelet count may all fall and require chemotherapy to be delayed or show the need for a blood transfusion. Ideally liver function tests and urea and electrolytes should also be monitored regularly, though this may not be possible in some centres.

Daily physical examination should be carried out looking for signs of pallor, infection, oral mucositis or bleeding. Evidence of peripheral neuropathy is uncommon with the use of vincristine but constipation and jaw pain are common complaints when it is given.

Some children may develop diarrhoea or typhlitis requiring appropriate rehydration and antibiotics. Others may have nausea and vomiting and will need fluids and encouragement to receive an adequate intake of fluids and calories. Naso-gastric feeds may be indicated though many mothers fear their placement as a sign of deteriorating well being of their child.

Complications

Burkitt's lymphoma tumours are very chemo-sensitive which means that with chemotherapy large tumours will rapidly get smaller producing large quantities of cell debris and waste products that are excreted through the kidneys. If hydration is inadequate and renal protection is not provided with a drug such as allopurinol, there is the risk of acute tumour lysis syndrome. In this syndrome the kidneys are damaged by high uric acid and phosphate loads; urine output is reduced and renal failure ensues. Intracellular potassium is released in to the blood with cell destruction and if serum potassium levels rise rapidly, ventricular fibrillation and cardiac arrest can occur with a sudden unexpected death shortly after starting chemotherapy. The prevention of tumour lysis syndrome in BL in resource-rich settings has been much improved with the availability of uric oxidase. Unfortunately the cost is prohibitive to its use in resource-poor settings.

Leucopenia makes a child vulnerable to infection and any fever must be identified and treated early. Mucositis is painful and makes feeding difficult. It also exposes the child to invasive infections. Anaemia and/or thrombocytopenia, if severe, will require blood transfusion and platelet transfusions if they are available. Children should sleep under bed nets on the ward and be kept well away from the children admitted with infections.

Outcomes

Outcomes are dependent on the stage of disease at presentation, the intensity of treatment given and the completion of a full course of treatment. Failure to complete treatment is a major problem in many places where endemic Burkitt's lymphoma is common. Guardians—usually the mothers—are far from home, may not have expected to be in hospital for long periods of time and have little financial means to make long journeys to and from hospital and home.

Stage 4 disease (in the CNS or bone marrow) has a long-term survival rate of about 10%; Stage One has a good prognosis in about 80–90% of cases.

Malnourished children may not tolerate the more intense regimens of chemotherapy and succumb to infections. Many children who present with paraplegia and incontinence will sadly not recover function; especially if their symptoms were present for several weeks prior to treatment. Nevertheless there are some children, who against all the odds, do very well and regain mobility and continence. It is always worthwhile to treat with the hope that such a recovery will be achieved. On discharge from hospital all children should be encouraged to sleep under a bed net and to receive cotrimoxazole prophylaxis for the first 4–8 weeks at home. Children with eBL are usually followed up for 1 year post treatment. If they remain disease free during this time period they are considered cured.

Relapse

The frequency of relapse will depend on the stage of presentation and the intensity of first-line treatment given. There are some tumours that do not respond to treatment or respond very little, and this is probably due to genetic factors that are not evident clinically. In the 178 patients given CPM monotherapy by Traoré et al., 83 achieved complete remission and of these, 23 relapsed (28%). Relapses principally occur within 6–12 months after diagnosis, as illustrated by the event-free survival curves found by Hesseling et al. (Fig. 6.10). Once the eBL patient is over a year beyond diagnosis and start of treatment, risk of relapse is less than 5%, as illustrated when children were still in complete remission a year after treatment in a study with long-term follow up reported from Ghana [63]. Relapses occur at the original site or not infrequently in the central nervous system, especially if CNS prophylaxis is suboptimal. In resource-rich countries, the treatment options for relapsed disease are restricted to high-dose myeloablative chemotherapy followed by allo- or autograft. Where CPM monotherapy or similar first-line chemotherapy has been used, there are various possible approaches using further CPM together with additional

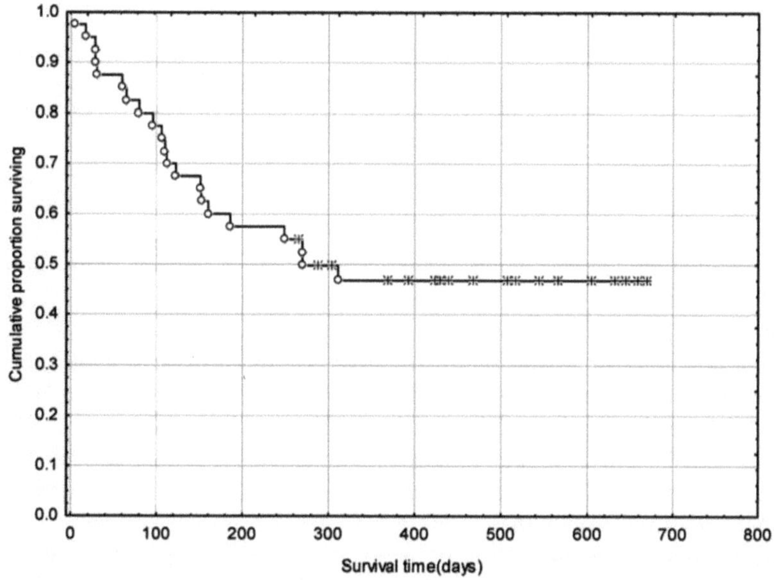

Fig. 6.10 Kaplan–Meir curve of event-free survival (0 treatment failed, ⁎ censored)

agents such as MTX, cytarabine arabinoside, etoposide and Ifosfamide/MESNA. Recent and ongoing eBL study methodologies and outcomes are summarised in Table 6.6. Depending on the setting 23–36% of relapsed or refractory disease may be salvaged after CPM monotherapy.

Play and School

Lengthy hospital stays are not conducive to happiness unless efforts are made to prevent children and parents getting bored and homesick. A play lady is a very important addition to the caring team. She can play with the children, help them with reading, writing, puzzles or drawing. She distracts them from discomfort or the anticipation of painful procedures. She can often talk with and listen to the older, (adolescent) child who is finding the whole business of illness, hospital stay, treatment and loss of self-control difficult and distressing.

School work for the older children keeps them up to date with their peers at school back at home and occupies the children. Limited and supervised television viewing is appreciated by both the children and their parents.

We have found that giving the guardians a small amount of money to go and buy some foodstuffs to cook together over the weekends is enjoyed, builds a community spirit, makes a change from the monotonous hospital diet and helps pass the time.

Future Directions

Future directions in treatment depend partially on general medical developments in endemic BL areas. If these improve, then access to health care with a reduction in late presentation with advanced disease, and improved supportive care will result in the possibility to deliver intense treatments. Ideally, one would hope that children will present earlier, in a better nutritional status and that improvement of supportive care would allow treatments comparable in intensity to treatments in high-income countries.

As the situation is now in many endemic areas, future directions should be sought that will benefit all children admitted to the hospital which include improvement of diagnostic facilities (ultrasonography, pathology, blood test and blood cultures). The same is true for improvement of palliative care that will be of wide benefit.

A few directions are foreseeable that are specific to Burkitt's lymphoma treatment. One is further risk-stratified treatment, attempting to avoid treatment-related mortality and also providing more intense treatment to those children who need it to survive (e.g. stage IV and resistant disease). With time, targeted therapy (e.g. rituximab) with reduced toxicity may become available at affordable prices and prove to be efficacious with tolerable toxicity in less resourced settings. Other options are to use adjuvant therapy such as sodium phenylbuturate. Sodium phenylbutyrate induces EBV lytic replication in susceptible B-lymphocyte cultures and may increase chemosensitivity to chemotherapy [64, 65].

References

1. Burkitt D (1958) A sarcoma involving the jaws in African children. Br J Surg 46(197): 218–223
2. O'Conor GT, Davies JN (1960) Malignant tumors in African children. With special reference to malignant lymphoma. J Pediatr 56:526–535
3. Epstein MA, Achong BG, Barr YM (1964) Virus particles in cultured lymphoblasts from Burkitt's lymhoma. Lancet 1(7335):702–703
4. Burkitt D (1962) A "tumour safari" in East and Central Africa. Br J Cancer 16:379–386
5. Burkitt D (1962) Determining the climatic limitations of a children's cancer common in Africa. Br Med J 2(5311):1019–1023
6. Cook-Mozaffari P, Newton R, Beral V et al (1998) The geographical distribution of Kaposi's sarcoma and of lymphomas in Africa before the AIDS epidemic. Br J Cancer 78(11):1521–1528
7. Rainey JJ, Mwanda WO, Wairiumu P et al (2007) Spatial distribution of Burkitt's lymphoma in Kenya and association with malaria risk. Trop Med Int Health 12(8):936–943
8. de-The G (1977) Is Burkitt's lymphoma related to perinatal infection by Epstein-Barr virus? Lancet 1(8007):335–338
9. Burkitt D (1963) A children's cancer dependent on environment. 17th Annual Symposium on Fundamental Cancer Research in Viruses, Nucleic Acids and Cancer, pp 615–629
10. Cardy AH, Sharp L, Little J (2001) Burkitt's lymphoma: a review of the epidemiology. Kuwait Med J 33:293–306
11. Orem J, Mbidde EK, Lambert B et al (2007) Burkitt's lymphoma in Africa, a review of the epidemiology and etiology. Afr Health Sci 7(3):166–175
12. Hesseling P, Molyneux E, Kamiza S et al (2009) Endemic Burkitt lymphoma: a 28-day treatment schedule with cyclophosphamide and intrathecal methotrexate. Ann Trop Paediatr 29(1):29–34
13. Magrath IT (1991) African Burkitt's lymphoma. History, biology, clinical features, and treatment. Am J Pediatr Hematol Oncol 13(2):222–246
14. Mbulaiteye SM, Biggar RJ, Bhatia K et al (2009) Sporadic childhood Burkitt lymphoma incidence in the United States during 1992–2005. Pediatr Blood Cancer 53(3):366–370
15. Mwando OW, Rochford R, Moorman AM et al (2004) Burkitt lymphoma in Kenya: geographical, age, gender and ethnic distribution. East Afr Med J 8:68–77
16. Owuru L, Yebonh FA, Osei-Akolo A (2010) Clinical and epidemiological characteristics of Burkitt's lymphoma: an eight year case study at Komfor Anokye teaching hospital Ghana. Br J Biomed Sci 87:9–14
17. Newton R, Ziegler J, Beral V et al (2001) A case–control study of human immunodeficiency virus infection and cancer in adults and children residing in Kampala, Uganda. Int J Cancer 92(5):622–627
18. Sinfield RL, Molyneux EM, Banda K et al (2007) Spectrum and presentation of pediatric malignancies in the HIV era: experience from Blantyre, Malawi, 1998–2003. Pediatr Blood Cancer 48(5):515–520
19. Orem J, Maganda A, Mbidde EK et al (2009) Clinical characteristics and outcome of children with Burkitt lymphoma in Uganda according to HIV infection. Pediatr Blood Cancer 52(4):455–458
20. Chintu C, Athale UH, Patil PS (1995) Childhood cancers in Zambia before and after the HIV epidemic. Arch Dis Child 73(2):100–104
21. Mutalima N, Molyneux E, Jaffe H et al (2008) Associations between Burkitt lymphoma among children in Malawi and infection with HIV, EBV and malaria: results from a case–control study. PLoS One 3(6):e2505
22. MacNeil A, Sumba OP, Lutzke ML et al (2003) Activation of the Epstein-Barr virus lytic cycle by the latex of the plant *Euphorbia tirucalli*. Br J Cancer 88(10):1566–1569
23. van den Bosch CA (2004) Is endemic Burkitt's lymphoma an alliance between three infections and a tumour promoter? Lancet Oncol 5(12):738–746

24. Tabuti JR, Dhillion SS, Lye KA (2003) Ethnoveterinary medicines for cattle (Bos indicus) in Bulamogi county, Uganda: plant species and mode of use. J Ethnopharmacol 88(2–3):279–286
25. Shiramizu B, Barriga F, Neequaye J et al (1991) Patterns of chromosomal breakpoint locations in Burkitt's lymphoma: relevance to geography and Epstein-Barr virus association. Blood 77(7):1516–1526
26. Pelicci PG, Knowles DM, Magrath I et al (1986) Chromosomal breakpoints and structural alterations of the c-myc locus differ in endemic and sporadic forms of Burkitt lymphoma. Proc Natl Acad Sci USA 83(9):2984–2988
27. Bellan C, Lazzi S, Hummel M et al (2005) Immunoglobulin gene analysis reveals 2 distinct cells of origin for EBV-positive and EBV-negative Burkitt lymphomas. Blood 106(3): 1031–1036
28. Mwando OW (2004) Aspects of epidemiological and clinical features of patients with central nervours system Burkitt's lymphoma in Kenya. East Afr Med J 8(suppl):897–903
29. Israels T, van de Wetering MD, Hesseling P (2009) Malnutrition and neutropenia in children treated for Burkitt lymphoma in Malawi. Pediatr Blood Cancer 53(1):47–52
30. Unicef (2011) The State of the World's Children 2011
31. Nelson M, Perkins SL, Dave BJ et al (2010) An increased frequency of 13q deletions detected by fluorescence in situ hybridization and its impact on survival in children and adolescents with Burkitt lymphoma: results from the Children's Oncology Group study CCG-5961. Br J Haematol 148(4):600–610
32. Jaffe ES, Harris NL, Stein H et al (2001) WHO classification. Tumours of haematopoietic and lymphoid tissues. Lyon
33. van Noorden S, Lampert IA, Xue SA et al (2011) Burkitt's lymphoma: maximising the use of fine needle aspirates by long-term preservation for diagnosis and research. Trans R Soc Trop Med Hyg 105(2):86–94
34. Hesseling P, Broadhead R, Mansvelt E et al (2005) The 2000 Burkitt lymphoma trial in Malawi. Pediatr Blood Cancer 44(3):245–250
35. Hesseling PB, Molyneux E, Tchintseme F et al (2008) Treating Burkitt's lymphoma in Malawi, Cameroon, and Ghana. Lancet Oncol 9(6):512–513
36. Patte C, Auperin A, Michon J et al (2001) The Societe Francaise d'Oncologie Pediatrique LMB89 protocol: highly effective multiagent chemotherapy tailored to the tumor burden and initial response in 561 unselected children with B-cell lymphomas and L3 leukemia. Blood 97(11):3370–3379
37. Oettgen HF, Burkitt D, Burchenal JH (1963) Malignant lymphoma involving the jaw in African children: treatment with Methotrexate. Cancer 16:616–623
38. Burkitt D, Hutt MS, Wright DH (1965) African lymphoma: preliminary observations on response to therapy. Cancer 18:399–410
39. Clifford P (1968) Treatment of Burkitt's lymphoma. Lancet 1(7542):599
40. Morrow RH, Pike MC, Kisuule A (1967) Survival of Burkitt's lymphoma patients in Mulago Hospital, Uganda. Br Med J 4(5575):323–327
41. Ziegler JL, Morrow RH, Fass L et al (1970) Treatment of Burkitt's tumor with cyclophosphamide. Cancer 26(2):474–484
42. Nkrumah FK, Perkins IV, Biggar RJ (1977) Combination chemotherapy in abdominal Burkitt's lymphoma. Cancer 40(4):1410–1416
43. Magrath I (1990) Small non-cleaved lymphoma. In: The non-Hodgkin's lymphoma. Edward Arnold, London, p 256
44. Murphy SB (1980) Classification, staging and end results of treatment of childhood non-Hodgkin's lymphomas, dissimilarities from lymphomas in adults. Semin Oncol 7:332–339
45. Patte C, Auperin A, Gerrard M et al (2007) Results of the randomized international FAB/LMB96 trial for intermediate risk B-cell non-Hodgkin lymphoma in children and adolescents: it is possible to reduce treatment for the early responding patients. Blood 109(7):2773–2780
46. Patte C, Michon J, Frappaz D et al (1994) Therapy of Burkitt and other B-cell acute lymphoblastic leukaemia and lymphoma: experience with the LMB protocols of the SFOP (French Paediatric Oncology Society) in children and adults. Baillieres Clin Haematol 7(2):339–348

47. Burkitt D (1967) Long-term remissions following one and two-dose chemotherapy for African lymphoma. Cancer 20(5):756–759
48. Ziegler JL, DeVita VT, Graw RG Jr et al (1976) Combined modality treatment of American Burkitt's lymphoma. Cancer 38(6):2225–2231
49. Link MP, Shuster JJ, Donaldson SS et al (1997) Treatment of children and young adults with early-stage non-Hodgkin's lymphoma. N Engl J Med 337(18):1259–1266
50. Ziegler JL, Bluming AZ (1971) Intrathecal chemotherapy in Burkitt's lymphoma. Br Med J 3(5773):508–512
51. Traore F, Coze C, Atteby JJ et al (2011) Cyclophosphamide monotherapy in children with Burkitt lymphoma: a study from the French-African Pediatric Oncology Group (GFAOP). Pediatr Blood Cancer 56(1):70–76
52. Hesseling PB, Njume E, Kouya F, Katayi T, Wharin P, Tamannai M, et al. The Cameroon 2008 Burkitt lymphoma protocol: improved event-free survival with treatment adapted to disease stage and the response to induction therapy. Pediatr Hematol Oncol 2012 Mar;29(2):119–129
53. Hesseling PB (2000) The SIOP burkitt lymphoma pilot study in Malawi, Africa. Med Pediatr Oncol 34(2):142
54. Harif M, Barsaoui S, Benchekroun S et al (2008) Treatment of B-cell lymphoma with LMB modified protocols in Africa – report of the French-African Pediatric Oncology Group (GFAOP). Pediatr Blood Cancer 50(6):1138–1142
55. El Kababri M, Mrimi F, Loumatine K (2009) Treatment of childhood Burkitt lymphoma in North Africa: a study of the French-African Pediatric Oncology Group (G.F.A.O.P.). Hematology Meeting Reports 3:5:88
56. Ahmad N, Zaidi A, Badar F et al (2010) Clinical characteristics and outcome analysis of pediatric B-cell non-Hodgkin's lymphoma. Experience with FAB-LMB 96 and UKCCSG B-cell NHL guidelines in a developing country. Asia Pac J Clin Oncol 6(1):49–56
57. Wessels G, Hesseling PB (2000) High-dose intense chemotherapy in South African children with B-cell lymphoma: morbidity, supportive measures and outcome. Med Pediatr Oncol 34:143–146
58. Moleti ML, Al-Hadad SA, Al-Jadiry MF et al (2011) Treatment of children with B-cell non-Hodgkin lymphoma in a low-income country. Pediatr Blood Cancer 56:560–567
59. Katona P, Katona-Apte J (2008) The interaction between nutrition and infection. Clin Infect Dis 46(10):1582–1588
60. Sala A, Pencharz P, Barr RD (2004) Children, cancer, and nutrition – a dynamic triangle in review. Cancer 100(4):677–687
61. Manary MJ (2006) Local production and provision of ready-to-use therapeutic food (RUTF) spread for the treatment of severe childhood malnutrition. Food Nutr Bull 27(3 Suppl):S83–S89
62. Collins JJ (2001) Cancer pain management in children. Eur J Pain 5(Suppl A):37–41
63. Nkrumah FK, Perkins IV (1976) Burkitt's lymphoma: a clinical study of 110 patients. Cancer 37(2):671–676
64. Phillips JA, Griffin BE (2007) Pilot study of sodium phenylbutyrate as adjuvant in cyclophosphamide-resistant endemic Burkitt's lymphoma. Trans R Soc Trop Med Hyg 101(12): 1265–1269
65. Stimson L, Wood V, Khan O et al (2009) HDAC inhibitor-based therapies and haematological malignancy. Ann Oncol 20(8):1293–1302
66. Pena A, Ortiz A, Gamboa A, Garrido C (2009) Preliminary results of a multicenter BFM-based study for B-cell malignancies in Central America. Hematology Meeting Reports 3:5:90
67. Klumb CE, Apa AG, Carrico MK (2009) Long-term outcome of children with B-non-Hodgkin's lymphoma: results from Brazilian National Cancer Institute. Hematology Meeting Reports 3:5:15
68. Chantada G, Zubizarreta P, Felice MS et al (2009) Results of a modified BFM strategy for the treatment of B-cell malignancies in Argentina. 3:5: 26
69. Woessmann W, Seidemann K, Mann G et al (2005) The impact of the methotrexate administration schedule and dose in the treatment of children and adolescents with B-cell neoplasms: a report of the BFM Group Study NHL-BFM95. Blood 105(3):948–958

Chapter 7
Non-endemic Burkitt's Lymphoma

Mwanda Walter Otieno

Introduction

There were, for about three decades and until the association and characterization of HIV/AIDS malignancies, two categories of Burkitt's lymphoma: endemic and non-endemic. The latter was described soon after the former. However, these two share many characteristics but vary in proportions and extent of the major defining features. Indeed the initial characteristics of the non-endemic Burkitt's lymphoma were epidemiological and could have fitted as a subclass of the Burkitt's disease due to exhibiting only proportions of the initially described entity.

Historical Perspective

There are clues that what is known to us today as BL was described as early as the turn of the twentieth century. In 1904, Sir Albert Cook described lesions of malignant tumors. While in Mengo Hospital in Uganda, he saw a little Mohammandan child with large malignant tumor.

The child's clinical description and the drawings are said to be still available in his clinical records, which are contained in case records of Mengo Hospital.

Early African carvings suggest that a tumor of similar descriptions had been present in the equatorial Africa for a long time. In Nigeria, case of round cell tumor in the jaw, orbit, and ovary was described in 1934.

In Lorenza Marquez, plaster models of patients who obviously had BL also suggested the existence of the tumor in Mozambique sometime long before Denis

M.W. Otieno (✉)
Department of Human Pathology, Hematology and Pediatric Oncology,
Kenyatta National Hospital, College of Health Sciences, University of Nairobi,
Nairobi, Kenya
e-mail: walter.mwanda@uonbi.ac.ke

E.S. Robertson (ed.), *Burkitt's Lymphoma*, Current Cancer Research,
DOI 10.1007/978-1-4614-4313-1_7,

Burkitt's description of lymphomatous lesions, which may have been BL. Several reports emanating from Ghana, Rwanda, Burundi, Cameroon, and other countries of the present central Africa States suggest the existence of BL decades prior to the initial description by Burkitt's. In 1948 Davis made remarks on the undue frequency of the tumor of reticuloendothelial system in Uganda. In 1953, lymphosarcoma of the ovary in young girls was described by Capponi, while Thjis in 1957 drew attention to the prevalence of neoplasma of the reticuloendothelial system in the Congo, now Democratic Republic of Congo. In the same year Burkitt's first, now historic description, defined the tumor as a round cell sarcoma recognizable by certain features and he stressed the high frequency of the tumor in children, but also pointed out that similar tumors were found in the abdominal viscera. After Burkitt's publication, numerous reports appeared in other parts of the world describing similar lymphomatous growths that were henceforth referred to as Burkitt's tumor. These culminated in the description in the two well-described types. It is not quite clear whether some of these early descriptions were all typical Burkitt's as it has now emerged that the distinctions purely on geographical and clinical parameters are not absolute. Indeed intermediate forms are described in some tropical countries and Brazil's series attest to this group. Purists would therefore use the terms African and American types for endemic and non-endemic BL, respectively, to avoid the gray area of possible intermediate type.

Current Concepts

Burkitt's lymphomas (BL) are malignant lymphoproliferative disorders. The French America British (FAB) cooperative group classified it as: high-grade malignant lymphoma, small cell, non-cleaved cell, diffused, malignant lymphoma. Little has changed in concept since these founding descriptions by Denis Burkitt's in 1958 and subsequent years by others. The observations lead to the consolidation into syndromes. The major ones include a peculiar age distribution, an unusual and characteristic anatomical distribution, and a limited geographical distribution which is unrelated to genetic factors. Since then, it has been demonstrated that the disease has typical catogenesis, cytologic, histologic, immunologic, biologic, clinical, and geographic distribution. For the non-endemic Burkitt's lymphoma (NEBL) features are usually contrasted and compared with endemic or African BL. The commonly notable synonyms are non-African, American (ABL), non-endemic (NEBL) temperate climate, non-tropical, atypical, and non-classical Burkitt's lymphoma. The majority would use either American-type Burkitt's lymphoma (ABL) or NEBL.

Geo-Demographic Features

Geographical characteristics of BL are the most distinctive features of this disease. Generally the sporadic forms are predominantly found in the temperate regions. There are, however, geographical regions, for example Brazil, a country that lies within the tropical latitudes that has features intermediate types of BL distribution. Comparatively, BL is rare in the temperate regions. In Europe, North and South America and Oceanic Age Standardized Rates (ASRs) in most populations are less than 1 per million in many countries. In the USA, malignant lymphoma accounts for only 10% of pediatric malignancies, being third in relative frequency after acute leukemia and brain tumors with BL comprising approximately 1–2% of all children tumors, and about one-fifth of childhood non-Hodgkin's lymphoma. The rate among US whites is approximately 2 per million, while that of the blacks is at 1.1 per million and accounts for only between 2.9 and 9.3% of all childhood cancers in countries of North America. American series vary also according to the investigating teams. Data from the Surveillance Epidemiology and End Results (SEER) study of the National cancer institute show an overall annual incidence of 1.4 per million among white male and 0.4 per million among white female between.

Other temperate countries also document nearly similarly low rates. In the continent of Asia, the levels are low and vary from country to country. For example in Japan, reported by Aya Hanai Isaburo Fujimoto on the age group 0–14, the ASR was 0.07 and with Crude Incidence (CI) of 0.07, while that of Seoul Korea Cancer Registry CI of 10. Kuwait Cancer registry, CI of 7.3, Philippines, Manila and Rizal Cancer registry CI was 0.3 and Singapore Cancer registry reported no BL. Nonetheless European experience with BL varies from one country to another. Danish Cancer registry estimates CI of 2.3. Finland cancer registry reported no BL till after 2000. Since then case reports show that 4–5 cases of Burkitt's lymphoma tumor are registered annually. While the national registry of childhood tumors, for England and Wales approximates CI of 0.5 and their counterpart in the United Kingdom Scotland had a CI of 0.4. The temperate regions in the in the Southern Hemisphere; Australian pediatric cancer registry documented CI of 1.8.

Age

The non-Hodgkin's lymphomas as a group account for about 7% of cancers in persons under 20 years of age. The BL constitute less than half of these lymphomas, for example Epidemiology and End Results (SEER) study of the National Cancer Institute show overall cases span a broad age group and only half were children. The mean age of onset is about 12 years. It accounts for a minor percentage of adult lymphoma, and its peak incidents occur in second and third decades of life.

Gender

The sporadic BL has an overall ratio of male to female of 3.5:1 but vary from one region to another. The USA, it is more common in male than in female children. Seoul Korea Cancer Registry documents M: F of 1:3 European experience with BL also showed some variations. Danish Cancer registry recorded M: F 1.6:1. While the national registry of childhood tumors, for England and Wales M: F 3:2. Data from the Surveillance Epidemiology and End Results (SEER) study of the National Cancer Institute show an overall annual of 1.4 per million among white male and 0.4 per million among white female between 1973 and 1981. In the Southern Hemisphere, Australian pediatric cancer registry shows M: F of 3:2. In Japan, reported by Aya Hanai Isaburo Fujimoto on the age group 0–14, M: F of 2:1.

Chromosomal

There are chromosomal translocations associated with BL disease. The sporadic form demonstrates these features only to some extent. The primary chromosome anomaly is the translocation t (8; 14) (q24; q32), found in 60–70% of the cases. Variant translocations having in common an 8q24 break, i.e., the t (8; 22) (q24; q11) and t (2; 8) (p12; q24) occur in approximately 10–15% and 2–5% of the cases, respectively. A minority of cases may carry a duplication of chromosome 1, involving the 1q21-25 segment as the only detectable chromosome lesion.

A common translocation t(8;14) and the consequent c-myc rearrangement and overexpression have been identified in BL. However, some not very strict associations between Sμ and Sα recombination was identified at 14q32, with near 5' or intronic c-myc recombination at 8q24. It seems probable that BL is composed of a mixture of molecular types and that the incidence of each subtype might depend upon environmental factors.

Cytology

Cytological features consistently found in slide preparations of tumor aspirates or tumor imprints stained by hematological stains include medium size lymphoid cells exhibiting no or very little morphologic heterogeneity, small to moderately plentiful bluish cytoplasm and some nuclear vacuoles. The blast cells in the peripheral blood and bone marrow display a basophilic cytoplasm with characteristic vacuolization, a picture indistinguishable from acute lymphoblastic leukemia (ALL) L3 of the FAB classification, which represents the leukemic counterpart of BL –type/like.

Histology

The features are characterized by monomorphic neoplastic lymphoid cell with interspersed histiocytes creating the typical starry sky appearance pattern. The lymphoma consists of a monomorphic infiltrate of the lymph node by medium-sized cells showing round nuclei with several nucleoli and basophilic cytoplasm. Numerous benign macrophages confer a histologic pattern referred to a starry sky. Involvement of the peripheral blood and bone marrow may occur.

Immunology

The cell markers are of B-cell characteristics. The malignant cells express surface immunoglobulins M (lgM) almost always in association with either the kappa or the lambda light chains. Also these cells express HLA-DR antigens and frequently express CALLA antigens and do not contain TdT a marker for T-cells.

Viral Linkage

The etiology of BL remains speculative but it is one of those malignancies for which the etiologic hypothesis has been focused on an infective agent based on its geographical pattern. The EBV determinants tend to be negative in the sporadic or American population with BL. Biopsy specimens from NEBL contain the EBV genome in only 15–20% of the cases. Other features noted are that only one-third or less of the American BL had an association with EBV, and 20% apparently had never even been infected with EBV. Ziegler 1981 had reported similar data earlier from non-endemic cases. Overall, the reported risk factors for BL in the industrialized countries may be quite different. Perhaps, the more recent observation on the occurrence of BL in conjunction with infection of which about 35–40% was also EBV positive.

Differences observed between ethnic groups in Singapore where the Chinese appeared to have a delayed infection rate compared to the Indians. A report from Brazil shows intermediate EBV markers between the regions of endemic and sporadic forms. Thus the proportion of cases of BL associated with EBV is lower in areas of low and intermediate incidence of the lymphoma and the subtypes of the virus involved may differ.

Clinical Manifestations

It is notable that due to the initial anatomic sites involved the sporadic BL is a highly aggressive disease with a propensity to invade the bone marrow and CNS, with a reported incidence of 30–38% and 13–17% of cases, respectively. Lymph nodes involvement is more common among adults than children. The jaw is infrequently involved in sporadic Burkitt's and the abdomen is the most common site, particularly the terminal ileum, cecum, and intra-abdominal lymph nodes. However, other anatomical sites namely the ovary, kidney, pancreas, liver, omentum, Waldeyer's ring, and breast are often involved. Breast involvement is observed almost exclusively in girls at the onset of puberty and in lactating women.

One-third of the patients have B symptoms at presentation, unexplained fever higher than 38 °C in the prior month, weight loss greater than 10% in the past 6 months, and recurrent drenching night in the prior month. Patients with abnormal diseases usually present with abdominal mass or pain, bowel obstruction, gastrointestinal bleeding, or a syndrome mimicking acute abdomen and constituting oncologic emergency.

The presentation is with abdominal swelling, often in the area of the ileocecal valve. About 90% of American children with Burkitt's lymphoma have abdominal tumors. Others may develop tumors in the testes, ovaries, skin, nasal sinuses, or lymph nodes. In adults, Burkitt's lymphoma frequently produces a bulky abdomen and may involve the liver, spleen, and bone marrow. Terminal BL disease often presents with bone marrow involvement. Other commonly encountered anatomic sites are liver, retroperitoneal nodes, and ultimately stomach and intestines and the only exceptionally involved sites are lymph nodes. Infrequent sites of involvement are bone, breasts, thyroid, parotid, and skin. Head and neck manifestations of Burkitt's lymphoma in less than a quarter of the reported cases and usually present as cervical adenopathy. Usual this subset with lymphoma of the head and neck presents with extranodal disease of the soft tissues or bone of the face.

Signs and Symptoms

The primary sites and other involved anatomical tissues generate the presenting features. This type of BL often affects the bowel and the lymph nodes in abdomen, causing symptoms such as pain, feeling sick, and diarrhea. It can sometimes cause intestinal obstruction and may in some cases be the initial presentation. Lymph nodes in the chest or throat can cause obstruction in these site, while different signs and symptoms depends on the part of the body involved by the BL. It may involve the bone marrow, spleen, and liver. Sometimes it may have already spread to the brain and spinal cord. BL often affects the bowel and the lymph nodes in the abdomen, causing symptoms such as pain, feeling sick, and diarrhea. BL can cause different symptoms depending on where else in the body it has spread. It may involve the bone marrow, spleen, and liver. Sometimes it may have already spread to the brain and spinal cord manifesting with central nervous signs and symptoms. It should be borne in mind that BL often presents as an emergency associated with abdomen obstruction, rupture of the viscera, peritonitis, central nervous system, brain, and spinal cord sudden affections, and rarely urinary tract acute obstructions. Most of these will also manifest with symptoms, known as B symptoms, include sweating at night, unexplained high temperatures, and weight loss.

Extensive involvement of the stomach may cause pain, vomiting on eating, and complicate with hematemesis. Two of these demonstrated abnormalities of CT examination manifested by either thickening of the gastric wall or thickening of the gastric folds, but the lesions are less well shown than the upper gastrointestinal series. Posterior mediastinal extension along the esophagus can exhibit with both abdominal and chest symptoms. Diffuse involvement of the upper abdomen manifest by obstructive symptoms in the paraesophageal region and partially obscured concomitant pleural effusion.

Tumor masses involving the pelvis may cause pain and mass effects on the tissues of rectum and urinary system.

Intra-abdominal tumors complicate with ascites, obstruction, infection, and may mimick a variety of diseases.

Ascites

Ascites is present on about 24%. Peritoneal tap in many instances has malignant BL cells. The ascites are generally mild to moderate in extent. Radiological examination usually required to define the location of small amounts of ascites particularly in the pararectal fossae. In larger ascetic collections tumor may be obscured. Massive ascites render discrimination of intra-abdominal masses extremely difficult, but such a quantity of ascites fluid. Usually ascites is associated with abnormal pelvis masses in most cases and concomitant pleural effusion is present in over 70% of such cases. Also a combination of ascites fluid and disseminated peritoneal neoplasm is found in most of the cases

Retroperitoneal

Retroperitoneal involvement, excluding kidney, is tend to accompany abdominal involvement. Diffuse retroperitoneal disease with anterior displacement of the kidney with unilateral hydronephrosis. In addition psoas mass and iliac adenopathy are commonly encountered findings.

Liver

Hepatic involvement is demonstrated usually before spleen in many cases. Lesions tend to be solitary in early phases of the disease.

Non-endemic Sites Commonly Involved Anatomical Sites

Site	Percentage
Abdomen	25.4
CNS	11.4
Jaw	11.4
Breast	20.2
Lymph nodes	11.4
Miscellaneous	20.2
	100

Miscellaneous sites include: skeletal system, bone, thyroid gland, and oral pharyngeal

Spleen

Of the tissues of the reticuloendothelial system spleen is rarely involved with 14% of patients having splenomegaly. In normal-sized spleen a focal lesion similar to lesion visualized in the liver is present.

Renal

Involvement of the kidneys is frequent and the enlargement when present represents BL involvement of the kidneys. In most cases the kidneys are mildly enlarged. Some of the cases in addition have unilateral primary renal involvement with perirenal extension. Encasement of the ipsilateral ureter by massive retroperitoneal neoplasm can lead to hydronephrosis.

Cases with massive tumor quickly lead to nephropathy. In most cases there is clinical evidence of elevated serum uric acid levels and decreased creatinine clearance.

Chest

Occasionally patients have mediastinal masses. The anterior mediastinal mass with a right cervical mass. A posterior mediastinal mass was an upward extension of a diffusely infiltrating upper abdominal mass and was manifested by widening of the posterior mediastinum. Pleural effusions are noted in some cases and these are associated with ascites. No pleural or parenchymal masses, or hilar adenopathy is observed to accompany these chest changes.

Miscellaneous

Bone lesion involving the right posterior iliac bone, the lower limb particularly the tibia, and the humerus is observed in about 4% of cases. Massive inguinal adenopathy and extending into the soft tissue of the thigh evolve rapidly in these cases.

Associations of Commonly Involved Anatomical Sites

There is apparent association between age and anatomic primary sites of the disease, although the feature is not as remarkable in non-endemic BL. The salient features are that stage A predominates in the early years 3–7. While from 8 to 15 years of age there is visible decrease in the stage A proportions. At 14 years the least is stage A with 11 %. In all age groups stage B is the least. Stage C appears to be increasing in proportion from age 5 years and 9 years and a rise again with a peak at I2 years followed by a slight decline and a rise. Stage D clearly shows a rising trend with advancing years. Starting with 20% at age 3 followed by 33% at 4 years, 39% at 10, peaks at 14 with 55% after the age of 16 years the predominant stages are C and D.

When all sites are considered at an initial evaluation and use of sensitive methods to detect involvement there are 38 sites and site combinations. Overall, in 63% are single sites consisting of any of the abdomen, maxilla, breast, mandibles, thyroid, oral pharyngeal, or skeletal involvement. In 37% of instances, more than anatomic site will be found involved. However, in adult cases there is no demonstrable actual single or isolated mandible, maxilla, skeletal, or miscellaneous sites as in those less than 16.

In adults the proportions of all involved sites, the order are abdomen, breast, miscellaneous and lymph nodes 11.4%, breast 20.2%, miscellaneous and lymph nodes 9.1%, in all there are seven sites involved compared to those in less than 16 years old. Furthermore in this age group the proportion distribution from lymph node enlargement is noted. Also observed are comparatively high CNS 11.4% proportions. Although BL in adults tend to present with more and diffuse site involvement, the breast has only occasionally been detected; however, cervical lymph node involvement is infrequent.

Staging

The most common system of staging for non-Hodgkin's lymphomas (NHL's) in adults and children, including Burkitt's lymphoma are the St Jude and Ann Arbor staging system for children and adults, respectively, describe how many groups of lymph nodes are affected, where they are in the body and involvement of other body organs such as the central nervous system, bone marrow, or liver is involved.

Stage I: The lymphoma is either limited to one group of lymph nodes either above or below the diaphragm, or is in an organ or part of the body other than the lymph nodes.

Stage II: The lymphoma is either in two or more lymph node groups on the same side of the diaphragm, or is in only one organ or site other than the lymph nodes but also involves surrounding lymph nodes.

Stage III: The lymphoma is present in groups of lymph nodes on both sides of the diaphragm. It may involve an organ or site outside the lymph nodes, the spleen, or both.

Stage IV: The lymphoma is disseminated with more organs outside the lymph nodes involved. There may or may not be involvement of lymph nodes that are remote from the affected organs.

In all the NEBL is a severe disease, affects older children and the adult populations. There are usually few or no stage A and B. The dominant stages are D and C. Indeed, the duration to presentation is shorter in stages C and D. The stages A and B tend to be detected at much earlier time due to conspicuousity of the sites.

It is fair to foresee more information coming about sporadic Burkitt's lymphoma and final finding of signatures that will obviate the descriptions in terms of largely geographical and clinical basis.

References

1. Blum KA, Lozanski G, Byrd JC (2004) Adult Burkitt leukemia and lymphoma. Blood 104:3009–3020
2. Kanbar AH (2012) Burkitt lymphoma and Burkitt-like lymphoma. http://emedicine.medscape.com/article/1447602-overview
3. Cuneo A, Castoldi GL (2001) Burkitt's lymphoma (BL). Atlas Genet Cytogenet Oncol Haematol. http://AtlasGeneticsOncology.org/Anomalies/BurkittID2077.html
4. Swerdlow SH, Campo E, Harris NL et al (eds) (2008) WHO classification of tumors of hematopoietic and lymphoma tissues, 4th edn. World Health Organization, Lyon
5. Kemeny MM, Magrath IT, Brennan MF (1982) The role of surgery in the management of American Burkitt's lymphoma and its treatment. Ann Surg 196(1):82–86
6. Burkitts D (1958) A sarcoma involving the jaws in African children. Br J Surg 46:218
7. Berarad CW, O'Connor GT, Thomas LB et al (1969) Histopathological definition of Burkitt's tumour. Bull World Health Organ 40(4):601–607
8. William RH, Pike MW, Smith PG, Day NE et al (1978) Space-time clustering of Burkitts Lymphoma in the West Nile District of Uganda: 1961–1975. Br J Cancer 37:109–118
9. Levine PH, Cho BR, Connelly RR et al (1975) The American Burkitt's lymphoma registry: a progress report. Ann Intern Med 83:31–36
10. Wang MB, Strasnick B, Zimmerman MC (1992) Extranodal American Burkitt's lymphoma of the head and neck. Arch Otolaryngol Head Neck Surg 118:193–199
11. Crawshaw J, Sohaib SA, Wotherspoon A, Shepherd JH (2007) Primary non-Hodgkin's lymphoma of the ovaries: imaging findings. Br J Radiol 90:155–158
12. Lister J, Miklos JA, Swerdlow SH, Bahler DW (1996) A clonally distinct recurrence of Burkitt's lymphoma at 15 years. Blood 88(4):1407–1410

Chapter 8
AIDS-Associated Burkitt's Lymphoma

Peter M. Mwamba and Scot C. Remick

Introduction

In the World Health Organization (WHO) classification of lymphoma three distinct clinical variants of Burkitt's lymphoma (BL) are recognized—endemic or classical BL, which is discussed in Chap. 6; sporadic BL discussed in Chap. 7; and herein epidemic or AIDS-related or other immunodeficiency-associated BL [1]. In 1981, the appearance in homosexual men of *Pneumocystis carinii* pneumonia on the West Coast and Kaposi's sarcoma on the East Coast in the USA heralded the onset of the AIDS epidemic [2, 3]. A year later the first cases of non-Hodgkin's lymphoma were described and it was soon appreciated that Burkitt's and Burkitt's-like and other high-grade lymphoma were seen in markedly increased incidence in this setting [4–6]. Accordingly, the case definition for AIDS surveillance immediately reflected the occurrence of B-cell and other indeterminate immunophenotypic non-Hodgkin's lymphoma including the cases of Burkitt's and Burkitt's-like lymphoma as meeting criteria for index AIDS-defining neoplasms by the U.S. Centers for Disease Control and Prevention [7]. Today Burkitt's and Burkitt's-like lymphoma represent significant causes of morbidity and mortality in patients with underlying HIV infection especially in the world's AIDS epicenters. Given this backdrop, this chapter will focus on the natural history of AIDS-associated BL in the resource-rich

Peter M. Mwamba and Scot C. Remick were supported in part by NIH grant nos.: D43 CA153707.

P.M. Mwamba
Haematology and Blood Transfusion, Department of Human Pathology,
University of Nairobi College of Health Sciences, Nairobi, Kenya
e-mail: pmmwamba@yahoo.com

S.C. Remick (✉)
Laurence and Jean DeLynn Chair of Oncology, Mary Babb Randolph Cancer Center,
West Virginia University, School of Medicine, Morgantown, WV, USA
e-mail: sremick@hsc.wvu.edu

E.S. Robertson (ed.), *Burkitt's Lymphoma*, Current Cancer Research,
DOI 10.1007/978-1-4614-4313-1_8, © Springer Science+Business Media New York 2013

(e.g., western world) versus the resource-constrained setting (e.g., sub-Saharan Africa), which presents special challenges to all types of investigators from epidemiologists, cancer virologists and researchers, physicians and other members of the health-care team taking care of these patients [8].

Epidemiology

Present estimates are that nearly 4% of AIDS patients in the USA have cancer and compared to the general population, HIV-infected individuals have a 77-fold increased risk of developing non-Hodgkin's lymphoma [9]. Despite a decline in incidence over the years, non-Hodgkin's lymphoma is now the most common malignancy diagnosed and most common cause of cancer mortality in HIV-infected individuals in the USA [9, 10]. Recent estimates in the USA also confirm that 5.5% of diffuse large B-cell lymphoma and 19.4% of BL cases occurred among persons with AIDS [11]. These lymphomas appear to be more common in males than in females, regardless of antiretroviral use, and there now appears to be a trimodal age-specific incidence pattern for BL in the USA, with the middle-age peak largely composed of cases with AIDS [9, 12]. After the widespread implementation of highly active antiretroviral therapy (HAART)/combination antiretroviral therapy (cART) [more contemporaneous terminology], the risk of non-Hodgkin's lymphoma decreased initially, especially in the western world, and has essentially remained stable since [13–15]. While distribution and access to cART in AIDS epicenters of the world such as sub-Saharan Africa is improving, the overall impact of such therapy on the incidence of AIDS-associated lymphoma including BL is less apparent. Until cART is widely disseminated and routinely available in sub-Saharan Africa, AIDS-related lymphoma and BL and other intermediate to high-grade lymphomas in particular remain significant causes of morbidity and mortality in this region of the world as well.

AIDS-Related Burkitt's Lymphoma in the Western World

Burkitt's lymphoma historically has been a rare tumor in the industrialized world. It is presently highly associated with AIDS, and among HIV-infected patients is on the order of 100-fold or higher incidence than in patients without HIV infection [9, 16, 17]. For the most part there is consistent epidemiologic data from prospective cohort and retrospective studies in the USA and Europe that the overall incidence of AIDS-related BL has either remained stable or declined from the pre-HAART to current HAART (cART) therapeutic eras [18–23]. In the large international collaborative study reported in 2000 on HIV infection and cancer [across three continents—United States, Europe, and Australia (notably Africa excluded) comprising nearly 48,000 HIV-infected cases and 2,702 tumors] there was no evidence that the incidence of BL had changed over time, though admittedly the number of BL cases was small [18]. In the EuroSIDA cohort, small retrospective German and Los Angeles, California studies the incidence of BL was reported to have decreased over time [19–22]. A single 2001 study in France, however, reported a trend (not statistically significant, $p=0.17$) of increased proportion of AIDS-associated BL cases from 17.7% in the pre-HAART to 26.8% in the HAART era [23].

AIDS-Related Non-Hodgkin's Including Burkitt's Lymphoma in Sub-Saharan Africa

In Uganda there is considerable published data from the Kampala Cancer Registry, which is the most mature tumor registry on the African continent. In 1989–1991, a decade after the onset of the AIDS epidemic, Kaposi's sarcoma was the most common cancer in men, the second most frequent in women, and there was a 40-fold increase in children [24, 25]. By the mid-to-late 1990s the incidence of non-Hodgkin's lymphoma had risen and it was recognized that HIV infection was significantly associated with increased risk of non-Hodgkin's lymphoma with an OR of 6.2 (95% CI 1.9–19.9) [26, 27]. Through 2002 the Uganda AIDS-Cancer Registry Match study reported that the increased risk of AIDS-defining neoplasms Kaposi's sarcoma, non-Hodgkin's lymphoma and cervical cancer remained high in HIV-infected cases [28]. Hodgkin's disease, an EBV-associated disease, was also noted for the first time to be seen in increased incidence in patients with underlying HIV infection [29]. By 2006, while the incidence of Kaposi's sarcoma declined in men, remained relatively constant in women, and rates of pediatric disease declined by a third, and the burden of AIDS-associated cancers, especially non-Hodgkin's lymphoma (precise histopathological characterization and specifically BL was not published) and cervical cancer, remained high [29]. A period prevalence study conducted in Nairobi, Kenya between1992 and 1996 clearly identified a threefold increase in the incidence of adult BL that was attributable to HIV infection [30].

Pathogenesis

The pathogenesis of lymphoma in the setting of underlying HIV infection is complex [8, 31]. There is likely an interaction between host factors—such as accompanying progressive immunodeficiency, which is the hallmark of untreated HIV infection—and molecular and genetic alterations, which may occur *de novo* or result from co-infection with EBV or human herpesvirus-8/Kaposi's sarcoma herpesvirus (KSHV) (see Table 8.1). Progressive immune suppression, chronic antigen stimulation, and resultant B-cell proliferation—initially polyclonal and proceeding to oligoclonal and monoclonal lymphoid expansion—are important for lymphomagenesis. Associated immune activation and dysregulation of cytokine modulatory pathways

Table 8.1 Immunological, molecular, and virological pathogenic determinants of AIDS-related lymphoma

	Burkitt's/ Burkitt-like	Large cell (centroblasts)	Immunoblastic (immunoblasts)	Primary CNS lymphoma
CD4 lymphocyte count	Usually normal to mild decrease	Decreased	Decreased	<50/μL
Relationship with germinal center	Germinal center B-cells	Germinal center B-cells	Post germinal center B-cells	Post germinal center B-cells
Histogenic profile	Ki67+ (very high proliferative index)	Bcl-6+/MUM1–/ CD138–	Bcl-6–/MUM1+/ CD138+	Bcl-6–/MUM1+/ CD138+
Molecular markers				
c-myc	>65–100%	30%	(–)	(–)
LMP-1	(–)	(–)	65–75%	90%
p53	50–60%	Rare	Rare	No data
EBV infection	30–50%	30%	>90%	100%

(especially interleukin-6 and interleukin-10); altered *bcl-6*, *p53*, and c-*myc* oncogene expression and coexisting viral infection(s) have all been implicated in the pathogenesis of lymphoma in this setting as well [32–40]. A proposed molecular and histogenic model of AIDS lymphoma pathogenesis identifies four major pathways [32]. In the first, BL is characterized by mild immunodeficiency, germinal center-derived B-cells, multiple genetic lesions, and a highly proliferative tumor. Large cell (centroblasts) and immunoblastic (immunoblasts) lymphoma, associated with intermediate immunodeficiency, are comprised of post-germinal center B-cells, which can be distinguished on the basis of *bcl-6* expression (large cell) and LMP-1 expression (immunoblastic). Primary CNS lymphoma can be considered a variant of immunoblastic lymphoma with severe immunodeficiency and ubiquitous association with EBV infection. Lastly, a fourth pathway is AIDS-associated primary effusion lymphoma, caused by KSHV infection and frequently associated with EBV infection as well.

Pathogenic Mechanisms in AIDS-Related Burkitt's Lymphoma

A defining feature of BL is the presence of a translocation between the c-*myc* gene and the *IgH* gene (found in 80% of cases [t(8;14)]) or between c-*myc* and the gene for either the kappa or lambda light chain (*IgL*) in the remaining 20% [t(2;8) or t(8;22), respectively] [41]. Other specific lymphoma-associated translocations, such as *IgH/bcl-2* and translocations involving *bcl-6*, are absent. In endemic BL, the breakpoint in c-*myc* is more than 100 kb upstream from the first coding exon, and the breakpoint in the *IgH* gene is in the joining segment. In sporadic and AIDS-associated BL, the breakpoint in c-*myc* is between exons 1 and 2, and the breakpoint in *IgH* is in the switch (Sμ) region, suggesting a different pathogenesis and that neoplastic transformation affects B cells at different maturational stages for these subtypes of BL [42]. There is evidence that the frequency of the c-*myc* translocation from chromosome 8 onto regulatory elements of immunoglobulin genes is increased in asymptomatic HIV-infected individuals compared to those who are not infected [43]. It has also been demonstrated that activation-induced cytidine deaminase (AID), an enzyme essential for antibody diversity in B cells, is markedly elevated in peripheral blood mononuclear cells of HIV-infected individuals who went on to develop non-Hodgkin's lymphoma compared to HIV-seronegative controls, with the highest levels seen in BL cases [44–46]. While increased c-*myc* translocation as well as AID over-expression appear to be demonstrably increased in HIV-infected individuals, the precise molecular events contributing to these cellular changes are unknown.

Degree of Immunosuppression in AIDS-Related Burkitt's Lymphoma

While immunodeficiency-associated BL occurs mainly in HIV-infected patients, it also occurs in allograft recipients (mostly solid organs but recipients of stem cells are rarely affected as well) and individuals with congenital immunodeficiency [47–49]. In the post-transplant setting, mean interval to onset of lymphoma in one series was reported as 4.5 years [49]. It is known that the degree of immune suppression is less in patients who develop AIDS-related BL compared to other histologic subtypes of non-Hodgkin's lymphoma in this setting [21, 22, 50–52]. The degree of immunosuppression in patients presenting with AIDS-related lymphoma, especially diffuse large B-cell lymphoma, has clearly lessened over time (i.e., median CD4+ lymphocyte counts are higher in the current cARV era), while median CD4+ lymphocyte counts in patients with AIDS-associated BL have largely remained unchanged [21, 22]. Numerous studies from sub-Saharan Africa have not reported an increase in endemic BL in HIV-infected children (the exception is a study reported by Newton et al. [27]); and not infrequently a decline in BL incidence has been observed with childhood HIV infection [53–57]. Taken together these observations are inconsistent with the notion that BL evolves in the backdrop of severe immunodeficiency that accompanies underlying HIV infection. Accordingly, it has been hypothesized that perhaps aberrant dysregulation of the immune response favoring a T-helper 2 (TH-2) dominant cytokine-driven profile that is stimulated by prolonged EBV-hyperproliferation of B-cells versus a weakened cell-mediated T-helper 1 (TH-1) profile that results in impaired tumor surveillance may be pathogenic [58].

Pathologic Features

With respect to morphology, the WHO Classification describes classic BL and two variants: Burkitt's lymphoma with plasmacytoid differentiation and atypical Burkitt's/Burkitt-like lymphoma [1]. Classic BL is found in cases of endemic BL and most cases of sporadic BL affecting children but in only a minority of adults with sporadic and immunodeficiency-associated BL. Neoplastic cells are uniform and medium-sized (their nuclei are no larger than the nuclei of admixed histiocytes), with round nuclei and several or multiple small basophilic nucleoli with moderately abundant cytoplasm. The classic "starry sky" pattern is derived from macrophages engulfing highly proliferative tumor cells. Burkitt's lymphoma with plasmacytoid differentiation and atypical BL both tend to have greater nuclear pleomorphism than classic BL, and both tend to have a smaller number of more prominent nucleoli. The plasmacytoid variant is highly associated with AIDS, makes up 20% of cases of non-Hodgkin's lymphoma, and in addition has monotypic cytoplasmic immunoglobulin. Atypical BL is further characterized by the translocation t(8;14)(q24;q32) or one of its variants, or rearrangement of the c-*myc* gene. Burkitt's lymphoma, regardless of subtype, typically expresses monotypic surface IgM; pan-B-cell antigens, including CD19, CD20, CD22, and CD79a; and co-expresses CD10, bcl-6, CD43, and p53, but not CD5, CD23, bcl-2, CD138, or TdT [39, 40]. The *sine qua non* is a proliferative fraction (e.g., Ki67) of essentially >95–100%; accordingly, the doubling time of the tumor is very short, between 24 and 48 h. Rare cases have been reported that lack surface immunoglobulin, including some occurring in allograft recipients [49, 59]. The immunophenotype suggests germinal center origin for this lymphoma. Chapter 2 provides additional details about the diagnosis and pathology of BL.

Clinical Manifestations

It was recognized early into the AIDS epidemic that the clinical course of AIDS-related non-Hodgkin's lymphoma was much more aggressive than patients without HIV infection. In general, AIDS-related non-Hodgkin lymphoma is characterized by higher grade (40–60%), extranodal disease (80%), advanced clinical stage (60–70%) often presenting with B symptoms (i.e., unexplained fever, night sweats, and weight loss in excess of 10% of normal body weight); and shortened survival (median 7–8 months) when compared with lymphomas in HIV-seronegative or indeterminate patients [8, 60]. At the time of clinical presentation prior to the cARV era, the median CD4 lymphocyte count was 100/μL. In the cARV era, patients are less immune suppressed with median CD4 lymphocyte counts ranging between 150 and 200/μL and higher. It is not uncommon for patients with AIDS-related BL to present with signs and symptoms of tumor lysis syndrome. In addition, the incidence of leptomeningeal involvement at the time of diagnosis of AIDS-related non-Hodgkin's lymphoma and over the course of disease appears to be declining as well. This could be attributable to the altered natural history of underlying HIV infection in the cARV era and perhaps less predominance of high-grade histologies (off-set by increase in intermediate-grade large-cell lymphoma). Though high-grade histology, especially BL, and lymphomas that harbor EBV, with bone marrow or disease involvement that impinges on or near the CNS such as paranasal sinuses and paraspinal masses are more likely to have leptomeningeal involvement [8, 60–62]. There remains a clear male predominance in AIDS lymphoma in the USA but in other regions of the world most affected by the epidemic such as sub-Saharan Africa, there is nearly an equal distribution of cases in men and women. This is reflective of the predominant heterosexual transmission of HIV infection in developing countries.

Presentation of AIDS-Related Burkitt's Lymphoma in Sub-Saharan Africa

Recent studies in Uganda have included a case–control study of non-Hodgkin's lymphoma (31 adult and 61 pediatrics cases identified between 1994 and 1998), and two others have reported the clinical characteristics and outcome of pediatric Burkitt's lymphoma (228 cases identified between 1994 and 2004) and adult non-Hodgkin's lymphoma (154 cases excluding BL identified between 2004 and 2008) in the backdrop of HIV infection for the first time [57, 63, 64]. In the case–control study, 92 cases had full phenotyping and documentation of EBV status, which were considered validated [57]. Burkitt's lymphoma and large B-cell lymphomas represented 71% of adult and BL represented 92% of pediatric cases validated, respectively [57]. EBV was present in 35% of adult of whom 34% were HIV-infected (vs. 20% of controls); and EBV was present in 91% of pediatric cases, of whom 4.9% were HIV-infected (vs. 5% controls) [57]. In another study of children with Burkitt's lymphoma, nearly one-third of cases were HIV-infected, the median age was 6.9 years, and over 60% were male [63]. HIV-infected children presented with more advanced stage, significant extrafacial (e.g., especially lymphadenopathy) and thoracic disease [63].

A Kenyan period prevalence study of adult BL in the backdrop of AIDS observed that the proportion of men (60%) was similar in HIV-seropositive versus seronegative cases; HIV-seropositive cases were significantly older at diagnosis (35 vs. 19.5 years); HIV-seropositive cases uniformly presented with B symptoms and advanced BL accompanied by diffuse lymph node involvement and extranodal presentations as well (see Figs. 8.1 and 8.2) as well [30]. What was striking in this study was the complete sparing of peripheral lymph nodes in HIV-seronegative adult BL cases, which is reminiscent of the "typical" pattern of clinical presentation in endemic disease. It was concluded that inclusion of AIDS-related BL in the differential diagnosis of the adult patient with unexplained fever and lymphadenopathy, which is often associated with *Myobacterium tuberculosis* and sexually transmitted diseases in Kenya and other parts of sub-Saharan Africa, warrants consideration. The corollary is that HIV infection is virtually excluded in an adult patient without peripheral lymphadenopathy and biopsy-proven BL [30].

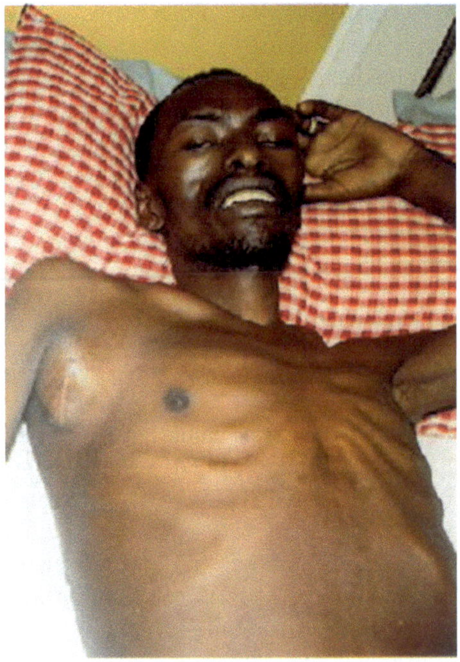

Fig. 8.1 Extensive peripheral lymphadenopathy and wasting in a Kenyan man with AIDS-related biopsy-proven Burkitt's lymphoma

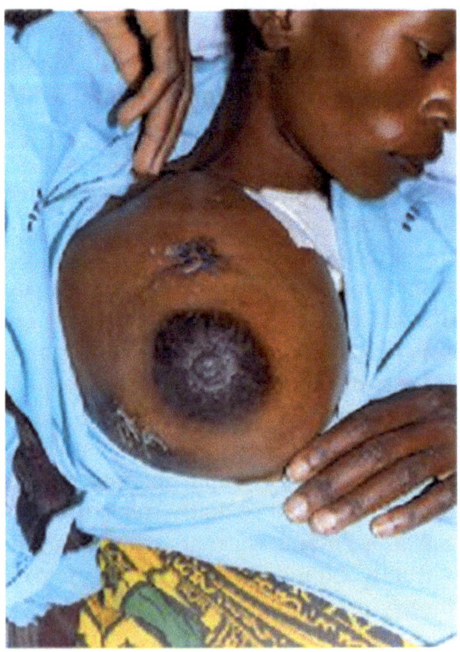

Fig. 8.2 A Kenyan woman with AIDS-related biopsy-proven Burkitt's lymphoma of the breast

Diagnosis and Staging

The diagnosis of AIDS-related non-Hodgkin's lymphoma including BL is established by pathological confirmation of malignant lymphoma on biopsy material of involved lymph node(s), bone marrow, or other extranodal site(s) and should include immunohistochemistry for confirmation of CD20 B-cell status of the tumor to guide selection of rituximab. In the resource-challenged setting diagnosis of BL is often made on fine needle aspiration of peripheral lesions alone and the inherent challenges of this approach are discussed in Chap. 2. Heightened clinical suspicion upon careful history taking for underlying risk behaviors for acquisition of HIV infection and physical examination for clinical signs and stigmata of HIV disease are critical to properly diagnose and sort out any association of HIV infection and malignant lymphoma. Routine HIV antibody testing is performed in patients with newly diagnosed non-Hodgkin's lymphoma.

Patients with AIDS-related BL are best staged according to the Ann Arbor staging criteria, which is adopted as an international staging classification scheme for non-Hodgkin's lymphoma [65]. Other staging schemes for endemic BL are discussed in this text (see Chap. 6). Clinical staging builds upon careful history and physical examination and incorporates laboratory investigations (including complete blood cell count and differential; serum electrolytes and chemistries, including lactate dehydrogenase with particular attention to metabolic parameters that are indicative of tumor lysis syndrome); body computed tomography of neck, chest, abdomen, and pelvis; (^{18}FDG)-positron emission tomography; bone marrow aspiration and biopsy; and examination of the cerebrospinal fluid for cytology and flow cytometry. Brain magnetic resonance imaging may help discern evidence of CNS involvement and echocardiography or other assessment of left ventricular function is obtained given the likely use of doxorubicin or other anthracycline-containing combination chemotherapy regimen. Lastly, assessment of HIV infection includes HIV serology, baseline determinations of CD4+ lymphocyte counts and HIV-1 plasma RNA levels (i.e., viral load).

Clinical Staging of AIDS-Related Burkitt's Lymphoma in Sub-Saharan Africa

In sub-Saharan Africa, reliance on physical examination is all the more important given the relative lack of computed tomography, magnetic resonance imaging, and positron emission tomography [8, 66, 67]. Although understaging of patients when compared to western and more resource-rich settings is likely this is, however, balanced by initial presentation at more advanced stages of disease than occurs in developed countries [66]. In this setting, physical examination becomes a reasonable and reliable instrument of assessment. In most situations, patients will also undergo chest radiography, abdominal ultrasonography, bone marrow aspiration biopsy, and cerebrospinal fluid cytology [66].

Therapeutic Approach

Endemic BL was one of the first malignancies shown to be curable with cytotoxic chemotherapy [68–71]. Sporadic and immunodeficiency-associated BL do not share endemic BL's exquisite sensitivity to chemotherapy, so that historically the prognosis has been poor, particularly among adults. Short-duration, high-intensity chemotherapy, sometimes combined with CNS prophylaxis, yielded excellent survival in children: patients with localized disease have a >90% 5-year survival rate [72] and children with widespread disease (including leukemic presentation) may achieve a >90% complete response rate (CR), with an event-free survival rate at 4 years of 65% in patients with leukemic presentation, and 79% for those presenting with stage IV lymphoma reported in one series [73]. When similar aggressive chemotherapeutic regimens have been administered to adults, good outcomes have been achieved, with CR rates of 65–100% and overall survival (OS) rates of 50–70% [74]. The institution of the CODOX-M/IVAC regimen (Magrath protocol)—two cycles of CODOX-M (cyclophosphamide, vincristine, doxorubicin, high-dose methotrexate, and intrathecal therapy) alternating with IVAC (ifosfamide with mesna, etoposide, high-dose cytarabine, and intrathecal therapy)—for high-risk disease, and for those with low-risk disease (e.g., one extranodal site or completely resected abdominal disease with normal LDH), three cycles of CODOX-M, represented a major step forward in the treatment of BL. Children and adults treated with this regimen had similar outcomes; the EFS rate at 2 years was 92% for the group as a whole [74]. The Dana-Farber Cancer Institute has treated patients with a modified Magrath regimen, aimed at decreasing toxicity while maintaining good outcome [75]. In this modification, the schedule of fractionated cyclophosphamide was altered and the vincristine dose was capped, but the dose of doxorubicin was escalated. In this cohort, there were no treatment-related deaths, one instance of severe mucositis, and no severe neurotoxicity. The 2-year event-free survival rate was 64% for all patients, 100% for low-risk patients, and 60% for high-risk patients [75]. Rituximab, a monoclonal anti-CD20 antibody, may improve outcome; a study of a small series from the M.D. Anderson Cancer Center used rituximab in conjunction with hyper-CVAD (hyperfractionated cyclophosphamide, vincristine, doxorubicin, and dexamethasone), with CNS prophylaxis, and achieved a CR rate of 89%; most patients had advanced-stage disease, and some were HIV-infected [76]. This backdrop provides the context for the evolution of treatment for AIDS-associated BL.

At the outset of the AIDS epidemic it was readily apparent that patients did not tolerate more aggressive or dose-intensive systemic therapy despite presenting with high-grade tumors including AIDS-associated BL and more advanced stage of disease when compared to HIV-seronegative or indeterminate cases of non-Hodgkin's lymphoma; all patients were generally treated in a similar manner regardless of histologic subtype; and prognosis was most dependent on the degree of immunosuppression with patients having demonstrably poorer outcomes with CD4+ lymphocyte counts <100/μL [8, 60, 77–79]. Thus, initial approaches incorporated dose-modified chemotherapeutic strategies, which over the first 15 years of the epidemic proved equally efficacious and markedly less toxic, especially with diminished myelotoxicity [80, 81]. It was also recognized that infusional versus bolus chemotherapy strategies (e.g., CDE—cyclophosphamide, doxorubicin, and etoposide or EPOCH—etoposide, prednisone, vincristine, cyclophosphamide, and doxorubicin) yielded better CR rates and survival outcomes [50, 82]. What is also intriguing by the published experience with infusional EPOCH regimen was the strategy of suspension of antiretroviral therapy over the course of chemotherapy to avoid increased risk of drug–drug interactions, potential for increased toxicity, and to enhance overall patient compliance [50]. The chemotherapy was also dose-adjusted on the basis of CD4 lymphocyte count in an attempt to individualize therapy. While this strategy (to suspend antiretroviral therapy) did not result in adverse clinical outcome (i.e., HIV-1 viral load and CD4 lymphocyte counts returned to baseline by 3 and 12 months, respectively), it should be carefully considered and requires larger, multi-center clinical trial(s) to firmly establish this approach. The role of rituximab has also been established in HIV-infected patients with CD20+ B-cell lymphomas despite initial observations (the addition of rituximab to standard-dose CHOP led to increased infectious complications and deaths attributable to sepsis) reported by the NCI-sponsored AIDS Malignancy Consortium (AMC 010 study) [83]. Confirmatory studies conducted by the AMC and others have proven the safety of adding rituximab to cytotoxic chemotherapy regimens for AIDS-related non-Hodgkin's lymphoma, including cases of BL and BL-like subtypes (reviewed in [60, 84]). Only recently, however, it has been recognized that in the cART era indeed outcomes are different between subtypes of AIDS lymphoma (see Fig. 8.3) and that patients with higher grade tumors, and BL in particular, do much worse and need to be treated with more aggressive systemic chemotherapy regimens [22]. It is no longer appropriate to treat all cases of AIDS-related lymphoma as constituting a single disease entity and into "one therapeutic basket" but rather lymphoma-specific features, especially tumor grade and likely other molecular markers in the not too distant future (e.g., CD20 and IRF4/MUM1-positive immunohistochemistry) need to guide the selection of chemotherapeutic regimens. In the not too distant future viral therapeutic targets will likely emerge in the clinic as well.

Recent reports of aggressive chemotherapy regimens specifically for AIDS-associated BL are now appearing [85, 86]. The French LMB86 protocol [which is a complex poly-drug cytotoxic chemotherapy containing regimen incorporating: (1) a cytoreductive phase with COP immediately followed by; (2) induction with two courses of COPDAM with doxorubicin and high-dose methotrexate; (3) consolidation phase with two courses of high-dose cytarabine and etoposide; and finally, (4) a maintenance phase with four courses of reduced dosages of the prior drugs] reported a 70% CR rate, median overall survival duration of 14.2 months, and 2-year disease-free and overall survival rates of 67.8 and 47.1%, respectively [85]. There were 7 (11%) treatment-related deaths, all patients experienced severe myelotoxicity, and 11 patients relapsed out of the 63 patients treated between November 1992 and January 2006. Low CD4+ lymphocyte counts and ECOG performance status of >2 were poor prognostic factors. Patients with 0 or 1 factor had a 60% 2-year survival rate, which contrasted with the 12% of patients who survived

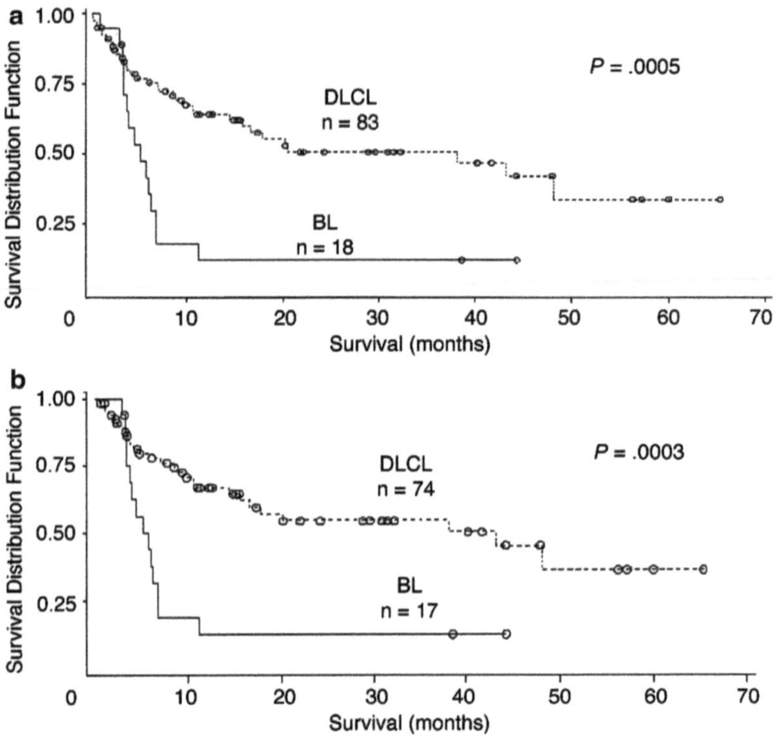

Fig. 8.3 First published report, albeit a retrospective study, of AIDS-related non-Hodgkin's lymphoma that demonstrated different survival outcomes among patients with intermediate grade (DLCL) and high-grade (BL) histology: (**a**) survival of all patients and (**b**) survival of patients treated with curative intent by pathologic type in the cART era; *BL* Burkitt's lymphoma and *DLCL* diffuse large-cell lymphoma [22]

2 years with both adverse prognostic factors [85]. The AMC recently reported its preliminary observations in 33 patients recruited from September 2006 to July 2010 incorporating further modifications of the Magrath regimen (R-CODOX-M/IVAC) for AIDS-associated BL [86]. In this study there was an acceptable safety and toxicity profile [39% of patients had grade 3 or 4 myelotoxicity, 61% had any grade 3 or 4 toxicity, there were 6 (18%) treatment-related deaths]; a 81.7% 1-year survival rate with a median survival duration of 35 months. The group also reported improved outcomes in patients whose tumors where IRF4/MUM1-positive, which is indicative of a post-germinal center activated B-cell negative by immunohistochemistry [86]. The rationale for several treatment modifications to the Magrath regimen specifically considered for AIDS-associated BL included: inclusion of rituximab for BL as a CD20+ lymphoma with high likelihood of improved efficacy without added toxicity; institution of infusion schedules of ifosfamide and etoposide rather than bolus administration given mounting evidence of improved outcomes with this strategy especially highly proliferative tumors and in HIV-infected patients; lessening toxicity

by reducing the dose of methotrexate (from total dose of 5,520 to 3,000 mg/m^2) while maintaining CNS penetration and during the CODOX-M portion of the regimen from day 10 (time of anticipated nadir) to day 15; and reducing neurotoxicity, which is especially troublesome to HIV-infected patients due to underlying HIV neuropathy or polypharmacy, by establishing a fixed ceiling dose of vincristine to a maximum of 2 mg. While comparative trials of BL chemotherapy regimens for patients with and without HIV infection have not been reported, the AMC experience appears to be less myelotoxic with improved overall survival duration. Further follow-up of this encouraging report are awaited.

Therapeutic Approach to AIDS-Related Burkitt's Lymphoma in Sub-Saharan Africa

There are limited published reviews on the clinicopathological spectrum of lymphoproliferative diseases encountered in this part of the world with or without the backdrop of underlying HIV infection and therapeutic outcome, including both prognostic and predictive indicators. Often these reviews focus more on the adoption of therapeutic approaches from the developed world that may or may not be suitable for the sub-Saharan African setting or report clinical experience in patients that are not HIV-infected (in a review from Cape Town, South Africa less than 2% of 512 consecutively treated lymphoma patients seen at a private sector academic center were HIV-infected) [87–90].

Other published reports have clearly identified the challenges in administering dose-intense chemotherapy to children with endemic Burkitt's lymphoma in other parts of sub-Saharan Africa [e.g., Malawi and International Society of Paediatric Oncology (SIOP) network], where 1-year event-free survival is 57% and treatment-related mortality is on the order of 30%, which contrasts with at 90% 1-year EFS rate in Europe and markedly diminished treatment-related mortality attributable to the requisite supportive care in the resource-rich environment to sustain children through prolonged periods of dose-intense myelosupppression [91–93]. In addition, a Ugandan study reported that the median survival of those patients presenting with non-Hodgkin's lymphoma in whom mortality status was confirmed was 2 months; of these 32% were HIV-seropositive; and median survival among patients with HIV infection receiving antiretroviral therapy was comparable to those without HIV infection [64]. In the majority of instances these patients were treated with standard CHOP combination chemotherapy and dose-adjusted CHOP based on CD4 lymphocyte count (<200 cells/μL) in HIV-infected patients [64]. Another Uganda study of pediatric BL reported that while treatment response rates (≤70%) were similar regardless of HIV-serostatus, median survival (11.79 months) in HIV-infected children was less than HIV-negative/indeterminate children (median survival not reached in HIV-negative children) [63]. In this report, no details were reported on the types of chemotherapy administered to these children. Inherent challenges remain in the administration of chemotherapy, supportive care, and follow-up of patients with non-Hodgkin's lymphoma in Uganda, which is akin to other resource-challenged areas in sub-Saharan Africa including anecdotal reports from Kenya with an established pediatric oncology unit [8, 64, 67, 94].

Given this backdrop the first prospective clinical trial of AIDS-related non-Hodgkin's lymphoma in sub-Saharan Africa utilizing a dose-modified oral chemotherapy regimen was reported in 2009 [66]. Important outcomes in 49 patients treated on this trial included overall objective response rate of 78%, median event-free and overall survival times of 7.9 months (95% CI, 3.3–13.0 months) and 12.3 months (95% CI, 4.9–32.4 months), respectively; and 33% of patients survived 5 years [66]. The regimen was well tolerated, had modest effects (decline) on CD4+ lymphocyte counts ($p=0.077$), and had negligible effects on HIV-1 viral replication. Four febrile neutropenia episodes (5% of cycles) and three treatment-related deaths (6% mortality rate) occurred. Importantly there was demonstrable activity in patients with high-grade tumors including three cases of verified AIDS-associated BL with survivals of 7.2, 12.3, and 14.8 months [66]. It was concluded that dose-modified oral chemotherapy is efficacious, has comparable outcome to that in the USA in the pre-cART setting, has an acceptable safety profile, and subsequent projects should focus on strategies to optimize combination antiretroviral therapy and chemotherapy and follow-up tissue diagnostic and correlative studies. The NCI-sponsored AIDS Malignancy Consortium plans shortly to launch a successor trial (AMC 068 protocol) of the dose-modified oral regimen in sub-Saharan Africa (in Eldoret, Kenya; Harare, Zimbabwe; Johannesburg, South Africa; and Kampala, Uganda) in which all patients will be treated with cART and the chemotherapy will be extended from a total course of 12–18 weeks (total of three cycles of therapy instead of two as in the original study). In the sub-Saharan setting, dose-modification of CHOP combination chemotherapy and/or utilization of more intensive chemotherapy regimens (including dose modification thereof) for AIDS-associated BL, especially patients with CD4+ lymphocyte counts <100 cells/μL seems prudent depending on drug supply and provision of supportive care in this setting [8, 66, 94]. It may also be clinically prudent to initiate antiretroviral therapy for patients once stabilized after their first course of chemotherapy if they are indeed cART naïve at time of BL diagnosis to limit potential risks of noncompliance with oral cART regimens and the nausea, vomiting seen with chemotherapy and the inherent debility of patients at time of presentation especially those with BL involvement of the gastrointestinal tract.

Summary and Ways Forward

AIDS-associated BL remains a significant cause of morbidity and mortality in HIV-infected patients. Since 1996, the treatment of HIV infection with cART has dramatically impacted patient outcomes with markedly improved overall survival, improved immune reconstitution and near complete suppression of HIV-1 viral replication. We have come full circle in treating AIDS-associated BL in the western world from less myelotoxic dose-modified strategies at the outset of the epidemic to more dose intense therapeutic regimens greatly afforded by improvements in antiretroviral therapy, better tolerance to cytotoxic chemotherapy, and incorporation of the CD20+ directed monoclonal antibody rituximab into front-line regimens. In the setting of widely accessible cART, it is imperative that the therapeutic approach be tailored to the subtype of lymphoma (e.g., BL and other high-grade subtypes versus diffuse large B-cell lymphoma and other intermediate-grade subtypes) rather than approaching AIDS-related lymphoma as a single disease entity. There is also less reliance on the prognostic impact of level of CD4+ lymphocyte counts at diagnosis in the current cART era. Identifying new agents, optimizing treatment within the context of cART, and determining biologic and virologic correlates of disease pathogenesis and of response to therapy in patients with AIDS-associated BL remain research priorities.

In sub-Saharan Africa and other developing countries, which bear the greatest burden of AIDS-associated BL, challenges still abound and concerted efforts need to be made to improve care in this setting. Clinical research should be prioritized so as to determine the best way to manage this disease by improving diagnostic capability and identifying pragmatic and better risk-adapted approaches for treatment and patient care. At the same time there are unprecedented opportunities for translational research to interrogate viral oncogenic pathways given the inherent increased rates of co-infection with viral pathogens such as HIV, EBV, and KSHV among others so unique in this part of the world. This may yield innovative viral-targeted therapeutic strategies and new insights into prevention efforts of AIDS-associated and other viral tumors in this setting altogether.

References

1. Swerdlow SH, Campo E, Harris NL, Jaffe ES, Pileri SA, Stein H, Thiele J, and Vardiman JW (2008). WHO classification of tumours of haematolpoietic and lymphoid tissues. In: WHO classification of tumours, vol. 2, 4th edn. IARC Press, Lyon
2. Centers for Disease Control (1981) Pneumocystis pneumonia—Los Angeles. MMWR Morb Mortal Wkly Rep 30:250–252
3. Centers for Disease Control (1981) Kaposi's sarcoma and pneumocystis Pneumonia among homosexual men—New York City and California. MMWR Morb Mortal Wkly Rep 30:305–308
4. Centers for Disease Control (1982) Diffuse and undifferentiated non-Hodgkin's lymphoma Kaposi's sarcoma and pneumocystis pneumonia among homosexual men—New York City and California. MMWR Morb Mortal Wkly Rep 30:305–308
5. Doll DC, List AF (1982) Burkitt's lymphoma in a homosexual. Lancet 1:1026–1027
6. Ziegler JL, Drew WL, Miner RC, Mintz L, Rosenbaum E, Gershow J, Lennette ET, Greenspan J, Shillitoe E, Beckstead J, Casavant C, Yamamato K (1982) Outbreak of Burkitt's-like lymphoma in homosexual men. Lancet 2:631–633
7. Centers for Disease Control (1985) Revision of the case definition of acquired immunodeficiency syndrome for national reporting—United States. MMWR Morb Mortal Wkly Rep 34:373–375
8. Mwanda (aka Otieno MW) WO, Banura C, Katongole-Mbidde E, Johnson JL, Ghannoum M, Dowlati A, Renne R, Arts E, Whalen C, Lederman MM, Remick SC (2002) Therapeutic

challenges of AIDS-related non-Hodgkin's lymphoma in the United States and East Africa. J Natl Cancer Inst 94:718–732
9. Shiels MS, Pfeiffer RM, Gail MH, Hall HI, Li J, Chaturvedi AK, Bhatia K, Uldrick TS, Yarchoan R, Goedert JJ, Engels EA (2011) Cancer burden in the HIV-infected population in the United States. J Natl Cancer Inst 103:753–762
10. Achenbach CJ, Cole SR, Kitahata MM, Casper C, Willig JH, Mugavero MJ, Saag MS (2011) Mortality after cancer diagnosis in HIV-infected individuals treated with antiretroviral therapy. AIDS 25:691–700
11. Shiels MS, Pfeiffer RM, Hall HI, Li J, Goedert JJ, Morton LM, Hartge P, Engels EA (2011) Proportions of Kaposi sarcoma, selected non-Hodgkin lymphomas, and cervical cancer in the United States occurring in persons with AIDS, 1980–2007. JAMA 305:1450–1459
12. Mbulaiteye SM, Anderson WV, Bhatia K, Rosenberg PS, Linet MS, Devsa SS (2010) Trimodal age-specific incidence patterns for Burkitt lymphoma in the United States, 1973–2005. Int J Cancer 126:1732–1739
13. Lim ST, Karim R, Tulpule A, Nathwani BN, Levine AM (2005) Prognostic factors in HIV-related diffuse large-cell lymphoma: before versus after highly active antiretroviral therapy. J Clin Oncol 23:8477–8482
14. Bower M, Palmieri C, Dhillon T (2006) AIDS-related malignancies: changing epidemiology and the impact of highly active antiretroviral therapy. Curr Opin Infect Dis 19:14–19
15. Bower M, Fisher M, Hill T, Bower M, Fisher M, Hill T, Reeves I, Walsh J, Orkin C, Phillips AN, Bansi L, Gilson R, Easterbrook P, Johnson M, Gazzard B, Leen C, Pillay D, Schwenk A, Anderson J, Porter K, Gompels M, Sabin CA, Steering Committee UKCHIC (2009) CD4 counts and the risk of systemic non-Hodgkin's lymphoma in individuals with HIV in the UK. Haematologica 94:875–880
16. Cote TR, Biggar RJ, Rosenberg PS, Devesa SS, Percy C, Yellin FJ, Lemp G, Hardy C, Geodert JJ, Blattner WA (1997) Non-Hodgkin's lymphoma among people with AIDS: incidence, presentation and public health burden. AIDS/Cancer Study Group. Int J Cancer 73:645–650
17. Morton LM, Wang SS, Devesa SS, Hartge P, Weisenburger DD, Linet MS (2006) Lymphoma incidence patterns by WHO subtype in the United States, 1992–2001. Blood 107:265–276
18. International Collaboration on HIV and Cancer (2000) Highly active antiretroviral therapy and incidence of cancer in human immunodeficiency virus-infected adults. J Natl Cancer Inst 92:1823–1830
19. Kirk O, Pedersen C, Cozzi-Lepri A, Antunes F, Miller V, Gatell JM, Katlama C, Lazzarin A, Skinhøj P, Barton SE, for the EuroSIDA Study Group (2001) Non-Hodgkin's lymphoma in HIV-infected patients in the era of highly active antiretroviral therapy. Blood 98: 3406–3412
20. Wolf T, Brodt HR, Fichtlscherer S, Mantzsch K, Hoelzer D, Helm EB, Mitrou PS, Chow KU (2005) Changing incidence and prognostic factors of survival in AIDS-related non-Hodgkin's lymphoma in the era of highly active antiretroviral therapy (HAART). Leuk Lymphoma 46:207–215
21. Levine AM, Seneviratne L, Espina BM, Wohl AR, Tulpule A, Nathwani BN, Gill PS (2000) Evolving characteristics of AIDS-related lymphoma. Blood 96:4084–4090
22. Lim ST, Karin R, Nathwani BN, Tulpule A, Espina B, Levine AM (2005) AIDS-related Burkitt's lymphoma versus diffuse large-cell lymphoma in the pre-highly active antiretroviral therapy (HAART) and HAART eras: significant differences in survival with standard chemotherapy. J Clin Oncol 23:4430–4438
23. Besson C, Goubar A, Gabarre J, Rozenbaum W, Pialoux G, Châtelet FP, Katlama C, Charlotte F, Dupont B, Brousse N, Huerre M, Mikol J, Camparo P, Mokhtari K, Tulliez M, Salmon-Céron D, Boué F, Costagliola D, Raphaël M (2001) Changes in AIDS-related lymphoma since the era of highly active antiretroviral therapy. Blood 98:2339–2344
24. Wabinga HR, Parkin DM, Wabwire-Mangen F, Mugerwa JW (1993) Cancer in Kampala, Uganda, in 1989–91: changes in incidence in the era of AIDS. Int J Cancer 54:26–36
25. Ziegler JL, Katongole-Mbidde E (1996) Kaposi's sarcoma in childhood: an analysis of 100 cases from Uganda and relationship to HIV infection. Int J Cancer 65:200–203

26. Wabinga HR, Parkin DM, Wabwire-Mangen F, Nambooze S (2000) Trends in cancer incidence in Kyadondo County, Uganda, 1960–1997. Br J Cancer 82:1585–1592
27. Newton R, Ziegler J, Beral V, Mbidde E, Carpenter L, Wabinga H, Mbulaiteye S, Appelby P, Reeves G, Jaffe H, and the Uganda Kaposi's Sarcoma Study Group (2001) A case–control study of human immunodeficiency virus infection and cancer in adults and children residing in Kampala, Uganda. Int J Cancer 92:622–627
28. Mbulaiteye SM, Katabira ET, Wabinga H, Parkin DM, Virgo P, Ochai R, Workneh M, Coutinho A, Engels EA (2006) Spectrum of cancers among HIV-infected persons in Africa: the Uganda AIDS-Cancer Registry Match Study. Int J Cancer 118:985–990
29. Parkin DM, Nambooze S, Wabwire-Mangen F, Wabinga HR (2010) Changing cancer incidence in Kampala, Uganda, 1991–2006. Int J Cancer 126:1187–1195
30. Mwanda WO, Remick SC, Whalen C (2001) Adult Burkitt's lymphoma in patients with and without human immunodeficiency virus infection in Africa. Int J Cancer 92:687–691
31. Cremer KJ, Spring SB, Gruber J (1990) Role of human immunodeficiency virus type 1 and other viruses in malignancies associated with acquired immunodeficiency disease syndrome. J Natl Cancer Inst 82:1016–1024
32. Carbone A (2003) Emerging pathways in the development of AIDS-related lymphomas. Lancet Oncol 4:22–29
33. Carbone A, Gloghini A, Larocca LM, Capello D, Pierconti F, Canzonieri F, Tirelli U, Dalla-Favera R, Gaidano G (2001) Expression profile of MUM1/IRF4, BCL-6, and CD138/syndecan-1 defines novel histogenetic subsets of human immune-deficiency virus-related lymphomas. Blood 97:744–751
34. Gaidano G, LoCoco F, Ye BH, Shibata D, Levine AM, Knowles DM (1994) Rearrangements of the bcl-6 gene in AIDS-associated non-Hodgkin's lymphoma: association with diffuse large-cell subtype. Blood 84:397–402
35. Gaidano G, Dalla-Favera R (1997) Molecular pathogenesis of AIDS-related non-Hodgkin's lymphoma. Adv Cancer Res 67:113–153
36. Gaidano G, Carbone A, Dalla-Favera R (1998) Genetic basis of acquired immunodeficiency syndrome-related lymphomagenesis. Monogr Natl Cancer Inst 23:95–100
37. Knowles DM (2003) Etiology and pathogenesis of AIDS-related non-Hodgkin's lymphoma. Hematol Oncol Clin N Am 17:785–820
38. Subar M, Neri A, Inghirami G, Knowles DM, Dalla-Favera R (1988) Frequent c-myc oncogene activation and infrequent presence of Epstein-Barr virus genome in AIDS-associated lymphoma. Blood 72:667–671
39. Ambinder RF (2001) Epstein-Barr virus associated lymphoproliferations in the AIDS setting. Eur J Cancer 37:1209–1216
40. Martinez-Maza O, Breen EC (2002) B-cell activation and lymphoma in patients with HIV. Curr Opin Oncol 14:528–532
41. Taub R, Kirsch I, Morton C, Lenoir G, Swan D, Tronick S, Aaronson S, Leder P (1982) Translocation of the c-myc gene into the immunoglobulin heavy chain locus in human Burkitt lymphoma and murine plasmacytoma cells. Proc Natl Acad Sci USA 79:7837–7841
42. Shiramizu B, Barriga F, Neequaye J, Jafri A, Dalla-Favera R, Neri A, Guttierez M, Levine P, Magrath I (1991) Patterns of chromosomal breakpoint locations in Burkitt's lymphoma: relevance to geography and Epstein-Barr virus association. Blood 77:1516–1526
43. Muller JR, Janz S, Goedert JJ, Potter M, Rabkin CS (1995) Persistence of immunoglobulin heavy chain/c-myc recombination-positive lymphocyte clones in the blood of human immunodeficiency virus-infected homosexual men. Proc Natl Acad Sci USA 92: 6577–6581
44. Epeldegui M, Breen EC, Hung YP, Boscardin WJ, Detels R, Martínez-Maza O (2007) Elevated expression of activation induced cytidine deaminase in peripheral blood mononuclear cells precedes AIDS-non-Hodgkin's lymphoma diagnosis. AIDS 21:2265–2270
45. Epeldegui M, Hung YP, McQuay A, Ambinder RF, Martinez-Maza O (2007) Infection of human B cells with Epstein-Barr virus results in the expression of somatic hypermutation-inducing molecules and in the accrual of oncogene mutations. Mol Immunol 44:934–942

46. Lenz G, Staudt LM (2010) Mechanisms of disease. Aggressive lymphomas. New Engl J Med 362:1417–1429
47. Gong JZ, Stenzel TT, Bennett ER, Lagoo AS, Dunphy CH, Moore JO, Rizzieri DA, Tepperberg JH, Papenhausen P, Buckley PJ (2003) Burkitt lymphoma arising in organ transplant recipients: a clinicopathologic study of five cases. Am J Surg Pathol 27:818–827
48. Xicoy B, Ribera JM, Esteve J, Brunet S, Sanz MA, Fernández-Abellán P, Feliu E (2003) Post-transplant Burkitt's leukemia or lymphoma. Study of five cases treated with specific intensive therapy (PETHEMA ALL-3/97 trial). Leuk Lymphoma 44:1541–1543
49. Blum KA, Lozanski G, Byrd JC (2004) Adult Burkitt leukemia and lymphoma. Blood 104:3009–3020
50. Little RF, Pittaluga S, Grant N, Steinberg SM, Kavlick MF, Mitsuya H, Franchini G, Gutierrez M, Raffeld M, Jaffe ES, Shearer G, Yarchoan R, Wilson WH (2003) Highly effective treatment of acquired immunodeficiency syndrome-related lymphoma with dose-adjusted EPOCH: impact of antiretroviral therapy suspension and tumor biology. Blood 101:4653–4659
51. Spina M, Tirelli U, Zagonel V, Gloghini A, Volpe R, Babare R, Abbruzzese L, Talamini R, Vaccher E, Carbone A (1998) Burkitt lymphoma in adults with and without human immunodeficiency virus infection: a single institution clinicopathologic study of 75 patients. Cancer 82:766–774
52. Levine AM, Sullivan-Hailey J, Pike MC, Rarick MU, Loureiro C, Bernstein-Singer M, Wilson E, Brynes R, Parker J, Rasheed S (1991) Human immunodeficiency virus-related lymphoma. Prognostic factors predictive of survival. Cancer 68:2466–2472
53. Chintu C, Athale UH, Patil PS (1995) Childhood cancers in Zambia before and after the HIV epidemic. Arch Dis Child 73:100–105
54. Chitsike I, Siziya S (1998) Seroprevalence of human immunodeficiency virus type I infection in childhood malignancy in Zimbabwe. Cent Afr J Med 44:242–245
55. Lazzi S, Ferrari F, Nyongo A, Palummo N, de Milito A, Zazzi M, Leoncini L, Luzi P, Tosi P (1998) HIV-associated malignant lymphomas in Kenya (Equatorial Africa). Hum Pathol 29:1285–1289
56. Lucas SB, Diomande M, Hounnou A, Beaumel A, Giordano C, Kadio A, Peacock CS, Honde M, De Cock KM (1994) HIV associated-lymphoma in Africa: an autopsy study in Cote d'Ivoire. Int J Cancer 59:20–24
57. Parkin DM, Garcia-Giannoli H, Raphael M, Martin A, Katongole-Mbidde E, Wabinga H, Ziegler J (2000) Non-Hodgkin lymphoma in Uganda: a case–control study. AIDS 14:2929–2936
58. Lubega J (2007) T-helper 1 versus T-helper 2 lymphocyte immunodysregulation is the central factor in the genesis of Burkitt lymphoma: hypothesis. Infect Agent Cancer 2:10. doi:10.1186/1750-9378-2-10, Available from: http://www.infectagentcancer.com
59. Burmeister T, Schwartz S, Horst HA, Rieder H, Gökbuget N, Hoelzer D, Thiel E (2005) Molecular heterogeneity of sporadic adult Burkitt-type leukemia/lymphoma as revealed by PCR and cytogenetics: correlation with morphology, immunology and clinical features. Leukemia 19:1391–1398
60. Yarchoan R, Uldrick TS, Little RF (2011) AIDS-associated lymphomas. In: Cancer: principles and practice of oncology, 9th edn. Lippincott, Williams & Wilkins, Philadelphia, pp 2099–2112
61. Scadden D (2000) Epstein-Barr virus, the CNS, and AIDS-related lymphomas: as close as flame to smoke. J Clin Oncol 18:3323–3324
62. Cingolani A, Gastaldi R, Fassone L, Pierconti F, Giancola ML, Martini M, De Luca A, Ammassari A, Mazzone C, Pescarmona E, Gaidano G, Larocca LM, Antinori A (2000) Epstein-Barr virus infection is predictive of CNS involvement in systemic AIDS-related non-Hodgkin's lymphomas. J Clin Oncol 18:3325–3330
63. Orem J, Maganda A, Katongole-Mbidde E, Weiderpass E (2009) Clinical characteristics and outcome of children with Burkitt's lymphoma in Uganda according to HIV infection. Pediatr Blood Cancer 52:455–458
64. Bateganya MH, Stanaway J, Brentlinger PE, Magaret AS, Wald A, Orem J, Casper C (2011) Predictors of survival after a diagnosis of non-Hodgkin lymphoma in a resource-limited

setting: a retrospective study on the impact of HIV infection and its treatment. J Acquir Immune Defic Syndr 56:312–319
65. Carbone PP, Kaplan HS, Musshoff K, Smithers DW, Tubiana M (1979) Report of the Committee on Hodgkin's disease staging classification. Cancer Res 49:2112–2135
66. Mwanda WO, Orem J, Fu P, Banura C, Kakembo J, Onyango CA, Ness A, Reynolds S, Johnson JL, Subbiah V, Bako J, Wabinga H, Abdallah FK, Meyerson H, Whalen CC, Lederman MM, Black J, Ayers LW, Katongole-Mbidde E, Remick SC (2009) Dose-modified oral combination chemotherapy in the treatment of AIDS-related non-Hodgkin's lymphoma in East Africa. J Clin Oncol 27:3480–3488
67. Krown S (2011) Cancer in resource-limited settings. J Acquir Immune Defic Syndr 56:297–299
68. Burkitt D, Hutt MSR, Wright DH (1965) The African lymphoma. Preliminary observations on response to chemotherapy. Cancer 18:399–410
69. Burkitt D (1967) Long-term remissions following one and two-dose chemotherapy for African lymphoma. Cancer 20:756–759
70. Ziegler JL, Magrath IT, Olweny CL (1979) Cure of Burkitt's lymphoma. Ten-year follow-up of 157 Ugandan patients. Lancet 2:936–938
71. Olweny CLM, Katongole-Mbidde E, Otim D, Lwanga SK, Magrath IT, Ziegler JL (1980) Long term experience with Burkitt's lymphoma in Uganda. Int J Cancer 26:261–266
72. Cairo MS, Sposto R, Perkins SL, Meadows AT, Hoover-Regan ML, Anderson JR, Siegel SE, Lones MA, Tedeschi-Bick N, Kadin ME, Kieldsberg CR, Wilson JF, Sanger W, Morris E, Krailo MD, Finlay JL (2003) Burkitt's and Burkitt-like lymphoma in children and adolescents: a review of the Children's Cancer Group experience. Br J Haematol 120:660–670
73. Bowman WP, Shuster JJ, Cook B, Griffin T, Behm F, Pullen J, Link M, Head D, Carroll A, Berard C, Murphy S (1996) Improved survival for children with B-cell acute lymphoblastic leukemia and stage IV small non-cleaved-cell lymphoma: a Pediatric Oncology Group study. J Clin Oncol 14:1252–1261
74. Magrath I, Adde M, Shad A, Venzon D, Seibel D, Gootenberg J, Neely J, Arndt C, Nieder M, Jaffe E, Wittes RA, Horak ID (1996) Adults and children with small non-cleaved-cell lymphoma have similar excellent outcome when treated with the same chemotherapy regimen. J Clin Oncol 14:925–934
75. Lacasce A, Howard O, Lib S, Fisher D, Weng A, Neuberg D, Shipp M (2004) Modified Magrath regimens for adults with Burkitt and Burkitt-like lymphomas: preserved efficacy with decreased toxicity. Leuk Lymphoma 45:761–767
76. Fayad L, Thomas D, Romaquera J (2007) Update of the M.D. Anderson Cancer Center experience with hyper-CVAD and rituximab for the treatment of mantle cell and Burkitt-type lymphomas. Clin Lymphoma Myeloma 8(Suppl 2):S57–S62
77. Stebbing J, Marvin V, Bower M (2004) The evidence-based treatment of AIDS-related non-Hodgkin's lymphoma. Cancer Treat Rev 30:249–253
78. Lim ST, Levine AM (2005) Recent advances in the acquired immunodeficiency syndrome (AIDS)-related lymphoma. CA Cancer J Clin 55:229–241, 260–261, 264
79. Mounier N, Spina M, Gisselbrecht C (2007) Modern management of non-Hodgkin's lymphoma in HIV-infected patients. Br J Haematol 136:685–698
80. Kaplan LD, Straus DJ, Testa MA, Von Roenn J, Dezube BJ, Cooley TP, Herndier B, Northfelt DW, Huang J, Tulpule A, Levine AM, for the NIAID Clinical Trials Group (1997) New Engl J Med 336:1641–1648
81. Ratner L, Lee J, Tang S, Redden D, Hamzeh F, Herndier B, Scadden D, Kaplan L, Ambinder R, Levine A, Harrington W, Grochow L, Flexner C, Tan B, Straus D, for the AIDS Malignancy Consortium (2001) Chemotherapy for human immunodeficiency virus-associated non-Hodgkin's lymphoma in combination with highly active antiretroviral therapy. J Clin Oncol 19:2171–2178
82. Sparano JA, Lee S, Chen MG, Nazeer T, Einzig A, Ambinder RF, Henry DH, Manalo J, Li T, Von Roenn JH (2004) Phase II trial of infusional cyclophosamide, doxorubicin, and etoposide

in patients with human immunodeficiency virus-associated non-Hodgkin's lymphoma: an Eastern Cooperative Oncology Group trial (E1494). J Clin Oncol 22:1491–1500
83. Kaplan LD, Lee JY, Ambinder RJ, Sparano JA, Cesarman E, Chadburn A, Levine AM, Scadden DT (2005) Rituximab does not improve clinical outcome in a randomized phase III trial of CHOP with or without rituximab in patients with HIV-associated non-Hodgkin's lymphoma. Blood 106:1538–1543
84. Sparano JA, Lee JY, Kaplan LD, Levine AM, Ramos JC, Ambinder RF, Wachsman W, Aboulafia D, Noy A, Henry DH, Von Roenn J, Dezube BJ, Remick SC, Shah MH, Leichman L, Ratner L, Cesarman E, Chadburn A, Mitsuyasu R, for the AIDS Malignancy Consortium (2010) Rituximab plus concurrent infusional EPOCH chemotherapy is highly effective in HIV-associated B-cell non-Hodgkin's lymphoma. Blood 115:3008–3016
85. Galicier L, Fieschi C, Borie R, Meignin V, Daniel MT, Gerard L, Oksenhendler E (2007) Intensive chemotherapy regimen (LMB86) for St. Jude stage IV AIDS-related Burkitt lymphoma/leukemia: a prospective study. Blood 110:2846–2854
86. Noy A, Kaplan L, Lee J, Cesarman E, Tam W (2011) Modified dose intensive R-CODOX-M/IVAC for HIV-associated Burkitt (BL) (AMC 048) shows efficacy and tolerability, and predictive potential of IRF4/MUM1 expression (2011). Presented at the 13th International Conference on Malignancies in AIDS and Other Acquired Immunodeficiencies, 7–8 November 2011, Bethesda, MD, p 38 (abstract nos. 014)
87. Sitas F, Pacella-Norman R, Carrara H, Patel M, Ruff P, Sur R, Jentsch U, Hale M, Rowji P, Saffer D, Connor M, Bull D, Newton R, Beral V (2000) The spectrum of HIV-1 related cancers in South Africa. Int J Cancer 88:489–492
88. Sissolak G, Abayomi EA, Jacobs P (2007) AIDS defining lymphomas in the era of highly active antiretroviral therapy (HAART) – an African perspective. Transfus Apher Sci 37:63–70
89. Sasco AJ, Jaquet A, Boidin E, Ekouevi DK, Thouillot F, LeMabec T, Forstin M-A, Renaudier P, N'Dom P, Malvy D, Dabis F (2010) The challenge of AIDS-related malignancies in sub-Saharan Africa. PLoS One 5(e8621):1–10
90. Sissolak G, Juritz J, Sissolak D, Wood L, Jacobs P (2010) Lymphoma – emerging realities in sub-Saharan Africa. Transfus Apher Sci 42:141–150
91. Hesseling PB, Molyneux E, Tchinsterne F, Welbeck J, McCormick P, Pritchard-Jones K, Wagner H-P (2008) Treating Burkitt's lymphoma in Malawi, Cameroon, and Ghana. Lancet Oncol 9:512–513
92. Hesseling PB, Broadhead R, Molyneux E, Borgstein E, Schneider JW, Louw M, Mansvelt EPG, Wessels G (2003) Malawi pilot study of Burkitt lymphoma treatment. Med Pediatr Oncol 41:532–540
93. Hesseling P, Broadhead R, Mansvelt E, Louw M, Wessels G, Borgstein E, Schneider J, Molyneux E (2005) The 2000 Burkitt lymphoma trial in Malawi. Pediatr Blood Cancer 44:245–250
94. Orem J, Mwanda WO, Remick SC (2006) Challenges and opportunities for treatment and research of AIDS-related malignancies in Africa. Curr Opin Oncol 18:479–486

Chapter 9
Diffuse Large B-Cell Lymphoma

Laura Pasqualucci

Introduction

Diffuse large B-cell lymphoma (DLBCL) represents the most common type of B-cell non-Hodgkin lymphoma (B-NHL) in the adult, comprising 30–40% of all new diagnoses and including cases that arise de novo as well as cases that result from the clinical evolution of more indolent B-NHL types (most commonly, follicular lymphoma and chronic lymphocytic leukemia) [1, 2]. While remarkable advances have been made over the past decade in our ability to diagnose and treat this disease, DLBCL remains an important clinical problem, with at least one-third of patients not being cured by currently available therapeutic approaches, including combination immuno-chemotherapy [3]. Such incomplete success is explained in part by the heterogeneity of these tumors, which can be appreciated from a morphologic, phenotypic, genetic, and clinical standpoint. Indeed, gene expression profile studies along with more recent genomic analyses have revealed the existence of several molecularly distinct DLBCL subtypes that reflect either the origin from B cells at various stages of differentiation or the coordinated expression of comprehensive transcriptional signatures. The identified subgroups not only differ in the expression of specific gene signatures, but also seem to rely on separate oncogenic mechanisms. Moreover, distinct phenotypic subtypes have been associated with different overall survival rates. Collectively, these observations provided a molecular framework for the development of rationally targeted therapeutic approaches. This chapter will focus on the molecular pathogenesis of the most common subtypes of DLBCL, with emphasis on the mechanisms of genetic lesion and on the nature of the involved genes/pathways in relationship with the normal biology of lymphocytes.

L. Pasqualucci (✉)
Institute for Cancer Genetics, Herbert Irving Comprehensive Cancer Center, Columbia University, 1130 St. Nicholas Avenue, New York 10032, NY, USA

Department of Pathology and Cell Biology, Columbia University, New York 10032, NY, USA
e-mail: lp171@columbia.edu

E.S. Robertson (ed.), *Burkitt's Lymphoma*, Current Cancer Research,
DOI 10.1007/978-1-4614-4313-1_9, © Springer Science+Business Media New York 2013

The Cell of Origin of DLBCL

Analogous to most other B-NHLs, DLBCL derives from the malignant transformation of mature B cells that have experienced the germinal center (GC) reaction and have undergone unique DNA modification events in order to produce highly efficient neutralizing antibodies. Thus, a fundamental concept for the understanding of the pathogenesis of DLBCL is the relationship between these tumors and the GC.

The Germinal Center and Its Master Regulator BCL6

The germinal center (GC) is a highly specialized microenvironment that forms in secondary lymphoid organs following the encounter of a naïve B-cell with a foreign antigen, in the context of signals provided by CD4+ T cells and antigen-presenting cells [4–6].

This structure, which represents the hallmark of T-cell-dependent immune responses, can be schematically divided into two anatomically well-recognizable areas, known as the dark zone and the light zone. In the dark zone, rapidly proliferating centroblasts (CBs) characterized by a doubling time of less than 12 h modify the variable region of their immunoglobulin genes (IgV) by the process of somatic hypermutation (SHM), which introduces not only mostly single nucleotide substitutions but also deletions and duplications in order to change the affinity of the antibody for the antigen [5–9]. CBs express elevated levels of BCL6 [7, 8], a potent transcriptional repressor [9] that modulates the expression of a broad set of genes involved in multiple biological functions, including signaling through the B-cell receptor (BCR) and CD40 receptor [10, 11], the control of apoptosis (via BCL2) [10, 12]; the response to DNA damage (by modulation of genes involved in both the sensing and execution of p53-dependent and -independent DNA damage responses) [13–16]; multiple cytokine and chemokine signaling pathways, such as those involved in interferon and TGFβ responses [10, 12]; and plasma cell differentiation, via suppression of the master regulator PRDM1 (also known as BLIMP1) (Fig. 9.1) [17–20]. Through these multiple functions, BCL6 plays a critical role in establishing the proliferative status of CBs while allowing the execution of DNA modification processes such as SHM and class-switch recombination, without eliciting DNA damage responses; additionally, BCL6 prevents the premature activation and differentiation of B cells prior to the selection for the survival of clones producing high affinity antibodies.

CBs then move to the light zone, where they are thought to cease proliferation and differentiate into centrocytes (CCs), which are re-challenged by the antigen through the interaction with CD4+ T-cells and follicular dendritic cells [4, 6]. Here, CCs expressing a BCR with reduced affinity for the antigen will be eliminated by apoptosis, while few cells with high affinity for the antigen will be stimulated by a variety of signals, including (but not limited to) the engagement of their BCR by the antigen itself, and the activation of the CD40 receptor by the CD40 ligand present

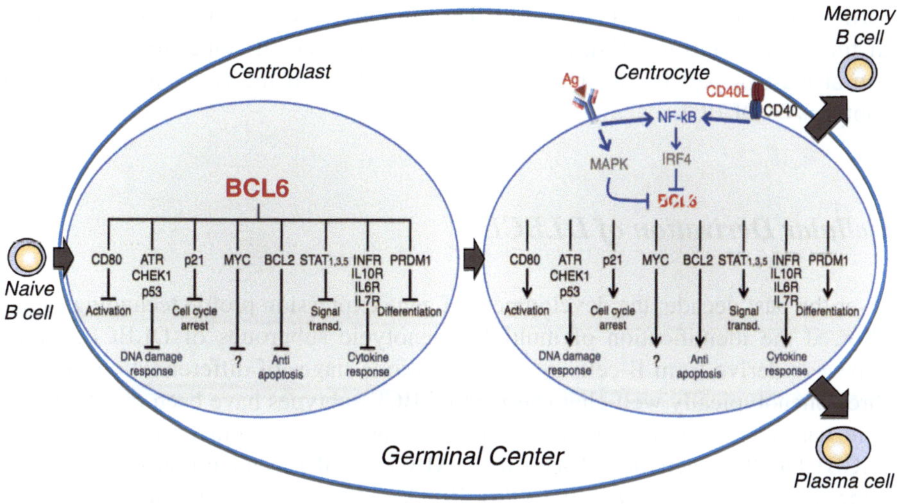

Fig. 9.1 *The germinal center reaction and its master regulator BCL6.* The figure shows a schematic representation of the germinal center reaction. Germinal centers form following antigenic stimulation of a naïve B-cell in the context of T-cell dependent responses, and can be schematically divided into a *dark zone* populated by proliferating centroblasts, and a *light zone* composed of smaller centrocytes. These two stages of B-cell differentiation are characterized by distinct biological programs that are largely governed by BCL6 (only representative targets shown). In proliferating centroblasts, BCL6 prevents premature response to signals that may cause exit from the GC before these cells have completed the remodeling of their Ig genes in order to produce high-affinity antibodies. BCL6 expression is subsequently downregulated in the light zone by a number of signals, including BCR cross-linking and engagement of CD40 by CD40L, thus restoring cellular programs that are required to proceed through terminal B-cell differentiation

on CD4+ T-cells (Fig. 9.1). These signaling cascades result in the downregulation of BCL6 expression, thereby allowing the restoration of DNA damage responses, as well as activation and differentiation capabilities, such that B cells can be selected for survival and differentiation into memory cells and plasma cells [4, 21]. In the GC, CCs also undergo class-switch recombination (CSR), a DNA remodeling event that confers distinct effector functions to the antibodies [22]. Both SHM and CSR represent B-cell-specific functions that modify the genome of these cells via mechanisms involving single- or double-strand breaks and depend on the activity of activation-induced cytidine deaminase (AID) [23–25], a DNA editing enzyme with important roles in the generation of genetic alterations associated with mature B-NHL.

This schematic description, which only partially reflects the complex dynamics of the GC reaction, is nonetheless useful to focus on two concepts that are key to the understanding of DLBCL pathogenesis, and B-NHL in general. First, the most frequent oncogenic events in DLBCL—namely chromosomal translocations and aberrant somatic hypermutation (ASHM)—result from mistakes in the AID-dependent machinery that normally diversifies the Ig genes during B lymphocytes differentiation, further supporting the GC origin of these tumors. Second, the definition of two distinct phases during GC development reflects stages of B-cell differentiation that can at least in part be recognized in the phenotype of the two major molecular subtypes of DLBCL.

Cellular Derivation of DLBCL

Over the past decade, the development of gene expression profile technologies has allowed the identification of multiple phenotypic subgroups of DLBCL, which appear to derive from B cells arrested at various stages of differentiation. At least three phenotypically well-characterized DLBCL subtypes have been recognized to date, based on similarities to their putative cell of origin: germinal center B-cell-like (GCB) DLBCL, activated B-cell-like (ABC) DLBCL, and primary mediastinal large B-cell lymphoma (PMBCL) [26–29]. An additional 15–30% of cases present signatures that are intermediate between the above categories and are thus termed unclassified [27].

GCB-DLBCLs are postulated to derive from a proliferating CB, as their expression profile is enriched in genes that are specific for GC B cells, e.g., BCL6 and CD10 [26], while lacking post-GC differentiation markers (Fig. 9.2). These tumors carry highly mutated Ig genes showing evidence of ongoing SHM [30], and express surface IgG in most cases, as an evidence of successful CSR [26].

The ABC-DLBCL subgroup displays a transcriptional signature that shares significant similarities to the one induced in BCR-activated peripheral blood B cells and in a small subset of plasmablastic B cells located in the GC light zone, and presumably poised to exit the GC [26] (Fig. 9.2). These cells have downregulated the GC-specific program and express genes (e.g., IRF4) that are necessary for terminal B-cell differentiation; however, they are precluded from exiting the GC due to genetic lesions that disrupt this pathway, namely PRDM1 loss or BCL6 translocations (see next section) [31–34]. ABC-DLBCLs are also characterized by constitutive activation of the NF-κB, BCR, and JAK/STAT signaling pathways [35]. Consistent with their derivation from a post-GC cell where the SHM machinery has been turned off, ABC-DLBCLs do not show ongoing SHM [36]. Interestingly, these tumors only rarely show evidence of legitimate CSR, a finding attributed to abnormalities in the regulation of this process [30, 37].

The third subtype of DLBCL, PMBCL, is postulated to arise from thymic medullary B cells [28, 29] and has been recently recognized as a separate clinicopathological entity in both the REAL and World Health Organization classifications [2] (Fig. 9.2). This disease, which typically involves the mediastinum and is most commonly observed in young female adults, shares significant histological, molecular, and clinical features with nodular sclerosis Hodgkin lymphoma (HL) [38], including the presence of an immune/inflammatory cell infiltrate with a distinctive cytokine profile, the decreased expression of BCR signaling pathway components, and the constitutive NF-κB activation [28, 29, 38].

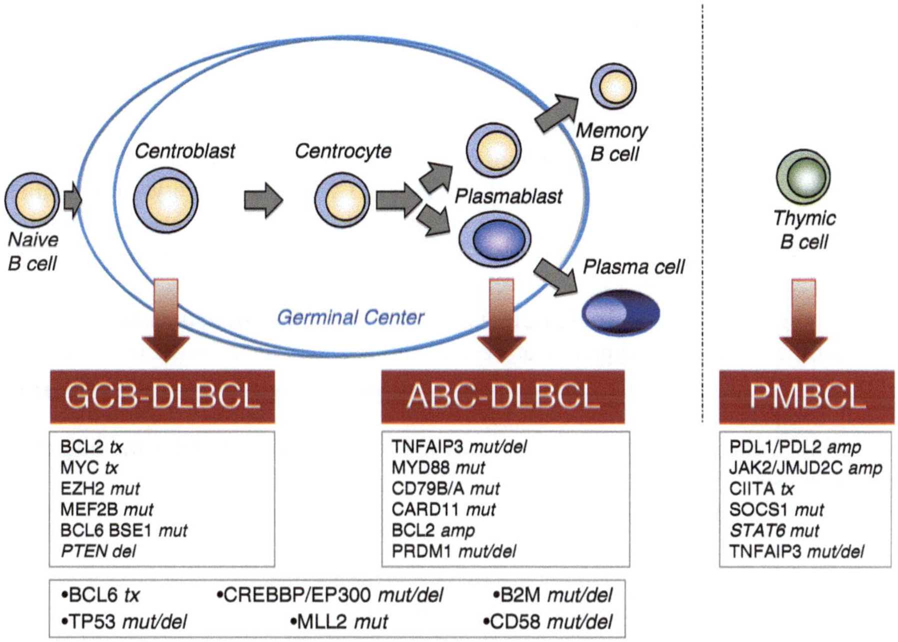

Fig. 9.2 *Postulated cellular origin of major DLBCL subtypes*. Schematic cartoon of the germinal center reaction, and its relationship with major DLBCL subtypes. GCB-DLBCLs express phenotypic similarities with proliferating centroblasts, while ABC-DLBCLs are related to a plasmablastic B cell. PMBCL is postulated to arise from a post-GC B cells in the thymic medulla. The most common genetic lesions that are associated with specific molecular subtypes (or shared by multiple subtypes) are indicated below. Abbreviations: Tx, translocation; BSE1, binding site in exon 1

Of note, several studies have shown that stratification according to gene expression profiles has prognostic value, and patients diagnosed with GCB-DLBCL display a better overall survival compared to ABC-DLBCL [39]. This prognostic advantage was also observed after the integration of the drug rituximab into standard combination therapies for DLBCL, although controversial findings have been reported in different studies [36, 40]. The distinction in GCB- and ABC-DLBCL has therefore not been officially incorporated into the WHO classification of lymphoid malignancies, mostly because it requires the use of sophisticated tools that are not routinely available in every diagnostic lab, and because it is imperfectly replicated by immunophenotyping or morphology [41, 42].

While the similarity to different stages of B-cell differentiation represents an important aspect in the phenotypic characterization of DLBCL, gene expression profile analyses also allowed the identification of three discrete subsets that reflect the coordinated expression of comprehensive consensus signatures defined by genes involved in oxidative phosphorylation, B-cell receptor/proliferation, and tumor microenvironment/host inflammatory response [43].

Classification of DLBCL

In addition to the "DLBCL, not otherwise specified" discussed here, updated 2008 WHO Classification of Tumours of Haematopoietic and Lymphoid tissues recognizes as separate categories a number of DLBCL subtypes and other "lymphomas of large B cells", as well as "borderline cases". The latter category, once termed "grey zone lymphomas" include those cases with overlapping morphologic and immunophenotypic features between DLBCL and classical Hodgkin lymphoma and between BL and DLBCL with MYC translocations or "double-hit" MYC and BCL2 translocations [2]. These rare tumors may resemble BL in their gene expression profile but exhibit atypical features, including a very aggressive clinical course that requires intensive chemotherapeutic regimens [44, 45]. Since this category likely comprises a biologically heterogeneous group of diseases, additional genetic and clinical characterization will be necessary for an improved understanding of its pathogenesis.

Mechanisms of Genetic Lesion in DLBCL

Common mechanisms of genetic lesion in DLBCL include chromosomal translocations leading to deregulated expression of proto-oncogenes, aberrant somatic hypermutation (ASHM), point mutations, and a variety of copy number aberrations [35, 46]. Of these, chromosomal translocations and ASHM are generated as by-products of the DNA remodeling reactions that are required for the assembly of functional BCR genes during B-cell development.

Chromosomal Translocations

DLBCL-associated chromosomal translocations represent reciprocal and balanced recombination events that occur between two specific chromosomes, most commonly without involving the coding regions of the affected genes, and are clonally represented in each tumor case. Although the precise molecular mechanisms that are responsible for the generation of translocations remain partially obscure, significant advances have been recently obtained in our understanding of the events that are required for their initiation. It is now well documented that chromosomal translocations in B cells occur at least in part as a consequence of mistakes during Ig gene rearrangements, including RAG-mediated V(D)J recombination (as it is in the case of BCL2 translocations and BCL1 translocations) and AID-mediated isotype class switching and somatic hypermutation (e.g., BCL6 translocations and MYC translocations) [47, 48]. In particular, in vivo studies using lymphoma-prone mouse models have conclusively demonstrated that the removal of the AID enzyme is sufficient to abrogate the generation of *MYC-IGH* translocations in normal B cells undergoing CSR [49–51], and to prevent the development of GC-derived lymphomas [52, 53].

The common denominator of all NHL-associated chromosomal translocations is the presence of a proto-oncogene in proximity to the chromosomal recombination sites. In contrast with acute leukemias, however, most chromosomal translocations in DLBCL do not affect the coding domain of the oncogene; instead, they cause alterations in its normal pattern of expression as a consequence of the juxtaposition of heterologous regulatory sequences derived from the partner chromosome. This process of proto-oncogene deregulation is referred to as *homotopic* when the involved proto-oncogene is tightly regulated in normal lymphoid cells and becomes constitutively expressed in the lymphoma cell, as it is the case for *BCL6* translocations. Conversely, the term *heterotopic* deregulation is used when the proto-oncogene is not expressed in the normal tumor counterpart and undergoes ectopic expression in the lymphoma. Paradigms of heterotopic deregulation in DLBCL are represented by translocations of the *MYC* and *BCL2* genes, both of which are not expressed in normal GC cells [10, 12, 21]. In most DLBCL-associated translocations, the heterologous regulatory sequences that are juxtaposed to the involved proto-oncogene and are responsible for its deregulation derive from antigen receptor loci that are expressed at high levels in GC/post-GC cells [47]. More promiscuous are the chromosomal translocations involving BCL6, which can be found juxtaposed to different promoter regions derived from over 30 distinct chromosomal sites in individual tumor cases [54–61].

Aberrant Somatic Hypermutation

The term aberrant somatic hypermutation (ASHM) defines a mechanism of genetic lesion that is predominantly associated with DLBCL (and, at lower frequencies, to a few other B-NHLs) and is due to the abnormal functioning of the physiologic SHM process that normally operates in the GC. In normal centroblasts, SHM is tightly regulated both spatially and temporally to introduce mutations only in the rearranged *IgV* genes [62] and in the 5′ region of a few other genes, including *BCL6, CD95* and the *CD79* components of the B-cell receptor [63–67] (although the functional role of the mutations found in these non-Ig loci remains unknown). Such restricted mutational activity in normal GC B cells, despite the ability of AID to bind multiple DNA sequences [63, 64] relies on high-accuracy repair mechanisms [65]. On the contrary, over half of DLBCL patients harbor multiple mutational events in numerous genes that are actively transcribed in B cells, including well-known proto-oncogenes such as *PIM1* and *MYC* [66]. Depending on the genomic configuration of the target gene, the mutations may affect untranslated as well as coding regions, potentially leading to alterations in gene expression or in key protein structural and functional properties [66]. This is the case of *MYC,* where a significant number of events lead to amino acid changes that have been experimentally shown to activate its oncogenic properties. Nonetheless, a comprehensive characterization of the potentially extensive genetic damage caused by ASHM is still lacking.

Oncogenic Mutations and Gene Amplifications

In addition to chromosomal translocations and ASHM, the structure of proto-oncogenes and/or their pattern of expression can be altered by gene copy number changes and somatic point mutations. To date, only a few genes have been identified as specific targets of chromosomal amplification in DLBCL, as exemplified by *BCL2, MYC, REL* [39, 67–69], and the genes encoding for the *PD-1* and *PD-2* ligands in PMBCL [70, 71]. However, the introduction of high resolution, genome-wide array-CGH and single nucleotide polymorphims (SNP) array technologies has revealed a more complex scenario, leading to the identification of additional chromosomal sites of amplification which may harbor important new oncogenic loci.

Somatic point mutations may alter the coding sequence of the target proto-oncogene and thus the biological properties of its protein product, as observed in *MYC* and *BCL2* [21, 72–74]. More recently, a number of genes involved in the activation of the NF-κB transcription complex have been found to harbor oncogenic point mutations which lead to constitutive activation of this signaling pathway in ABC-DLBCL [35, 75, 76]. Mutations of the *RAS* genes, a very frequent alteration in human neoplasia, are virtually absent in lymphomas [77].

Loss of Tumor Suppressor Genes

In addition to the *TP53* gene, possibly the most common target of genetic lesions in human cancer [78], several genes have been recently identified as targets of biallelic or monoallelic loss in DLBCL. Analogous to other tumors, the mechanisms responsible for inactivation of tumor suppressor genes in DLBCL entail point mutation of one allele with genetic deletion or mutation of the second allele. Two such genes lie on the long arm of chromosome 6, a region long known to be deleted in a large percentage of aggressive lymphomas, and generally associated with poor prognosis [79, 80]: the *PRDM1/BLIMP1* gene on chromosomal region 6q21, which is biallelically inactivated in ~25% of ABC-DLBCL cases [31, 32, 34], and the *TNFAIP3* gene on chromosome 6q23, which encodes for the negative NF-κB regulator A20 and is commonly lost in both ABC-DLBCL and PMBCL (besides a few other lymphoma types) [75, 81–83]. More recently, monoallelic inactivating mutations and deletions of the acetyltransferase genes *CREBBP* and *EP300* have been reported in a significant proportion of DLBCL and FL, suggesting a role as haploinsufficient tumor suppressors [84]. Furthermore, one or both alleles of the *MLL2* gene, encoding for a histone trimethyltransferase, are targeted by disruptive mutations in over 30% of DLBCL [84, 85]. Other tumor suppressor genes that are homozygously deleted in a discrete fraction of DLBCL include *CDKN2A* and *CDKN2B* [86] and the immune regulatory genes *B2M* and *CD58* [85], while loss of *PTEN* is observed in rare cases [86].

Molecular Pathogenesis of DLBCL

Recent genome-wide efforts have led to a better definition of the multitude of genes and pathways that are disrupted by genetic lesions in DLBCL. Consistent with the phenotypic heterogeneity of this neoplasm, the catalogue of structural alterations that have been identified to date is remarkably diverse, including alterations that are common to all DLBCL subgroups, as well as lesions that are preferentially or exclusively associated with individual DLBCL categories (Fig. 9.2). These observations revealed the involvement of distinct oncogenic pathways that in turn may influence treatment outcome. The following section will focus on well-characterized genetic lesions as related to the three main subtypes of DLBCL, defined by cell of origin.

Alterations Common to Various DLBCL Subtypes

Chromosomal Translocations of *BCL6*

Up to 35% of all DLBCL cases harbor chromosomal translocations involving the *BCL6* proto-oncogene on band 3q27 [80, 87, 88], with a twofold higher frequency in the ABC-DLBCL subtype [89] (Table 9.1). These rearrangements juxtapose the intact coding domain of *BCL6* downstream and in the same transcriptional orientation to heterologous sequences derived from the partner chromosome, including the *IG* heavy and light chain loci, and at least 20 other chromosomal sites [54–61]. The majority of these translocations result in a fusion transcript in which the promoter region and the first non-coding exon of *BCL6* are replaced by sequences derived from the partner gene [55, 90]. Since the common denominator of these alternative promoters is a broader spectrum of activity throughout B-cell development, including expression in the post-GC differentiation stage, the translocation is thought to prevent the downregulation of BCL6 expression that is normally associated with differentiation into post-GC cells (e.g., by abrogating IRF 4 binding sites in its promoter) [33]. Deregulated expression of a normal *BCL6* gene product may play a critical role in tumorigenesis by enforcing the proliferative phenotype typical of GC cells, while attenuating DNA damage-induced responses and blocking terminal B-cell differentiation, as confirmed by a mouse model in which deregulated BCL6 expression causes DLBCL [91].

Inactivation of Acetyltransferase Genes

Recent studies have revealed the presence of mutations and/or deletions inactivating the acetyltransferase genes *CREBBP* and, less frequently, *EP300* in nearly 40% of all DLBCL cases, with some preference for the GCB-DLBCL subtype [92]. *CREBBP* and *EP300* encode for ubiquitously expressed transcriptional activators

Table 9.1 Most common genetic lesions in DLBCL

Genetic lesion	Frequency	Functional consequences	Gene function/mechanism of transformation
Shared lesions			
MLL2 mutations	32%	Loss of function	H3K4 methyltransferase/epigenetic reprogramming
CREBBP/EP300 mutations/ deletions	22–40%	Loss of function	Epigenetic reprogramming; impaired p53 activation and BCL6 inactivation
BCL6 translocations	25–40%	Transcriptional deregulation	Enhanced proliferation; impaired DNA damage responses, block in differentiation
B2M mutations/ deletions	29%	Loss of function	Reduced tumor cell immunogenicity; downregulation of HLA class I
CD58 mutations/ deletions	21%	Loss of function	Reduced tumor cell immunogenicity
GCB-DLBCL			
BCL2 translocations	30–40%	Transcriptional deregulation	Enhanced resistance to apoptosis
MYC translocations	10%	Transcriptional deregulation	Enhanced proliferation and growth, DNA replication
EZH2 mutations	22%	Gain of function	H3K27 methyltransferase/epigenetic reprogramming
BCL6 mutations in BSE1	20%	Loss of BCL6 autoregulation	Enhanced proliferation; impaired DNA damage responses, block in differentiation
MEF2B mutations	8%	Unclear	
ABC-DLBCL			
BCL2 amplification	30%	Increased gene dosage	Enhanced resistance to apoptosis
PRDM1 mutations/ deletions	25%	Loss of function	Block in terminal B-cell differentiation
MYD88 mutations	29%	Gain of function	Constitutive activation of NF-κB and JAK-STAT signaling
TNFAIP3 mutations/ deletions	20%	Loss of function	Constitutive activation of NF-κB signaling due to loss of negative regulation
CD79B/CD79A mutations	20%	Gain of function	Constitutive activation of NF-κB and BCR signaling
CARD11 mutations	9%	Gain of function	Constitutive activation of NF-κB signaling
PMBCL			
REL amplification	75%	Increased gene dosage	Constitutive activation of NF-κB signaling
JAK2 amplification	63%	Increased gene dosage	Activation of JAK-STAT pathway
JMJD2C amplification	63%	Increased gene dosage	Histone modification/Epigenetic reprogramming
PDL1, PDL2 amplification	63%	Increased gene dosage	T-cell exhaustion; Reduced tumor cell immunogenicity
SOCS1 mutations/ deletions	45%		Enhanced JAK2 signaling due to impaired JAK2 degradation
STAT6 mutations	36%	Unclear	Activation of JAK-STAT pathway?
CIITA translocations	38%	Overexpression of fusion protein	Reduced tumor cell immunogenicity; downregulation of HLA class II

GCB germinal center B-cell-like, *ABC* activated B-cell-like, *PMBCL* primary mediastinal B-cell lymphoma, *BSE1* BCL6 binding sites in exon 1

that modify lysine residues on numerous histone and non-histone proteins, and are thus involved in multiple signaling and developmental pathways. In most DLBCLs, these lesions are heterozygous and are associated with the expression of the residual normal allele, thus suggesting a role as haploinsufficient tumor suppressor genes. Indeed, a dose-dependent effect of CREBBP expression has been documented by the observation that a rare genetic disease known as Rubinstein-Taybi syndrome is due to CREBBP and, more rarely, EP300 haploinsufficiency. While the functional consequences of these alterations are likely to be broad, *CREBBP* mutations were shown to impair the ability of this enzyme to acetylate the known substrates BCL6 [93] and p53 [94, 95], leading to constitutive activation of the oncoprotein and to decreased p53 tumor suppressor function [92]. Since the balance between the activities of these two genes is critical for the regulation of DNA damage responses during *Ig* gene remodeling processes in the GC [13, 14], one consequence of BCL6 activity overriding p53 would be an increased tolerance for DNA damage in the context of impaired apoptotic and cell cycle arrest responses. Given the broad involvement of histone acetyltransferases in gene transcriptional regulation, additional studies will be required to dissect the entire set of cellular targets/pathways that are critically affected by acetyltransferases reduction in lymphoma. Importantly, the identification of mutations in *CREBBP* and *EP300* may have direct therapeutic implications in view of current attempts to use histone deacetylase inhibitors as anticancer drugs.

Inactivating Mutations of *MLL2*

The most commonly mutated gene that emerged from recent unbiased genome sequencing efforts in DLBCL is the mixed-lineage leukemia 2 (*MLL2)* gene [84, 85]. *MLL2* encodes for a histone H3K4 methyltransferase involved in the control of gene transcription via PolII-dependent activation of target genes. In approximately 32% of DLBCL cases (as well as in almost 89% of FL cases), either one or both *MLL2* alleles are targeted by somatic mutations, introducing stop codons, out-of-frame insertions/deletions, and alterations at consensus splice sites [84, 85]. These variants are predicted to generate truncated proteins that lack the entire C-terminal cluster of conserved domains (including the SET domain) or significant portions of it, thus abrogating its enzymatic activity. Missense mutations, the significance of which is still unknown, have also been reported in a smaller proportion of cases. While the precise mechanism of transformation imposed by *MLL2* mutations has not been investigated yet, the multitude of genes that are normally influenced by its methyltransferase activity suggest a multifaceted role for MLL2 inactivation in DLBCL.

Loss of Immunomodulatory Genes

A set of lesions recurrently observed in DLBCL involve immune recognition and antigen-presenting functions. Inactivating mutations and focal deletions of the *B2M* locus, mostly biallelic, occur in ~29% of cases [85]. These lesions abrogate the expression of β2-microglobulin, a polypeptide found in association with the major histocompatibility complex (MHC) class I on the surface of nearly all nucleated cells, and required for the proper recognition by cytotoxic T lymphocytes (CTL) [96]. In an additional 45% of cases, the B2M protein is either not expressed or aberrantly localized, suggesting the involvement of alternative genetic or epigenetic mechanisms of inactivation [97]. Since the assembly of the class I human leukocyte antigen complex (HLA-I) plays an essential role in antitumor immunosurveillance, these lesions are thought to facilitate lymphomagenesis by allowing the escape of the cancer cell from immune recognition by CTLs. Homozygous deletions and truncating mutations are also commonly detected in the *CD58* gene [85], a member of the immunoglobulin superfamily that functions as the ligand of the CD2 receptor, present on T cells and most natural killer (NK) cells, and participates in their adhesion and activation [98]. Notably, loss of B2M/HLA-I and CD58 expression is often concurrent in the same DLBCL cases [97], suggesting that these two lesions have been selected for their ability to interfere with the interaction between tumor cells and the microenvironment, thus allowing the combined escape from CTL- and NK-mediated immunosurveillance mechanisms.

ASHM

Over half of all DLBCL patients present evidence for an aberrant activity of the SHM mechanism, irrespective of their subgroup classification [66]. The number and identity of the genes that accumulate mutations in their coding and non-coding regions due to this mechanism varies in different cases and is still largely undefined. However, preferential targeting of individual genes has been observed in the two main DLBCL subtypes, with mutations of *MYC* and *BCL2* being found almost exclusively in GCB-DLBCL, and mutations of *PIM1* showing significantly higher frequencies in ABC-DLBCL. ASHM may therefore contribute to the heterogeneity of DLBCL via the alteration of different cellular pathways in different cases.

GCB-DLBCL ASSOCIATED LESIONS

Chromosomal Translocations of *BCL2*

The t(14;18) translocation, resulting in the deregulated expression of the antiapoptotic BCL2 oncoprotein, is almost exclusively found in GCB-DLBCL (~30–40% of cases) (Table 9.1). BCL2 is a known target of BCL6, which binds to its promoter sequences via the transcriptional coactivator Miz1 and prevents its expression in GC B cells [10, 12, 21], presumably to facilitate apoptosis. This mechanism is disrupted in tumors carrying the t(14;18) translocation, which removes the BCL6-binding sequences in the BCL2 promoter while bringing the *BCL2* coding sequences under the control of potent regulatory elements from the Ig locus. BCL2 expression is also detected in a large fraction of DLBCL cases lacking *BCL2* translocations, as the results of several mechanisms including deregulation of Miz1, ASHM of the *BCL2* promoter sequences, and mutations in the *BCL2* coding sequence [21]. Increased levels of BCL2 provide a survival advantage to the tumor cells and have been associated with an inferior outcome in DLBCL [99].

Chromosomal Translocations of *MYC*

In 10–14% of GCB-DLBCL cases, chromosomal translocations of *MYC* cause its ectopic expression by joining its coding exons to the Ig heavy or light chains loci, and by allowing the escape from BCL6 mediated transcriptional repression [21, 39, 100–102]. Notably, the presence of MYC translocations has been linked with worse prognosis, possibly due to the potent activity of this known proto-onocogene in promoting cell proliferation and DNA replication [103].

Mutations of the *EZH2* Gene

Heterozygous mutations of the polycomb-group oncogene *EZH2* have been reported in 21.7% of GCB-DLBCL [104]. *EZH2* encodes for a histone methyltransferase that is responsible for trimethylating Lys27 of histone H3 (H3K27me3). *EZH2* mutations replace a single evolutionary conserved residue (Tyr641) within the protein SET domain, and have been shown to alter the catalytic specificity of the mutant EZH2 enzyme for its substrates, leading to increased levels of H3K27me3 [105, 106]. However, the precise role of these mutations in malignant transformation has not been elucidated yet.

Mutations in the BCL6 Autoregulatory Motifs

Consistent with their derivation from a GC B-cell, up to 75% of all DLBCLs harbor mutations in the BCL6 5′ sequences [63, 107, 108], which reflect the physiologic activity of the SHM mechanism operating in GC B-cells [63, 64, 67]. However, a distinctive set of mutations have been observed only in GCB-DLBCL, suggesting a specific role in the pathogenesis of these tumors [89, 109, 110]. These mutations affect two BCL6 binding sites within the first non-coding exon of the gene and disrupt an autoregulatory circuit through which the BCL6 protein controls its own expression levels, leading to its transcriptional deregulation [109, 110]. In a smaller fraction of cases, mutations interfere with IRF4 mediated downregulation of BCL6, suggesting that the overall fraction of cases carrying BCL6 abnormalities may be even higher. Further efforts will be necessary to characterize the full extent of mutations deregulating BCL6 expression in DLBCL.

Other Lesions

Mutations and deletions of the *TP53* tumor suppressor gene are predominantly restricted to DLBCL cases derived from the transformation of FL and chronic lymphocytic leukemia [111–113], and are therefore commonly associated with chromosomal translocations of *BCL2* and with a GCB-DLBCL phenotype [113]. In approximately 9% of DLBCLs, missense mutations target the Myocyte Enhancer Factor 2B (*MEF2B*) gene [84, 85], which encodes for a member of the MADS/MEF2 family of DNA binding proteins and is thought to cooperate with histone modifying enzymes to regulate gene expression [107]. Inhibition of the tumor suppressor *PTEN* via mutually exclusive deletions of chromosome 10q and amplifications of the miR-17-92 micro-RNA cluster have been also preferentially reported in GCB-DLBCL [35, 86], where they favor the activation of the phosphatidylinositol 3 kinase (PI3K)/AKT pathway.

ABC-DLBCL ASSOCIATED LESIONS

Alterations in NF-κB Pathway Components

A prominent feature of ABC-DLBCL, also shared by PMBCL and Hodgkin Lymphoma, is the presence of constitutive activation of the NF-κB transcription complex, which can be appreciated in most, if not all cases [108]. A genetic explanation to this phenotypic trait has been provided by the recent discovery of structural alterations affecting multiple positive or negative regulators of this signaling pathway. Up to 30% of ABC-DLBCLs harbor biallelic mutations and/or focal deletions that inactivate the *TNFAIP3* gene, encoding for the negative regulator A20 [75, 81]. A tumor suppressor role for A20 in ABC-DLBCL is supported by the observation that reconstitution of A20-null cell lines with wild-type A20 proteins induces apoptosis and blocks proliferation, in part due to suppression of NF-κB activity [75, 81]. Loss of A20 may thus contribute to DLBCL development by preventing the termination of NF-κB responses. In an additional ~10% of cases, the *CARD11* gene is targeted by oncogenic mutations that cluster in the coiled-coil domain, enhancing the ability of this adaptor molecule to transactivate NF-κB target genes [75, 76]. Less commonly, mutations were found in a variety of other genes encoding for NF-κB components, overall accounting for over half of all ABC-DLBCL cases [75] and suggesting that yet unidentified lesions may be responsible for the NF-κB activity observed in the remaining fraction of cases.

Alterations in BCR Signaling

In addition to constitutive NF-κB activity, ABC-DLBCLs display evidence of chronic active BCR signaling. Activation of this pathway is required for the survival

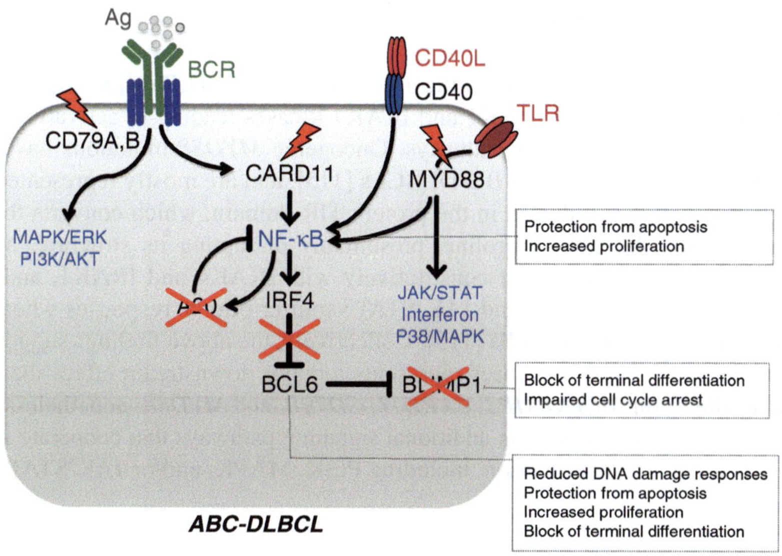

Fig. 9.3 *Disrupted signaling pathways in ABC-DLBCL.* In normal B cells, a variety of signals, including engagement of the BCR by the antigen, interaction of the CD40 receptor with the CD40L presented by T-cells, and stimulation of Toll-like receptors activate the NF-κB transcription complex, leading to the upregulation of numerous target genes (shown are IRF4 and A20). IRF4 downregulates the expression of BCL6, terminating the germinal center programme and allowing the release of PRDM1/BLIMP1, another master regulator required for plasma cell differentiation. The A20 negative regulator terminates NF-κB responses via a negative feedback loop. In ABC-DLBCL, multiple genetic lesions converge on this pathway and disrupt it at multiple levels in different cases. These observations suggest a model in which structural alterations in various NF-κB pathway components promote lymphomagenesis by favoring the anti-apoptotic and pro-proliferative functions of NF-κB while blocking terminal B-cell differentiation through mutually exclusive alterations deregulating BCL6 or inactivating BLIMP1

of ABC-DLBCL cells, possibly because of its ability to induce of NF-κB (via the CBM complex) and PI3K [114]. Indeed, more than 20% of ABC DLBCL biopsy samples have selected gain-of-function somatic mutations affecting the immunoreceptor tyrosine-based activation motif (ITAM) signaling modules of *CD79B* and *CD79A* [114]. These mutations appear to promote chronic BCR signaling by attenuating the phosphorylation and activation of the Lyn kinase, which is necessary for internalization of the surface BCR and serves as a negative feedback regulator of this cascade. As a consequence, ABC-DLBCL cases with *CD79B* mutations display greater abundance of BCR on their surface [114]. Interestingly, *CD79A* and *B* mutations and *CARD11* mutations tend to be mutually exclusive, indicating that they may represent alternative mechanisms converging on the same pathway (Fig. 9.3).

Mutations of the *MYD88* Gene

MyD88 is an adaptor molecule in the Toll-like receptor (TLR) signaling pathway, which associates with the IRAK1 and IRAK4 kinases leading to activation of the NF-κB and type I interferon pathways. Oncogenic *MYD88* mutations have been reported in up to 20–39% of ABC-DLBCLs [115], and are mostly represented by a single amino acid substitution in the protein TIR domain, which converts the leucine at position 265 into a proline, presumably disrupting its structure. Mutant L265P MyD88 alleles interact constitutively with IRAK4 and IRAK1, and were able to activate both NF-κB and JAK/STAT3 transcriptional responses when reintroduced into heterologous cells [115]. Collectively, the above findings suggest that deregulation of NF-κB responses represents a major downstream effect shared by genomic alterations of *TNFAIP3*, *CARD11*, *CD79B*, and *MYD88*; nonetheless, individual lesions may impinge on additional signaling pathways that cooperate in promoting malignant transformation, including PI3K, MAPK, and/or JAK/STAT.

Inactivation of PRDM1

More than 75% of all ABC-DLBCL cases lack expression of the PRDM1/BLIMP1 protein. In up to 25% of cases, this is due to genetic alterations that disrupt the *PRDM1* locus on chromosomal band 6q21, including truncating mutations, missense mutations, and genomic deletions [31, 32, 34]. In an additional large proportion of cases, PRDM1 is transcriptionally repressed through constitutively active, translocated BCL6 alleles [31, 32, 34]. The *PRDM1* gene encodes for a zinc finger transcriptional repressor that is expressed in a subset of GC B-cells undergoing plasma cell differentiation and in all plasma cells [116, 117]. Since the PRDM1 protein constitutes an essential requirement for terminal B-cell differentiation [118], one mechanism by which PRDM1 inactivation contributes to lymphomagenesis is by blocking post-GC B-cell differentiation, as demonstrated in mouse models where conditional ablation of this gene in GC B cells leads to the development of DLBCL [31, 119] Notably, translocations deregulating the *BCL6* gene are virtually never found in PRDM1 mutated DLBCL cases [34, 35], suggesting that BCL6 deregulation and PRDM1 inactivation represent alternative oncogenic mechanisms converging on the same pathway (Fig. 9.3).

Other Lesions

Additional ABC-DLBCL-specific structural alterations include amplifications of the *BCL2* locus, observed in more than one-third of the cases [39, 120, 121]; deletions or lack of expression of the *CDKN2A* and *CDKN2B* tumor suppressor genes [86, 107]; and mutations of the *ATM* gene, which have been reported at smaller frequencies [122, 123].

PMBCL

A genetic hallmark of both PMBCL and HL is the amplification of chromosomal region 9q24, detected in nearly 50% of patients [70, 71]. This relatively large interval encompasses multiple genes of possible pathogenetic significance, including the gene encoding for the *JAK2* tyrosine kinase and the *PDL1* and *PDL2* genes, which encode for inhibitors of T-cell responses [70, 71]. Amplifications of the *PDL1* locus have been linked to impaired antitumor immune responses in several cancers. Moreover, elevated expression levels of these genes may in part explain the unique features of these lymphoma types, which are characterized by a significant inflammatory infiltrate. Other lesions affecting regulators of immune responses in PMBCL include genomic rearrangements and mutations of the MHC class II transactivator gene *CIITA* [124]. These rearrangements cause the downregulation of surface HLA class II expression, which is associated with reduced tumor cell immunogenicity [124]. PMBCL also shares with HL the presence of genetic lesions affecting the NF-κB pathway and the deregulated expression of receptor tyrosine kinases [83, 125–127].

Concluding Remarks

During the past decade, our understanding of the pathogenesis of DLBCL has improved dramatically. Genome-wide expression profiling has demonstrated the degree of heterogeneity of DLBCL and opened the way to a better definition of the molecular mechanisms underlying diverse subtypes of the disease. More recently, powerful genomic technologies such as high-density genome-wide single nucleotide polymorphism array analyses and massively parallel sequencing, applied to whole genomes/exomes/transcriptomes, have allowed the identification of previously unsuspected genes and pathways that are disrupted by genetic alterations in DLBCL, further improving our understanding of the disease. These discoveries will be essential for the development of new diagnostic tests that may allow the stratification of patients according to different prognostic groups as well as the design of more effective therapeutic approaches aimed at targeting specific signaling pathways in distinct disease categories.

References

1. A clinical evaluation of the International Lymphoma Study Group classification of non-Hodgkin's lymphoma. The Non-Hodgkin's Lymphoma Classification Project. Blood 89:3909–3918 (1997)
2. Swerdlow SH et al (2008) WHO classification of tumours of haematopoietic and lymphoid tissues. IARC, Lyon

3. Abramson JS, Shipp MA (2005) Advances in the biology and therapy of diffuse large B-cell lymphoma: moving toward a molecularly targeted approach. Blood 106:1164–1174
4. Klein U, Dalla-Favera R (2008) Germinal centres: role in B-cell physiology and malignancy. Nat Rev Immunol 8:22–33
5. MacLennan IC (1994) Germinal centers. Annu Rev Immunol 12:117–139
6. Rajewsky K (1996) Clonal selection and learning in the antibody system. Nature 381:751–758
7. Klein U et al (2003) Transcriptional analysis of the B cell germinal center reaction. Proc Natl Acad Sci U S A 100:2639–2644
8. Cattoretti G et al (1995) BCL-6 protein is expressed in germinal-center B cells. Blood 86:45–53
9. Chang CC, Ye BH, Chaganti RS, Dalla-Favera R (1996) BCL-6, a POZ/zinc-finger protein, is a sequence-specific transcriptional repressor. Proc Natl Acad Sci U S A 93:6947–6952
10. Basso K et al (2010) Integrated biochemical and computational approach identifies BCL6 direct target genes controlling multiple pathways in normal germinal center B cells. Blood 115:975–984
11. Niu H, Cattoretti G, Dalla-Favera R (2003) BCL6 controls the expression of the B7-1/CD80 costimulatory receptor in germinal center B cells. J Exp Med 198:211–221
12. Ci W et al (2009) The BCL6 transcriptional program features repression of multiple oncogenes in primary B cells and is deregulated in DLBCL. Blood 113:5536–5548
13. Phan RT, Dalla-Favera R (2004) The BCL6 proto-oncogene suppresses p53 expression in germinal-centre B cells. Nature 432:635–639
14. Phan RT, Saito M, Basso K, Niu H, Dalla-Favera R (2005) BCL6 interacts with the transcription factor Miz-1 to suppress the cyclin-dependent kinase inhibitor p21 and cell cycle arrest in germinal center B cells. Nat Immunol 6:1054–1060
15. Ranuncolo SM et al (2007) Bcl-6 mediates the germinal center B cell phenotype and lymphomagenesis through transcriptional repression of the DNA-damage sensor ATR. Nat Immunol 8:705–714
16. Ranuncolo SM, Polo JM, Melnick A (2008) BCL6 represses CHEK1 and suppresses DNA damage pathways in normal and malignant B-cells. Blood Cells Mol Dis 41:95–99
17. Keller AD, Maniatis T (1991) Identification and characterization of a novel repressor of beta-interferon gene expression. Genes Dev 5:868–879
18. Turner CA Jr, Mack DH, Davis MM (1994) Blimp-1, a novel zinc finger-containing protein that can drive the maturation of B lymphocytes into immunoglobulin-secreting cells. Cell 77:297–306
19. Shaffer AL et al (2000) BCL-6 represses genes that function in lymphocyte differentiation, inflammation, and cell cycle control. Immunity 13:199–212
20. Tunyaplin C et al (2004) Direct repression of prdm1 by Bcl-6 inhibits plasmacytic differentiation. J Immunol 173:1158–1165
21. Saito M et al (2009) BCL6 suppression of BCL2 via Miz1 and its disruption in diffuse large B cell lymphoma. Proc Natl Acad Sci U S A 106:11294–11299
22. Liu YJ et al (1996) Sequential triggering of apoptosis, somatic mutation and isotype switch during germinal center development. Semin Immunol 8:169–177
23. Longerich S, Basu U, Alt F, Storb U (2006) AID in somatic hypermutation and class switch recombination. Curr Opin Immunol 18:164–174
24. Muramatsu M et al (2000) Class switch recombination and hypermutation require activation-induced cytidine deaminase (AID), a potential RNA editing enzyme. Cell 102:553–563
25. Revy P et al (2000) Activation-induced cytidine deaminase (AID) deficiency causes the autosomal recessive form of the hyper-IgM syndrome (HIGM2). Cell 102:565–575
26. Alizadeh AA et al (2000) Distinct types of diffuse large B-cell lymphoma identified by gene expression profiling. Nature 403:503–511
27. Wright G et al (2003) A gene expression-based method to diagnose clinically distinct subgroups of diffuse large B cell lymphoma. Proc Natl Acad Sci U S A 100:9991–9996

28. Savage KJ et al (2003) The molecular signature of mediastinal large B-cell lymphoma differs from that of other diffuse large B-cell lymphomas and shares features with classical Hodgkin lymphoma. Blood 102:3871–3879
29. Rosenwald A et al (2003) Molecular diagnosis of primary mediastinal B cell lymphoma identifies a clinically favorable subgroup of diffuse large B cell lymphoma related to Hodgkin lymphoma. J Exp Med 198:851–862
30. Lossos IS et al (2000) Ongoing immunoglobulin somatic mutation in germinal center B cell-like but not in activated B cell-like diffuse large cell lymphomas. Proc Natl Acad Sci U S A 97:10209–10213
31. Mandelbaum J et al (2010) BLIMP1 is a tumor suppressor gene frequently disrupted in activated B cell-like diffuse large B cell lymphoma. Cancer Cell 18:568–579
32. Pasqualucci L et al (2006) Inactivation of the PRDM1/BLIMP1 gene in diffuse large B cell lymphoma. J Exp Med 203:311–317
33. Saito M et al (2007) A signaling pathway mediating downregulation of BCL6 in germinal center B cells is blocked by BCL6 gene alterations in B cell lymphoma. Cancer Cell 12:280–292
34. Tam W et al (2006) Mutational analysis of PRDM1 indicates a tumor-suppressor role in diffuse large B-cell lymphomas. Blood 107:4090–4100
35. Lenz G, Staudt LM (2010) Mechanisms of disease: aggressive lymphomas. N Engl J Med 362:1417–1429
36. Lenz G et al (2008) Stromal gene signatures in large-B-cell lymphomas. N Engl J Med 359:2313–2323
37. Lenz G et al (2007) Aberrant immunoglobulin class switch recombination and switch translocations in activated B cell-like diffuse large B cell lymphoma. J Exp Med 204:633–643
38. Steidl C, Gascoyne RD (2011) The molecular pathogenesis of primary mediastinal large B-cell lymphoma. Blood 118:2659–2669
39. Rosenwald A et al (2002) The use of molecular profiling to predict survival after chemotherapy for diffuse large-B-cell lymphoma. N Engl J Med 346:1937–1947
40. Nyman H et al (2007) Prognostic impact of immunohistochemically defined germinal center phenotype in diffuse large B-cell lymphoma patients treated with immunochemotherapy. Blood 109:4930–4935
41. Choi WW et al (2009) A new immunostain algorithm classifies diffuse large B-cell lymphoma into molecular subtypes with high accuracy. Clin Cancer Res 15:5494–5502
42. Hans CP et al (2004) Confirmation of the molecular classification of diffuse large B-cell lymphoma by immunohistochemistry using a tissue microarray. Blood 103:275–282
43. Monti S et al (2005) Molecular profiling of diffuse large B-cell lymphoma identifies robust subtypes including one characterized by host inflammatory response. Blood 105:1851–1861
44. Dave SS et al (2006) Molecular diagnosis of Burkitt's lymphoma. N Engl J Med 354:2431–2442
45. Hummel M et al (2006) A biologic definition of Burkitt's lymphoma from transcriptional and genomic profiling. N Engl J Med 354:2419–2430
46. Dalla-Favera R, Pasqualucci L (2010) Molecular genetics of lymphomas. In: Mauch PM, Armitage JO, Coiffier B, Dalla-Favera R, Harris NL (eds) Non-Hodgkin's lymphoma. Lippincott Williams & Wilkins, Philadelphia, pp 825–843
47. Kuppers R, Dalla-Favera R (2001) Mechanisms of chromosomal translocations in B cell lymphomas. Oncogene 20:5580–5594
48. Nussenzweig A, Nussenzweig MC (2010) Origin of chromosomal translocations in lymphoid cancer. Cell 141:27–38
49. Ramiro AR et al (2004) AID is required for c-myc/IgH chromosome translocations in vivo. Cell 118:431–438
50. Robbiani DF et al (2008) AID is required for the chromosomal breaks in c-myc that lead to c-myc/IgH translocations. Cell 135:1028–1038

51. Franco S et al (2006) H2AX prevents DNA breaks from progressing to chromosome breaks and translocations. Mol Cell 21:201–214
52. Pasqualucci L et al (2008) AID is required for germinal center-derived lymphomagenesis. Nat Genet 40:108–112
53. Takizawa M et al (2008) AID expression levels determine the extent of cMyc oncogenic translocations and the incidence of B cell tumor development. J Exp Med 205:1949–1957
54. Akasaka H et al (2000) Molecular anatomy of BCL6 translocations revealed by long-distance polymerase chain reaction-based assays. Cancer Res 60:2335–2341
55. Chen W, Iida S, Louie DC, Dalla-Favera R, Chaganti RS (1998) Heterologous promoters fused to BCL6 by chromosomal translocations affecting band 3q27 cause its deregulated expression during B-cell differentiation. Blood 91:603–607
56. Ye BH et al (1993) Alterations of a zinc finger-encoding gene, BCL-6, in diffuse large- cell lymphoma. Science 262:747–750
57. Ye BH, Rao PH, Chaganti RS, Dalla-Favera R (1993) Cloning of bcl-6, the locus involved in chromosome translocations affecting band 3q27 in B-cell lymphoma. Cancer Res 53:2732–2735
58. Yoshida S et al (1999) Identification of heterologous translocation partner genes fused to the BCL6 gene in diffuse large B-cell lymphomas: 5'-RACE and LA - PCR analyses of biopsy samples. Oncogene 18:7994–7999
59. Baron BW et al (1993) Identification of the gene associated with the recurring chromosomal translocations t(3;14)(q27;q32) and t(3;22)(q27;q11) in B-cell lymphomas. Proc Natl Acad Sci U S A 90:5262–5266
60. Kerckaert JP et al (1993) LAZ3, a novel zinc-finger encoding gene, is disrupted by recurring chromosome 3q27 translocations in human lymphomas. Nat Genet 5:66–70
61. Miki T et al (1994) Molecular cloning of the breakpoint for 3q27 translocation in B-cell lymphomas and leukemias. Blood 83:217–222
62. Neuberger MS (2008) Antibody diversification by somatic mutation: from Burnet onwards. Immunol Cell Biol 86:124–132
63. Pavri R et al (2010) Activation-induced cytidine deaminase targets DNA at sites of RNA polymerase II stalling by interaction with Spt5. Cell 143:122–133
64. Yamane A, Resch W, Casellas R (2011) Deep-sequencing identification of the genomic targets of the cytidine deaminase AID and its cofactor RPA in B lymphocytes. Nat Immunol 12:62–69
65. Liu M et al (2008) Two levels of protection for the B cell genome during somatic hypermutation. Nature 451:841–845
66. Pasqualucci L et al (2001) Hypermutation of multiple proto-oncogenes in B-cell diffuse large-cell lymphomas. Nature 412:341–346
67. Houldsworth J et al (1996) REL proto-oncogene is frequently amplified in extranodal diffuse large cell lymphoma. Blood 87:25–29
68. Houldsworth J et al (2004) Relationship between REL amplification, REL function, and clinical and biologic features in diffuse large B-cell lymphomas. Blood 103:1862–1868
69. Rao PH et al (1998) Chromosomal and gene amplification in diffuse large B-cell lymphoma. Blood 92:234–240
70. Green MR et al (2011) Integrative analysis reveals selective 9p24.1 amplification, increased PD-1 ligand expression, and further induction via JAK2 in nodular sclerosing Hodgkin lymphoma and primary mediastinal large B-cell lymphoma. Blood 116:3268–3277
71. Rui L et al (2011) Cooperative epigenetic modulation by cancer amplicon genes. Cancer Cell 18:590–605
72. Bhatia K et al (1993) Point mutations in the c-Myc transactivation domain are common in Burkitt's lymphoma and mouse plasmacytomas. Nat Genet 5:56–61
73. Bhatia K et al (1994) Mutations in the coding region of c-myc occur frequently in acquired immunodeficiency syndrome-associated lymphomas. Blood 84:883–888
74. Tanaka S, Louie DC, Kant JA, Reed JC (1992) Frequent incidence of somatic mutations in translocated BCL2 oncogenes of non-Hodgkin's lymphomas. Blood 79:229–237

75. Compagno M et al (2009) Mutations of multiple genes cause deregulation of NF-kappaB in diffuse large B-cell lymphoma. Nature 459:717–721
76. Lenz G et al (2008) Oncogenic CARD11 mutations in human diffuse large B cell lymphoma. Science 319:1676–1679
77. Neri A, Knowles DM, Greco A, McCormick F, Dalla-Favera R (1988) Analysis of RAS oncogene mutations in human lymphoid malignancies. Proc Natl Acad Sci U S A 85:9268–9272
78. Hollstein M, Sidransky D, Vogelstein B, Harris CC (1991) p53 mutations in human cancers. Science 253:49–53
79. Gaidano G et al (1992) Deletions involving two distinct regions of 6q in B-cell non-Hodgkin lymphoma. Blood 80:1781–1787
80. Offit K, Wong G, Filippa DA, Tao Y, Chaganti RS (1991) Cytogenetic analysis of 434 consecutively ascertained specimens of non-Hodgkin's lymphoma: clinical correlations. Blood 77:1508–1515
81. Kato M et al (2009) Frequent inactivation of A20 in B-cell lymphomas. Nature 459:712–716
82. Novak U et al (2009) The NF-{kappa}B negative regulator TNFAIP3 (A20) is inactivated by somatic mutations and genomic deletions in marginal zone lymphomas. Blood 113:4918–4921
83. Schmitz R et al (2009) TNFAIP3 (A20) is a tumor suppressor gene in Hodgkin lymphoma and primary mediastinal B cell lymphoma. J Exp Med 206:981–989
84. Morin RD et al (2011) Frequent mutation of histone-modifying genes in non-Hodgkin lymphoma. Nature 476:298–303
85. Pasqualucci L et al (2011) Analysis of the coding genome of diffuse large B-cell lymphoma. Nat Genet 43:830–837
86. Lenz G et al (2008) Molecular subtypes of diffuse large B-cell lymphoma arise by distinct genetic pathways. Proc Natl Acad Sci U S A 105:13520–13525
87. Lo Coco F et al (1994) Rearrangements of the BCL6 gene in diffuse large cell non-Hodgkin's lymphoma. Blood 83:1757–1759
88. Offit K et al (1989) t(3;22)(q27;q11): a novel translocation associated with diffuse non-Hodgkin's lymphoma. Blood 74:1876–1879
89. Iqbal J et al (2007) Distinctive patterns of BCL6 molecular alterations and their functional consequences in different subgroups of diffuse large B-cell lymphoma. Leukemia 21:2332–2343
90. Ye BH et al (1995) Chromosomal translocations cause deregulated BCL6 expression by promoter substitution in B cell lymphoma. EMBO J 14:6209–6217
91. Cattoretti G et al (2005) Deregulated BCL6 expression recapitulates the pathogenesis of human diffuse large B cell lymphomas in mice. Cancer Cell 7:445–455
92. Pasqualucci L et al (2011) Inactivating mutations of acetyltransferase genes in B-cell lymphoma. Nature 471:189–195
93. Bereshchenko OR, Gu W, Dalla-Favera R (2002) Acetylation inactivates the transcriptional repressor BCL6. Nat Genet 32:606–613
94. Tang Y, Zhao W, Chen Y, Zhao Y, Gu W (2008) Acetylation is indispensable for p53 activation. Cell 133:612–626
95. Gu W, Roeder RG (1997) Activation of p53 sequence-specific DNA binding by acetylation of the p53 C-terminal domain. Cell 90:595–606
96. Cresswell P, Ackerman AL, Giodini A, Peaper DR, Wearsch PA (2005) Mechanisms of MHC class I-restricted antigen processing and cross-presentation. Immunol Rev 207:145–157
97. Challa-Malladi M, Lieu Y, Pasqualucci L, Dalla-Favera R (2011) Inactivating mutations of immunomodulatory genes. Cancer Cell (in press)
98. Moingeon P et al (1989) CD2-mediated adhesion facilitates T lymphocyte antigen recognition function. Nature 339:312–314
99. Barrans S et al (2010) Rearrangement of MYC is associated with poor prognosis in patients with diffuse large B-cell lymphoma treated in the era of rituximab. J Clin Oncol 28:3360–3365

100. Iqbal J et al (2004) BCL2 translocation defines a unique tumor subset within the germinal center B-cell-like diffuse large B-cell lymphoma. Am J Pathol 165:159–166
101. Kawasaki C et al (2001) Rearrangements of bcl-1, bcl-2, bcl-6, and c-myc in diffuse large B-cell lymphomas. Leuk Lymphoma 42:1099–1106
102. Ladanyi M, Offit K, Jhanwar SC, Filippa DA, Chaganti RS (1991) MYC rearrangement and translocations involving band 8q24 in diffuse large cell lymphomas. Blood 77:1057–1063
103. Dominguez-Sola D et al (2007) Non-transcriptional control of DNA replication by c-Myc. Nature 448:445–451
104. Morin RD et al (2010) Somatic mutations altering EZH2 (Tyr641) in follicular and diffuse large B-cell lymphomas of germinal-center origin. Nat Genet 42:181–185
105. Yap DB et al (2011) Somatic mutations at EZH2 Y641 act dominantly through a mechanism of selectively altered PRC2 catalytic activity, to increase H3K27 trimethylation. Blood 117:2451–2459
106. Sneeringer CJ et al (2010) Coordinated activities of wild-type plus mutant EZH2 drive tumor-associated hypertrimethylation of lysine 27 on histone H3 (H3K27) in human B-cell lymphomas. Proc Natl Acad Sci U S A 107:20980–20985
107. Potthoff MJ, Olson EN (2007) MEF2: a central regulator of diverse developmental programs. Development 134:4131–4140
108. Davis RE, Brown KD, Siebenlist U, Staudt LM (2001) Constitutive nuclear factor kappaB activity is required for survival of activated B cell-like diffuse large B cell lymphoma cells. J Exp Med 194:1861–1874
109. Pasqualucci L et al (2003) Mutations of the BCL6 proto-oncogene disrupt its negative autoregulation in diffuse large B-cell lymphoma. Blood 101:2914–2923
110. Wang X, Li Z, Naganuma A, Ye BH (2002) Negative autoregulation of BCL-6 is bypassed by genetic alterations in diffuse large B cell lymphomas. Proc Natl Acad Sci U S A 99:15018–15023
111. Ballerini P et al (1993) Multiple genetic lesions in acquired immunodeficiency syndrome-related non-Hodgkin's lymphoma. Blood 81:166–176
112. Gaidano G et al (1991) p53 mutations in human lymphoid malignancies: association with Burkitt lymphoma and chronic lymphocytic leukemia. Proc Natl Acad Sci U S A 88:5413–5417
113. Lo Coco F et al (1993) p53 mutations are associated with histologic transformation of follicular lymphoma. Blood 82:2289–2295
114. Davis RE et al (2010) Chronic active B-cell-receptor signalling in diffuse large B-cell lymphoma. Nature 463:88–92
115. Ngo et al (2011) Oncogenically active MYD88 mutations in human lymphoma. Nature 470:115–119
116. Angelin-Duclos C, Cattoretti G, Lin KI, Calame K (2000) Commitment of B lymphocytes to a plasma cell fate is associated with Blimp-1 expression in vivo. J Immunol 165:5462–5471
117. Cattoretti G et al (2005) PRDM1/Blimp-1 is expressed in human B-lymphocytes committed to the plasma cell lineage. J Pathol 206:76–86
118. Shapiro-Shelef M et al (2003) Blimp-1 is required for the formation of immunoglobulin secreting plasma cells and pre-plasma memory B cells. Immunity 19:607–620
119. Calado DP et al (2010) Constitutive canonical NF-kappaB activation cooperates with disruption of BLIMP1 in the pathogenesis of activated B cell-like diffuse large cell lymphoma. Cancer Cell 18:580–589
120. Iqbal J et al (2006) BCL2 expression is a prognostic marker for the activated B-cell-like type of diffuse large B-cell lymphoma. J Clin Oncol 24:961–968
121. Monni O et al (1997) BCL2 overexpression associated with chromosomal amplification in diffuse large B-cell lymphoma. Blood 90:1168–1174
122. Gronbaek K et al (2002) ATM mutations are associated with inactivation of the ARF-TP53 tumor suppressor pathway in diffuse large B-cell lymphoma. Blood 100:1430–1437

123. Bai M et al (2001) Low expression of p27 protein combined with altered p53 and Rb/p16 expression status is associated with increased expression of cyclin A and cyclin B1 in diffuse large B-cell lymphomas. Mod Pathol 14:1105–1113
124. Steidl C et al (2011) MHC class II transactivator CIITA is a recurrent gene fusion partner in lymphoid cancers. Nature 471:377–381
125. Mestre C et al (2005) Homozygous deletion of SOCS1 in primary mediastinal B-cell lymphoma detected by CGH to BAC microarrays. Leukemia 19:1082–1084
126. Melzner I et al (2005) Biallelic mutation of SOCS-1 impairs JAK2 degradation and sustains phospho-JAK2 action in the MedB-1 mediastinal lymphoma line. Blood 105:2535–2542
127. Weniger MA et al (2006) Mutations of the tumor suppressor gene SOCS-1 in classical Hodgkin lymphoma are frequent and associated with nuclear phospho-STAT5 accumulation. Oncogene 25:2679–2684

Chapter 10
Epstein–Barr Virus and Burkitt's Lymphoma

Shuvomoy Banerjee, Hem Chandra Jha, Qiliang Cai, and Erle S. Robertson

Historical Overview

Almost 50 years ago, Burkitt's lymphoma (BL) was initially described in association with the first human tumour virus, Epstein–Barr virus (EBV) discovered in BL tumour samples [1]. Since then, the role of EBV in BL pathogenesis has become more enigmatic in the field of cancer Biology. In the middle of the last century, Denis Burkitt, an English surgeon was working in central Africa in the Kampala region of Uganda and equatorial Africa. He observed the occurrence of a malignant tumour in children with lesions in the face, as well as upper and lower jaws. He also noted that some children had huge abdominal masses, sometimes accompanied by disease in the facial bones, although there was usually no lymph node involvement. This typical malignant syndrome was initially thought to be a sarcoma [2, 3], but later characterized as a lymphoma, now referred to as BL. Interestingly, the lymphoma was found to occur throughout tropical Africa except at high altitudes or in some areas where the climate was relatively cool. Importantly, he also realized that BL was an independent clinical entity with a particular geographical distribution [4]. On safari, together with Ted Williams and Cliff Nelson, he identified epidemiological features of this disease which was associated with high incidence in the low lands with tropical climate and its absence in the high lands with little rainfall [5, 6]. This phenomenon led to the hypothesis that malaria, a disease associated with the arthropod borne parasite, was involved in the pathogenesis of this disease. These geographic and climatic associations strongly suggested a compatibility with *Plasmodium falciparum*.

S. Banerjee • H.C. Jha • Q. Cai • E.S. Robertson (✉)
Department of Microbiology, Perelman School of Medicine, University of Pennsylvania, Philadelphia, PA, USA
e-mail: erle@mail.med.upenn.edu

E.S. Robertson (ed.), *Burkitt's Lymphoma*, Current Cancer Research,
DOI 10.1007/978-1-4614-4313-1_10,

In 1961, Denis Burkitt made the acquaintance of Anthony Epstein, a young experimental pathologist. He shipped samples of the lymphoma to him at his lab in England. Epstein and his colleagues Barr and Achong identified the virus that is now known as Epstein– Barr virus (EBV). This was the first description of a virus involved in the pathogenesis of a tumour in humans. In present-day Africa, BL continues to account for a large portion of childhood malignancies [7].

Werner and Gertrude Henle, two virologists at the Children's Hospital in Philadelphia, became interested in this novel virus and developed serological techniques to detect the virus in the human population [8]. Surprisingly, they found that Epstein–Barr virus was not only restricted to BL patients as initially believed, but also proved to be prevalent in 95% of the adult population [4]. In the African population, the virus appeared to be detected in the younger age groups, significantly earlier than seen in the USA and Europe where seroconversion was often delayed to adolescence [4]. Furthermore, African children with BL displayed particularly high antibody titers to EBV [9]. In 1968, based on the seroepidemiological studies, the Henles identified EBV as the causal agent of an acute disease, now reffered to as infectious mononucleosis [10]. Infectious mononucleosis is characterized by fever and swollen lymph nodes and an abnormal increase in mononuclear leucocytes or monocytes in the bloodstream [10]. Volker Diehl, the Henles and John Pope in Brisbane, independent of each other demonstrated that EBV has the ability to transform primary human B cells into B blasts [10–12], which, upon a crisis and telomere stabilization [13] grew out into continuously proliferating immortalized B-cell lines. Later, zur Hausen et al. also established the association between EBV and African Burkitt's lymphoma as well as nasopharyngeal carcinoma [14]. These studies strongly suggested that the EBV genome is present in tumour cells of these cancers in vivo and that the virus also has strong transforming potential in vitro.

Geographical Distribution

BL are commonly distinguished on the basis of a number of factors including, geographical location, EBV incidence, clinical features, age and sex ratio [15]. Typically, one form is called "endemic" or African form, found in equatorial Africa and Papua New Guinea region, and another represents the "sporadic" form which was found in Northern part of America, Northern and Eastern Europe and the Far East. An "intermediate" form may also be considered which occurs mainly in Southern Europe, the Middle East and some parts of South America [16].

The Zone of High Risk

The zone of highest risk for BL appears to be between 10° north and 10° south of the equator and in Papua New Guinea, where the prevalence of this malignancy is very common in relation to other types of childhood cancers [17]. In general, the proportion of lymphomas which accounts for BL is very high in these regions; in Papua New Guinea, 58% (1979–1988), and in Nigeria, Uganda and Malawi (1985–1995) 67–70% of lymphomas are considered BL [18]. Interestingly, the frequency of BL may vary substantially, even within high-risk areas. It was reported that occurrence of BL was preferentially found in lowland areas, warm, humid regions of Western Kenya which is divided into three provinces, two of which are primarily hot, moist, tropical savannahs (known as Nyanza and Western provinces), and the other is predominantly highland area and semi-arid regions (known as Rift Valley Province) [19]. Overall, BL accounted for one third (201/600) of solid tumours of those under 15 years, but the proportion varied in each province. For example, it accounted for 52% of neoplasms in Nyanza province, 31% in the Western province and 23% in the Rift Valley [19]. The incidence of BL is also relatively infrequent in other upland areas within the high-risk zone, such as Rwanda, Burundi and the plateaux of Zambia and Zimbabwe [20].

The Zone of Intermediate Risk

Southern Europe, North Africa and Asia as far west as Iraq and Kuwait are designated as intermediate-risk regions [21]. In countries like Spain, France and Portugal BL accounts for 15–46% of lymphomas, and for 25–33% of lymphomas in the Middle East [22]. Denmark and the Netherlands may also fall into the intermediate risk zone [23].

The Zone of Low Risk

Most of the Northern and Eastern Europe, and Northern parts of South America were recognized as the zone of low risk. The incidence of BL also appears to be rare in certain regions of Asia including the eastern zone of Pakistan; Bangladesh, China, Singapore and Vietnam with minimal report of cases of BL. Importantly, some Asian registries tend to show lower childhood cancer incidence rates than registries from America, Europe or Australia [24].

Signs and Symptoms of Burkitt's Lymphoma

BL is a B-cell malignancy of the lymphatic system. This neoplastic condition can be presented with several signs and symptoms which may vary from patient to patient. The symptoms will also vary in intensity and frequency between different individuals. They include painless swelling of lymph nodes in the groin, neck, underarm, abdomen or chest, recurring infections, fever, itchy skin, sore throat, loss of appetite and weight loss, a feeling of fullness in the groin area, fatigue and pain in the joints and bones [25]. These signs and symptoms of BL typically can be similar to those of other medical problems, especially blood disorders, making this type of cancer difficult to diagnose.

Staging of Burkitt's Lymphoma

It is critical to determine the anatomical sites of involvement in patients with such malignant lymphomas when radiotherapy is considered the treatment of choice as the treatment field must encompass the sites of known disease. Recent correlations between the type of histology and the extent of clinical disease have greatly facilitated the choice and sequence of staging procedures for BL [26]. Generally, childhood lymphomas belong to three major histological categories, undifferentiated (either the Burkitt or the non-Burkitt type); "histiocytic" or large-lymphoid-cell types; and lymphoblastic lymphoma [27]. The first two types typically involve the head and neck region as well as the lymph nodes and abdominal viscera, and the third type, even though commonly involving the mediastinum, may involve only the lymph nodes, either in a localized or generalized distribution [28]. Simply stated, patients with childhood lymphomas, including Burkitt's, can be subdivided into two clinical stages: those with a small tumour burden and those with a large tumour burden [29].

Clinicopathologic Features of Burkitt's Lymphoma

There are three distinct epidemiological forms of BL that are well established. The high-incidence "endemic" form typically presents as a jaw or abdominal tumour in children in equatorial Africa where malaria is holoendemic, and is 100% EBV genome positive [30]. Elsewhere, the occurrence of BL as a "sporadic" form in children is related to the degree of EBV association in different geographical areas [30]. It is therefore possible that chronic immune stimulation from other parasitic infections may also increase BL incidence which preferentially involves EBV-associated disease. Interestingly, a third, adult form of the disease, AIDS-associated BL, has proven to be very common among HIV-infected individuals with about 30–40% of these tumours positive for EBV [30]. According to WHO report, BL can be classified into classic, and two variant categories which depend upon their cellular morphology that are BL with plasmacytoid differentiation and atypical Burkitt's/Burkitt-like lymphoma [31]. Classic BL is associated with some cases of endemic BL and mostly in sporadic BL. For diagnostic purposes, it is very important to review the morphological features of BL, as defined in the 2001 WHO leukaemia/

lymphoma classification: medium-sized cells with round nuclei, fine granular chromatin, relatively clear para-chromatin, centrally situated multiple basophilic nucleoli, deeply basophilic cytoplasm, usually containing lipid vacuoles, and a high mitotic rate [31, 32]. BL, regardless of subtype, typically expresses monotypic surface IgM, pan-B-cell antigens, including CD19, CD20, CD22 and CD79a, and also co-expresses CD10, Bcl-6, CD43 and p53, but not CD5, CD23, Bcl-2, CD138 or TdT [31, 33]; consequently, the doubling time of the tumour is very short, between 24 and 48 h. In rare cases, Burkitt's lymphoma lacks surface immunoglobulin [34], including some occurring in allograft recipients [35]. The immuno-phenotyping study suggests follicle centre origin for this lymphoma. Some additional characteristics feature of BL as seen on Pap-stained smears that include coarse nuclear chromatin and multiple nucleoli [36, 37]. Another atypical Burkitt/Burkitt-like lymphoma has some of the above features, but with greater occurrence of pleomorphism in nuclear size and shape, and fewer, more prominent nucleoli [31].

Pathogenesis of Epstein–Barr Virus (EBV)-Associated Burkitt's Lymphoma

Even after intensive research in the field of viral oncology for over 40 years, the precise contributions of EBV in the pathogenesis of BL have yet to be fully realized. EBV-infected cells display predominantly three different types of latency based on the EBV-encoded protein and RNA expression. Type I latency is characterized by an almost exclusive expression of EBV-encoded nuclear small non-polyadenylated RNA (EBER) molecules and EBV-encoded nuclear antigen (EBNA) 1. Type II latency shows additional expression of latent membrane proteins (LMP). Type III latency displays expression of EBV nuclear antigen 2–6 by virtue of differential promoter usage [38]. Generally, BL cells usually display latency type I but may convert to latency type III in cell culture condition [39]. Table 10.1 shows some of the described roles of the EBV latent antigens and their interacting host factors which are likely to be important for progression of BL.

Role of Major EBV Gene Products in Burkitt's Lymphoma

EBNA1

Studies have suggested that BL is a tumour derived from cells containing EBV maintained as a persistent latent infection [65]. Some findings also indicated that BL has the Ig gene somatic mutations of a memory B cell [66], and that EBV persists

Table 10.1 The EBV latent antigens and their associated cellular proteins important for their activities in BL cells

EBV latent antigens	Associated cellular proteins	Functions	References
EBNA1	PKR, H2B, Rag-1, Bcl2, CD25	Essential for B-cell immortalization, inhibition of apoptosis, genome maintenance	[40–45]
EBNA2	CD21, CD23, c-Fgr, RBP-JK, Spi, PU-1	Transcriptional co-activator that up regulates expression of viral (LMP1) and cellular genes (c-myc)	[46–50]
EBER's	c-Myc, ribosomal protein L22	Enhanced immunogenicity, Inhibition of apoptosis, IL-10 production, BCL2L11 (BIM) down-regulation	[51–53]
BART's	miRBART 2, miRBART5, PUMA, p53, BIM, c-Myc	Protein product may modify Notch signaling	[54–56]
EBNA3A and 3C	Bcl2, BIM	Essential for B-cell immortalization, stabilizing c-Myc, cyclin D1 and Mdm2	[57]
LMP1	CD40, ICAM1, NFkB, c-JUN, JNK, STAT	Essential for B-cell immortalization, MAPK and Wnt signaling	[58–60]
LMP2A	AKT, mTOR, PI3K, c-Myc, p53	Drives EBV in to latency, blocks BCR, AKT, mTOR and PI3K signaling pathway	[61–64]

This table shows the important functions of EBV latent antigens and associated host factors in Burkitt's lymphoma cells. *EBNA* Epstein–Barr virus nuclear antigen, *EBER* EBV-encoded RNA, *BART* BamHI-A rightward transcript, *LMP1* latent membrane proteins1, *PKR* protein kinase RNA-activated, *H2B* histone H2B, *RAG1* V(D)J recombination-activating protein 1, *BCL2* B-cell lymphoma 2, *CD* cluster of differentiation, *c-FGR* Gardner–Rasheed feline sarcoma viral (v-fgr) oncogene homolog, *RBP-JK* recombination signal binding protein for immunoglobulin kappa J region, *Spi*, Salmonella pathogenicity island 1, *PU.1* transcription factor PU.1, *c-MYC* v-myc avian myelocytomatosis viral oncogene homolog, *miR-BART* micro-RNA BamHI-A rightward transcript, *PUMA* p53 upregulated modulator of apoptosis, *BIM* BCL2-like 11, *ICAM1* inter-cellular adhesion molecule1, *NFkB* nuclear factor kappa-light-chain-enhancer of activated B cells, *c-jun* jun proto-oncogene, *JNK* c-Jun N-terminal kinases, *STAT* signal transducer and activator of transcription, *AKT* protein kinase B, *mTOR* mammalian target of rapamycin, *PI3K* phosphatidylinositol 3-kinases, *MDM2* mouse double minute 2, *MAPK* mitogen-activated protein (MAP) kinases, *NOTCH* Notch (*Drosophila*) homolog, *Wnt* proto-oncogene Int-1 homolog, *BCR* breakpoint cluster region

in resting memory B cells in the peripheral blood [67, 68]. BL also showed a unique pattern of viral latent protein expression, with expression of the EBV-encoded nuclear antigen (EBNA) 1 protein, as the predominant latent antigen necessary for maintenance and replication of the viral genome [69]. EBNA1 is produced from a transcript of EBNA1 (Q-K), originating from a unique Qp promoter [70]. EBNA1 is ultimately to be a predominant target for cytotoxic T lymphocytes and previous studies suggested that only EBNA1 is expressed in the progenitor of BL cell type [65]. Recent genetic studies revealed that infection of B cells with derivatives of EBV lacking EBNA1, induced their proliferative capacity but with less potency when compared to wild-type EBV [40]. This indicated that the functions of EBNA1 can provide activities important for driving initiation and maintenance of the proliferative state of EBV infected B cells. Other studies investigating EBV-infected B cells demonstrated inhibition of EBNA1-induced apoptosis [41]. Interestingly, in Burkitt's lymphoma cells, expression of the two small, non-translated EBERs were shown [71]. These viral RNAs can inhibit apoptosis induced by interferon treatment through a mechanism involving inhibition of RNA-dependent protein kinase (PKR) [72]. EBNA1 inhibition in Burkitt's lymphoma cells showed no alteration in the level of EBERs detected and further supports a role for EBNA1 in inhibition of apoptosis [41].

EBNA2

In lymphoblastoid cell lines, only a subset of viral genes is expressed. They code for six nuclear proteins, three membrane proteins and two small non-polyadenylated nuclear RNAs [73, 74]. The latent genes required for transformation is still a subject of intense investigation. The EBV nuclear antigen 2 (EBNA2) is deleted in the transformation-defective virus P3HR 1 [73]. The two forms EBNA2A and EBNA2B found in the different strains of the virus and share about 50% homology [75]. EBNA2 was detected as the first viral gene expressed together with EBNA-LP, after infection of primary B cells [73, 76]. It functions as a transcriptional activator of different latent viral as well as cellular proteins including the viral Cp, LMP1 and LMP2, and cellular CD21, CD23 and c-fgr genes [46, 47, 77–87]. EBNA2 exerts its trans-activating function by binding to RBP-JK in complex with its cognate DNA sequence [48, 50, 88, 89], and through interaction with transcription factors of the ETS gene family members including, Spi-1 and PU-1 [82, 90]. In vitro transformation of primary B cells is strictly dependent on EBNA2 [91, 92]. However, EBNA2 is not predominantly expressed in BL tumours [93], although some studies have shown EBNA2 expressed in BL tumours [94]. Therefore, the role of EBNA2 in BL is still significant. Studies have shown that EBNA2 down-regulates the surface expression of IgM and transcription of the Ig-μ locus [73]. BL cells with t(8;14) translocations showed down-regulation of Ig- and μ expression was observed in association with concomitant transcriptional shut-down of the c-myc gene [73]. This finding revealed the dysregulation of c-Myc under the control of the Ig heavy chain locus in these cells [73]. Additionally, the function of EBNA2 as a negative regulator of Ig-I transcription provided an explanation for the growth inhibitory effect of EBNA2 in Burkitt's cells carrying a t(8;14) translocation [73].

EBERs

EBERs 1 and 2 were identified as small, non-coding, non-polyadenylated RNAs expressed during EBV latent infection [95]. They are generally abundant but their mechanism of action in EBV mediated B-cell transformation remains poorly understood. Reports have suggested that the EBERs have anti-apoptotic effects on infected cells but these results are still controversial. Currently, it was suggested that EBERs may furnish B cells with a degree of protection from the pro-apoptotic activity of alpha-interferon; however, the contribution of EBERs to the pathogenesis of BL is still unclear [96]. The genes coding for the non-polyadenylated RNAs EBER1 and EBER2, 173 and 169 nucleotides, respectively, are highly expressed in all EBV-associated tumours [97] and may contribute to EBV-mediated oncogenesis. However, studies by Swaminathan et al. demonstrated that they were not essential for in vitro transformation. Independent studies by Takada and Sample investigated the oncogenic potential of the parental EBV-positive BL cells using individual EBV genes. In this study, they used loss variants of EBV-positive BL cell lines as recipients. Interestingly, they concluded that EBNA1 alone is not sufficient to reconstitute resistance of the cells to apoptotic stimuli and that the EBERs are partially responsible for the onset of tumorigenesis [98]. Further, Niller et al. demonstrated a c-MYC binding site in the EBER promoter and suggested that the probable role of c-MYC is to induce expression of EBERs as cooperative partners which promotes oncogenesis [51, 99] . Importantly, it was also reported that EBER2, but not EBER1 contributes to B-cell immortalization [100]. Often, EBERs are found in complexes with the La protein, the auto-antigen in lupus erythematosis, and the ribosomal protein L22 [101], but the functional relationship with EBV-mediated B-cell transformation has not been elucidated.

BARTs

BamHI-A rightward transcripts are lower in abundance in EBV-immortalized cells and BL cells expressing latency I pattern [102] as well as in fresh BL biopsies [103]. BHRF1 is also expressed in BL cells with Wp-restricted latency [104]. This is the primary transcript which gives rise to miR-BHRF-1–3 [97]. Three viral BHRF1-micro-RNAs were also detected in BL cells with latency I at low levels due to residual Cp promoter activity [105]. Interestingly, Pratt et al. showed a correlation between viral micro-RNA expression and maintenance of the viral genome in that three BL lines (Akata, MutuI and Daudi) spontaneously lost their viral genomes with the low expression levels of viral micro-RNAs [97]. This finding suggested that viral micro-RNAs may exhibit a maintenance function for survival or growth of BL cells in vitro and potentially also in vivo [106]. To determine the role of viral micro-RNAs in regulation of viral and cellular gene expression, as well as cellular micro-RNA expression, primary B cells were infected with EBV. Global down-regulation of cellular micro-RNAs was observed with the exception of miR-155 which was found up-regulated in EBV-immortalized B cells [107]. The results suggested that the viral latency III program induces miR-155 which globally regulates the T helper and germinal centre response [54]. Recently, targets of two other viral BART-derived micro-RNAs have been described. Among them, miRBART2 targets BALF5, the gene coding for the viral DNA polymerase [55], and miR-BART5 which targets PUMA [56], a pro-apoptotic protein and target of p53 that strongly cooperates with Bim in driving lymphomagenesis [108]. This observation is significant in regards to c-MYC/Bim/PUMA signaling in EBV-associated BL with implications for pathogenesis [109].

EBNA3

The three EBV latency-associated proteins, EBNA3A, EBNA3B and EBNA3C, are a family of latent antigens which share limited but significant amino-acid sequence homology predominantly in their amino terminal regions [110]. They have the same gene structure and are arranged in tandem in the EBV genome [109]. Recently, it was shown that BL cells latently infected with EBV provide significant protection from programmed cell death induced by a variety of cytotoxic agents [57, 94, 111]. Studies on EBV latent gene expression patterns in various EBV-positive BL-derived cell lines suggested that the EBNA3 family might play a crucial role in B-cell survival and transformation. Delecluse et al. generated recombinant viruses using a bacterial artificial chromosome (BAC) system to evaluate the contribution made by each of the EBNA3 proteins in B-cell survival [57]. EBV recombinants were produced with deletions in the individual EBNA3 genes and, importantly, viruses in which the deleted EBNA3 gene was restored to the wt viral genome (revertants) [57]. These viruses were used to infect EBV-negative BL cells. Several experiments with EBNA3-knockout (KO) viruses in BL31 cells after exposure to different cytotoxic drugs revealed that cell survival was dependent on both EBNA3A and EBNA3C, which correlated with a significant down-regulation of the three isoforms of Bim, BimEL (extra-long), BimL (long) and BimS (short) [57]. These findings suggest a model which described the contribution of EBV to the pathogenesis of BL. EBV nuclear proteins, EBNA3A and EBNA3C (but not EBNA3B) are necessary to establish LCLs [112], and their expression may be involved in the resistance of BL cells to cytotoxic drugs. The regulation of Bim was observed predominantly at the RNA level, with little evidence of post-translational Bim stabilization by EBV [113]. The molecular mechanism by which Bim is regulated has not been completely elucidated.

LMP1

The Epstein–Barr virus latent membrane protein 1 (LMP1) is critical for EBV-induced B-cell immortalization and transformation [114]. Expression of LMP1 induces phenotypic changes of B cells and also activates cellular genes like CD40 or ICAM1/CD54, NFkB, c-jun N-terminal-kinase (JNK), and the STAT signaling pathway [113]. This protein is abundantly expressed during the lytic cycle of viral replication [115]. LMP1 possesses six hydrophobic transmembrane domains in its protein structure that enable ligand-independent aggregation in the plasma membrane important for altering cell growth and cellular gene activation [116]. This cellular gene activation is permitted through two major effector domains like, C-terminal activation regions (CTAR) 1 and 2 [117, 118]. The C-terminal activation region1 contributes to the initial induction of lymphocyte transformation and NFkB activation and also interacts with tumour necrosis factor receptor-associated factor (TRAF) [119]. It was also reported that CTAR2 is critical for long-term growth of lymphoblastoid cell lines [118]. This domain was proved to interact with TNF receptor-associated death domain protein (TRADD) and is essential for activation of NFkB and JNK [117, 120]. EBV suppresses the cellular apoptotic program important for establishment of latent infection and the development of viral associated neoplasia. Furthermore, expression of LMP1 in BL cell lines leads to increased mRNA levels of bfl-1, the cellular anti-apoptotic gene [121]. Moreover, ectopic expression of Bfl-1 in an EBV-positive cell line induces a latency type 1 program and protects against apoptosis induced by growth factor deprivation [122]. A recent report demonstrated that LMP1 can activate the bfl-1 promoter activity through interactions with components of the tumour necrosis factor receptor (TNFR)/CD40 signaling pathway in BL-derived cell lines [122].

LMP2A

LMP2A influences the balance of survival factors in B lymphocytes and may contribute functionally to BL-associated pathogenesis. Low levels of LMP2A transcripts were detected in fresh tumour biopsies supporting the hypothesis that LMP2A protects B cells from apoptosis which is induced by deregulated c-MYC in human BL cell lines [123]. Additionally, studies using transgenic mice revealed a functional role for LMP2A in development of BL [124]. It was reported that LMP2A induces a BCR-like signal in absence of functional BCR [63]. Previous studies have shown that LMP2A plays a major role in activation of PI3K/Akt/mTOR signaling pathway [125]. Akt was identified as one of the downstream targets of LMP2A in B cells [126], and LMP2A expression induces PI3K dependent AKT phosphorylation [127]. Additionally, expression of c-Myc in association with LMP2A increases the probability of acquiring a mutation in p53 in EBV-positive cells [123]. Therefore, LMP2A is probably an important component of the missing link between EBV and BL. Moreover, LMP2A was found to increase the pro-survival levels of Bcl family members in B lymphocytes [123].

Cellular Factors That Contribute to Lymphomagenesis

Translocation of c-Myc and Burkitt's Lymphoma Pathogenesis

c-Myc is a major transcription factor which plays a crucial role in many cellular processes like-growth, proliferation and apoptosis [128, 129]. Interestingly, c-Myc-induced apoptosis was found as a key phenomenon in BL cells as c-Myc expression levels above a threshold induces apoptosis of these cells [130]. However, c-Myc potently drives S phase progression in somatic cells [131]. Therefore, c-myc expression is tightly regulated and immediately sensitive to external stimuli. In case of normal cells, c-Myc exerts pro-proliferative effects by the upregulation of cyclins including, D and E and down-regulation of p27 [30]. In addition, over-expression of c-Myc in B cells leads to induction of p53 or ARF and results in induction of apoptosis [132]. It was also demonstrated that in mouse cells, the product of CDKN2A (INK4a-ARF) locus, p19ARF80 stabilizes p53 by forming a complex with and antagonizing MDM2, a key negative regulator of p53 [133, 134]. In human, the p14ARF protein is a homolog of the ARF protein [135]. Interestingly, deregulation of c-Myc is implicated in a number of human malignancies which occurs through gene translocation or amplification, mRNA stabilization, enhanced translation or protein stabilization [136]. Different forms of BL are strongly associated with specific chromosomal translocations that result in the juxtaposition of the c-myc locus on chromosome 8 and various immunoglubulin (lg) loci located on chromosome 14, 22, or 2 [137, 138]. These chromosomal translocations lead to deregulated expression of the c-myc gene [139, 140], because of structural alterations present in the 5′ regulatory portion of the translocated gene [141, 142]. Additionally, a number of transcriptional regulatory factors from the lg loci also influence c-myc expression [139]. Deregulated expression of the c-myc gene plays a pathogenic role in BL and in analogous B-cell tumours in several animal species [143]. This was also shown in studies, involving the transfection of an activated c-myc gene into murine B lymphocytes [144], and in vivo studies using transgenic mice carrying activated c-myc genes in their B cells [145]. Those experiments indicate that c-myc activation per se does not lead to transformation, and that additional, most likely genetic, alterations are required for tumour development. Lombardi et al. observed that EBV infection and c-myc activation are sufficient for tumorigenic conversion of human B cells in vitro, strongly supporting the hypothesis that these same two pathogenic steps may be involved in the in vivo development of BL [146]. It is well established that higher levels of c-Myc expression facilitates enhanced protein synthesis and energy metabolism, reduction of cell adhesion, stimulation of angiogenic property, promotes genomic instability and metastasis potential towards lymphomagenesis [147]. This growth promoting activity of c-Myc is counteracted by its capacity to induce programmed cell death via activation of ARF [148]. ARF stabilizes p53 by antagonizing MDM2, which results in transcriptional activation of the pro-apoptotic targets of p53 like, NOXA, PUMA and BAX [149]. The majority of BL tumours and derived cell lines carry mutations that result in deregulation of the p53/MDM2/ARF signaling pathway [149] and threonine 58 mutation blocks the ability of c-Myc protein to induce the expression of the apoptotic BCL-2 family member BIM [131]. BIM interacts with the anti-apoptotic protein BCL-2, inhibiting its function and appears to be an important regulator of apoptosis [150]. The exact mechanism by which MYC activates BIM is not fully understood and recent studies demonstrated that EBV-infected cell lines express lower levels of BIM than parental lines, suggesting that a latent EBV product blocks apoptosis by down-regulating the expression of BIM [151]. Interestingly, the anti-apoptotic kinase, PIM-1 was also reported to be hyperactive in BL and induces MDM2 in these cells resulting in the destabilization of p53 [152]. Importantly, BL cells with inactivating TP53 mutations appear to be devoid of MYC mutations [108]. Furthermore, once inactivating TP53 mutations are present there is no longer a requirement for further lesions in MYC to block apoptosis. Additionally, mutations that disrupt the nuclear localization signal of RB-related genes like, RBL2 (RB2/p130) have also been reported in endemic BL, which correlates with increased cellular proliferation [153], and alterations in p130 may drive proliferation prior to translocation of the MYC gene [131].

Deregulation of p53 and Burkitt's Lymphoma

Deregulation of c-myc appears to be one of the essential features of BL. Additional genetic and epigenetic alterations have been detected in BL tumours or derived cell lines that affect the p53 and Rb signaling pathways and are thought to be crucial in pathogenesis of this disease [154]. Thirty percent of endemic BL tumours and up to 70% of long-established BL cell lines carry p53 mutations [154]. Furthermore, those endemic BLs carrying wild-type p53 frequently carry some genetic alterations at other genes involved in the p53 and RB pathways, such as over-expression of the MDM2, silencing of p16INK4A through promoter methylation and deletion, and in a few cases inactivation of the tumour suppressor p14ARF through homozygous deletion [155]. Over-expression of MDM2, due to enhanced translation, results in inactivation of wild-type p53 in BL cells [156]. These findings strongly suggest that disruption of the p53 signaling pathway contributes to BL development [154, 157, 158]. In EBV-negative BL cells, reactivation of p53, by reducing MDM2 protein levels, led to apoptosis [158]. Moreover, nutlin-3, a potent antagonist of MDM2, activates the p53 signaling pathway in BL cell lines harbouring wild-type p53, regardless of EBV status. Nevertheless, nutlin-3 strongly induced apoptosis in EBV-negative or latency I-associated EBV-positive BL cells, whereas latency III-associated EBV-positive BL cells were more resistant [158].

Rb Function is Dysregulated in BL Cells

The Rb/p105 gene is a well-known prototypical tumour suppressor gene identified as one of the first genes which belongs to the retinoblastoma (RB) family [159]. The Rb family consists of pRb/p105, p107 and pRb2/p130 which are structurally and functionally related [160]. These proteins have major roles in gene regulatory networks that govern the cellular response to anti-mitogenic signals. The deregulation of these proteins contribute towards the malignant transformation of cells [161]. Interestingly, pRb/p105 is expressed frequently in BL; however, the Rb pathway is inactivated in a large fraction of BL tumours [159]. In most cases, inactivation of p16 by promoter methylation, homozygous deletion or point mutations have been observed [154]. Moreover, some reports have been shown that the pRb-related protein pRb2/p130 is mutated in its nuclear localization signal in BL cell lines as well as in primary tumours [153]. This fact allows for the possibility that inactivation of pRb2/p130 renders BL cells more susceptible to malignant transformation by activated c-Myc [162]. Additionally, missense mutations of c-Myc have altered interactions with p107 during lymphomagenesis [163]. It should be noted, however, that analysis of AIDS-related lymphomas revealed no mutations in the RB2/p130 gene [164] and a high percentage of cells, expressing nuclear pRb2/p130 have enhanced proliferative activity [164]. These observations suggest that a potent, molecular mechanism of Rb regulation is linked to viral-mediated oncogenesis in BL cells.

Deregulation of Cellular Signaling Pathways Associated with Burkitt's Lymphoma

EBV viral onco-proteins are capable of altering a number of cellular signal transduction pathways. These EBV latent proteins play prominent roles in deriving virus-mediated oncogenesis. They can trigger several signaling cascades which alter cellular growth and survival. These viral oncoproteins can stimulate a number of signal transduction pathways such as, NF-kB, JNK, JAK/STAT, PI3K/Akt, ERK1/2, and p38 mitogen-activated protein kinase (MAPK) [165]. Additionally, they can regulate downstream genes which are functionally related to different biological processes. These deregulated cellular signaling can contribute to the development of BL. Here we will discuss the molecular interactions of EBV latent proteins with cellular host factors (Fig. 10.1), which contribute significantly to the modulation of cellular signal transduction pathways.

JAK-STAT Signaling

The EBV latency antigens, EBNA-1, EBNA-2 and LMP-1, have been shown to play critical roles in B-lymphocyte transformation [91, 167]. The LMP1 protein is composed of a short cytoplasmic N-terminus domain of 24 amino acids, six transmembrane domains of 186 amino acids and also a cytoplasmic C-terminus domain of 200 amino acids [168]. The six transmembrane domains are essential for LMP-1 aggregation in the cell membrane as well as cellular signal transduction [169]. The long cytosolic C-terminal domain contains the C-terminal activating regions (CTAR)-1 and -2 [170]. These domains play a major role in LMP1 contribution to EBV mediated B-cell transformation and immortalization [117]. Interestingly, the region between CTAR-1 and -2 (CTAR-3) was also found to induce the JAK/STAT signaling pathway [171]. LMP-1 mimics a constitutively active tumour necrosis factor receptor (TNF-R), and by this constitutive activation contributes to B-cell

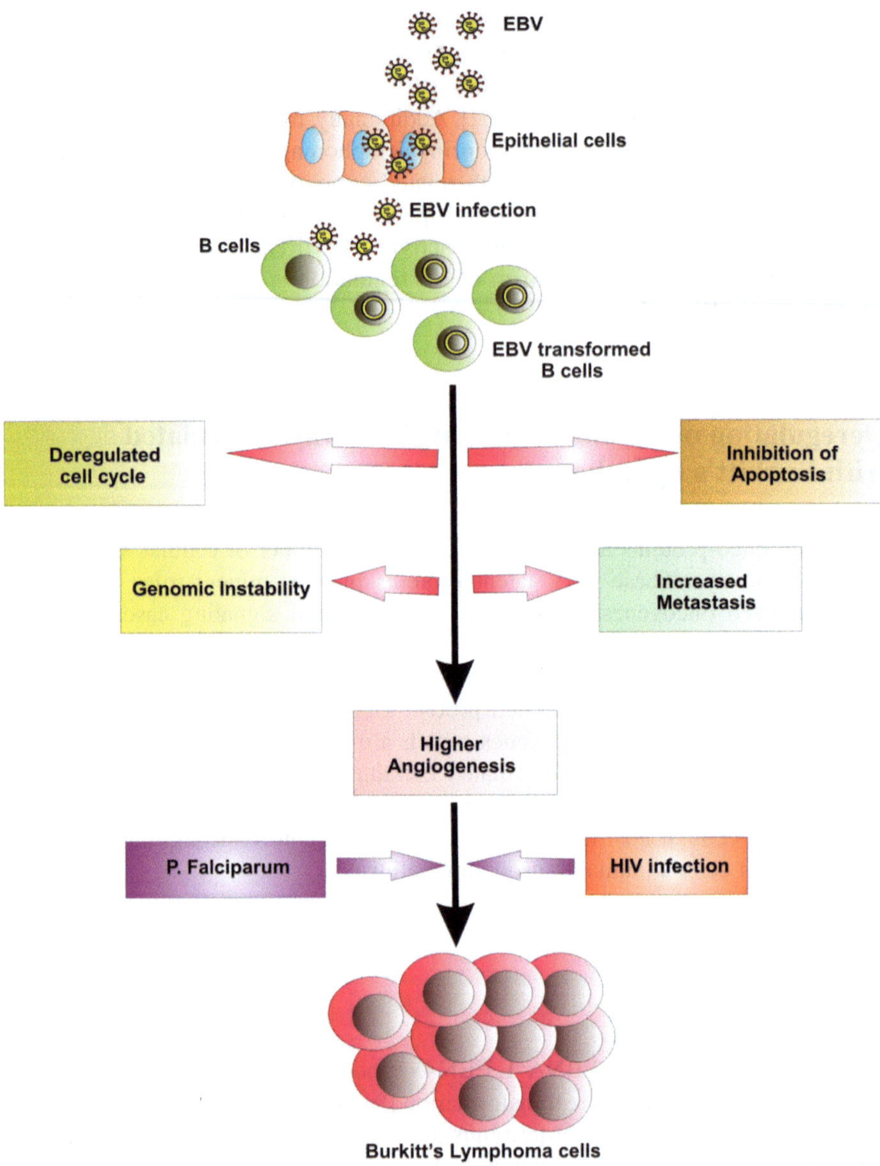

Fig. 10.1 EBV latency proteins modulate major cellular signal transduction pathways [166]. Viral proteins interact with different cellular proteins to deregulate their signaling cascades. This eventually leads to the formation of Burkitt's lymphoma by abnormal cell proliferation and inhibition of the apoptotic process

immortalization and transformation [113, 172]. Interestingly, IL-21 can also induce the JAK/STAT signaling pathway and so regulate expression of the EBV latency proteins EBNA2 and LMP1 in BL cell line Jijoye, as well as in B95-8 transformed lymphoblastoid cells [173]. They also suggested that intact JAK/STAT signaling was required for IL-21-mediated regulation of EBNA2 and LMP1 expression in EBV positive cells [173].

MAPK Kinase Pathway

Three genetically distinct groups of mitogen-activated protein kinase (MAPK), including ERK, JNK/SAPK and p38 MAPK, were identified in mammalian cells all activated by a kinase cascade [174]. Recent studies revealed that activation of the ERK cascade is generally responsible for survival or proinflammatory processes, whereas JNK signaling exerts the apoptotic response [175]. These MAPK pathways are implicated in regulation of stress-induced apoptosis [176]. Both JNK and p38 are activated in response to a variety of stress agents including ionizing radiation [177]. Importantly, some reports have provided evidence to show that EBV-positive BL is associated with high levels of MAPK activation and high levels of ROS generation when compared with EBV-negative BL [178]. Latent EBV can be reactivated by different stimuli, including tumour promoters, *n*-butyrate and antibodies against cell surface immunoglobulins (sIg) [179]. Cross-linking with sIg can induce MAPK signaling pathways through phosphorylation of MAPK [180]. Phosphorylation of MAPK triggers intracellular signaling cascades which are involved in proliferation, differentiation and apoptosis of B-cells [181, 182]. Notably, LMP1 and LMP2A can both modulate the signaling activities of MAPK in BL cell lines [183].

PI3K/Akt Pathway

The serine/threonine kinase Akt or PKB promotes cellular proliferation, survival and apoptosis in a wide range of cell types [184]. Akt is a well-known downstream effector molecule of PI3-kinase [185]. Akt phosphorylates a number of signaling molecules involved in a number of major cellular processes [186, 187]. Akt phosphorylates the Bcl-2 family member BAD, to promote cellular survival [186]. Thus, PI3-K/Akt signaling pathway is involved in regulation of cell proliferation and survival in a wide range of different malignancies. In EBV-immortalized B-cells, PI3-K/Akt signal transduction also plays a crucial role in both cell survival and proliferation [188]. PI3-K/Akt pathway activation cooperates with EBV proteins in B-cell transformation. Latent membrane protein (LMP) 2A activates the PI3-K/Akt pathway and inhibits TGF-beta-induced apoptosis in BL and gastric carcinoma cell lines [189]. LMP2A can also contribute to EBV-associated neoplasia by regulating β-catenin signaling pathways [127]. LMP1 can also promote cell survival through these pathways. In the context of EBV lytic infection, BRLF1, but not BZLF1 has a contributory role in PI3-K/Akt activation and studies have also demonstrated that PI3-K is a major determinant of responsiveness to the B-cell antigen receptor (BCR)-mediated

EBV activation [189]. These findings provide important evidence for the role of PI3-K/Akt signaling pathway in EBV-mediated growth and survival of BL cells.

Notch Signaling

Signal transduction through members of the Notch signaling pathway has multiple roles in cell fate determination. This family of proteins is conserved in evolution from nematodes to human [190]. The Notch signaling pathway in mammals includes four different receptors, Notch1-4, and five ligands including Jagged1, 2 and Delta-like1, 3, 4 [191]. The Notch receptor is activated by direct interaction with its ligands expressed on neighbouring cells [192]. Sequentially, the intracellular domain of the Notch receptor (NIC) is released from the membrane after receptor cleavage which is executed by the ADAM/TACE protease and gamma-secretase complexes [193]. NIC translocates to the nucleus and associates with the transcription repressor RBP-Jk, which results in transactivation of the RBP-Jk responsive promoter through recruitment of the co-activators of the Mastermind-like (MAML) family [194]. The N-terminal Delta-Serrate-Lag2 (DSL) domains are extracellular domains which are essential for Notch-binding [195].

Notch signaling is linked to multiple functions during mammalian haematopoiesis and lymphopoiesis [196]. One important function is the regulation of T-cell commitment from a common lymphoid precursor at the expense of B-cell development in the thymus [149]. Notch signaling also controls marginal zone B-cell differentiation in the spleen [56] and deregulated Notch signaling plays a pivotal role in T-cell malignancies [197]. Importantly, EBV antigens have derived strategies for usurping this function of Notch. Involvement of EBV protein EBNA2 with the transcription factor RBP-Jk was shown to be essential for B-cell transformation [198, 199]. EBNA2 activates B cells by up-regulating the B-cell activation markers CD21 and CD23 [199]. Thus, deregulated Notch signaling may promote the immortalization of B cells through usurpation of RBP-Jk interaction. Notch-1 can mimic EBNA2's ability to activate CD21 expression and down-regulate Igμ transcription in BL cell lines infected with a mutant EBV lacking EBNA2 [200]. Interestingly, CD23 and LMP1 were not activated by Notch-1 [200], and activated Notch-1 can transiently maintain the proliferation of LCLs [201]. These LCLs do not have EBNA2 but express viral oncoprotein LMP1 suggesting that activated Notch-1 can partially substituted for EBNA2 [202].

Wnt Signaling

Activation of the wnt/wingless signaling cascade is an important contributor to a number of malignancies. β-catenin, the downstream transcriptional regulatory factor is a critical component of the wnt signaling pathway [203]. To activate transcription, β-catenin is stabilized and translocated to the nucleus where it binds to other transcription factors, like-T-cell factor (Tcf), or lymphocyte enhancer factor (Lef) [204]. In *Xenopus laevis* and *Drosophila melanogaster*, β-catenin–Tcf/Lef complexes regulate a number of processes involved in their development. In mammalian systems, β-catenin–Tcf/Lef complexes have been shown to regulate the expression of c-*myc* and cyclin D1 [205], as well as genes important for cell growth and tumour progression, such as MMP7 [206], gastrin [207], connexin [208] and WISP proteins [209]. β-Catenin has significant roles in regulation of leukemic cell adhesion, proliferation and survival [210]. Moreover, the specific roles of β-catenin are linked to lymphocyte proliferation and the development of lymphomas but the underlying mechanisms are yet to be fully explored. β-Catenin activity is tightly regulated by targeted ubiquitination and proteasomal degradation by glycogen synthase kinase-3β (GSK-3β) [211]. Studies have revealed that during EBV type I latency, when EBNA1 is predominantly expressed; β-catenin is degraded via a proteasome-dependent process [212]. However, β-catenin was found stabilized in type III latency, in which all EBV latent proteins are expressed [213]. Interestingly, bone marrow B cells from LMP2A transgenic mice showed a significant induction of TCF mRNA expression, compared with B cells from non-transgenic littermates, signifying that LMP2A activates the Wnt signaling pathway in vivo [209]. It is also interesting that BCR activation induces β-catenin activity by inhibiting GSK-3β, which indicates that LMP2A exploits normal B-cell signaling to mimic an activated BCR [214]. Therefore, LMP2A utilizes ubiquitination to regulate the turnover of β-catenin or other proteins which are involved in Wnt signaling to maintain B-cell survival during EBV latency [132].

EBV-Mediated Genomic Instability Contributes to Progression of Burkitt's Lymphoma

Genomic instability is considered a hallmark of malignant transformation and tumour progression. It promotes the fixation of multiple genetic changes required for evolution of a pre-malignant cell clone to invasive cancers [212, 215]. This requires an increased rate of mutations combined with failure to correct mutagenic lesions through the inactivation of DNA repair pathways. Two types of genetic alterations are commonly seen in cancerous cells, these are microsatellite instability (MIN) and chromosome instability (CIN) [216]. Chromosomal aberrations such as the reciprocal translocations, deletions, inversions and duplications can be transmitted to progeny, while non-clonal aberrations, including di-centric chromosomes, rings, fragments, satellite associations, double minutes and chromatid gaps are often lethal and are therefore generated de novo at each cell cycle [148]. Interestingly, clonal and non-clonal chromosomal aberrations have been observed in EBV-positive BL [217, 218], and cells carrying EBV are also associated with a 3–10-fold increase of di-centric chromosomes, chromosome fragments and chromatid gaps by scoring non-clonal chromosomal aberrations in metaphase plates from EBV-positive and negative BL cell lines [219]. A distinct role for the virus was suggested by comparison of paired EBV-negative and in vitro EBV-converted cells line. Most importantly, non-clonal chromosomal aberrations were decreased in EBV-loss variants of EBV-positive BLs and reappeared in their converted sublines, suggesting that the phenotype is reversible and, hence, dependent on the expression of one or more viral products [148].

Other Risk Factors Associated with Burkitt's Lymphoma Progression

Malaria

Extensive studies on EBV associated lymphomagenesis revealed that EBV and *P. falciparum* infections are two important polymicrobial stimuli which are important for malignant progression in endemic BL [220–222]. However, reports have indicated that the presence of holoendemic malaria is associated with increased risk of endemic BL in equatorial Africa rather than EBV infection in early stage of life [223]. Recently, two hypothetical models were proposed to explain the impact of holoendemic malaria on EBV latency and immunity in children. These are suppression of EBV-specific T-cell immunity and the expansion of the latently infected B-cell pool [224]. In 1983, Moss and colleagues first observed impaired EBV-specific T-cell responses in adults living in malaria prone holoendemic regions of Papua New Guinea [225]. Additionally, EBV loads are higher in areas of holoendemic malaria compared to areas where malaria is sporadic [226]. Furthermore, an increased persistence in children is seen with a history of severe malaria due to higher viral reactivation [227]. Endemic BL also appears in elderly individuals who have migrated from malaria-free high altitude region to lower, malaria-endemic region [228], and EBV viral load in blood is reported to be highest in children from malaria endemic areas [226]. There are three possible consequences for EBV and malaria infections in BL: (a) EBV infection occurs first followed by malarial infection; (b) EBV infection and malarial infection occurs simultaneously; (c) Malarial infection is followed by EBV infection. Moreover, the highest parasitic loads were found in very young children [224]. Recently, studies have shown that the malaria parasite *P. falciparum* can directly activate B cells via a cysteine-rich inter-domain region 1α (C1DR1α) on the *P. falciparum* erythrocyte membrane protein 1 (PfEMP1), which binds to surface Ig [229]. The activation of B cells by C1DR1α and subsequent protection from apoptosis has been postulated to play a role in enhancing survival of GC B cells bearing oncogenic mutations [131]. It was generally thought that the association between malaria and BL arises from a combination of immunosuppression and B-cell activation. Interestingly, cytotoxic T-cell-mediated control over the outgrowth of EBV-infected B cells is impaired during acute malaria infection [230]. This suggested that peripheral EBV loads may reach levels five times higher during acute malaria compared to healthy individuals [226]. The findings of Whittle and co-workers also demonstrated that peripheral blood lymphocytes from adults and children with acute malaria were unable to control outgrowth of EBV-transformed cells in colony regression assays in vitro [231], and *P. falciparum* may stimulate EBV latently infected memory B cells via Toll like receptor-9 engagement [224]. Furthermore, the expression of interleukin-10 (IL-10) was increased after *P. falciparum* infection leading to TLR9 induction in naïve B cells [232]. Kataaha and co-workers observed that addition of P. falciparum extracts to peripheral blood lymphocytes ex vivo increased the efficiency of EBV-induced cell transformation [233]. Thus, *P. falciparum* infection is an additional factor which can contribute to endemic BL pathogenesis (Fig. 10.1). In addition the influence of malaria in stimulating B-cell expansion is only one contributor; however, there is the possibility that mosquito-borne arboviruses are another risk factor for endemic BL [235].

AIDS

Burkitt and Burkitt-like/atypical BL are the largest group of HIV-associated non-Hodgkin lymphomas, comprising up to 35–50% of these neoplasms in some cases [236]. According to pathological classifications, BL was placed as the second most common subtype after immunoblastic DLBCL [237]. The diagnosis of Burkitt or Burkitt-like lymphoma requires a medium-sized CD10-positive B-cell population with a high proliferative rate and demonstration of c-Myc translocation [238]. Involvement of peripheral blood was found to be less common in HIV-infected patients compared with HIV-negative patients in BL [239]. The cell population in BL was observed as characteristically uniform in nature, with indistinct nucleoli, whereas Burkitt-like lymphomas display a greater degree of nuclear pleomorphism and may comprise more prominent nucleoli [237]. A subset of BL may show unique plasmacytoid differentiation, a morphological variation that appears only in AIDS patients [237]. In the plasmacytoid variant, the cells have eccentrically placed nuclei and abundant cytoplasm which contains immunoglobulin [237]. HIV-associated BL is characterized by multiple genetic lesions. The relative significance of each in the pathogenesis of this lymphoma is not fully understood. Additionally, the translocations involving c-Myc, point mutations within the regulatory regions associated with c-Myc, and within the p53 gene are common [240]. Male predominance was observed in sporadic BL (sBL) and AIDS-related BL, suggesting that males may be genetically predisposed to BL, and is independent of the geographic origin of the cases, and of antecedent illnesses, including EBV, malaria, or human immunodeficiency virus [241]. BL tumours make up about 30% of AIDS-associated lymphomas and EBV is more often found in HIV-associated BL tumours than in sporadic BL tumours [74]. In Western nations, 30–40% of HIV-associated BL tumour cells harbour EBV and the presence of EBV-encoded RNA (EBER) was observed by in situ hybridization technique in tumour cells in about 30% cases of BL [98]. Similar to sporadic or epidemic forms of BL, or in HIV-associated EBER-positive disease, the major viral antigens LMP-1 and EBNA-2 are not typically detected [237]. This phenomenon is in contrast to EBER-positive immunoblastic DLBCL and PEL, which shows the expression of these EBV-associated viral oncogenes [237]. Thus EBV may have distinctly different roles in oncogenesis in these different types of lymphomas. It is also interesting that although BL is common in HIV-infected patients, it is not associated with other forms of immunosuppression [242]. This may indicate that the oncogenic properties of HIV itself can play a greater role in pathogenesis of this highly aggressive tumour when compared with EBV, or that there are additional mechanisms yet to be uncovered. Deregulation of cell cycle protein functions has been implicated in the development of BL. Inactivating mutations of the tumour suppressor gene RBL2 (Rb2/p130) were frequently found in endemic and sporadic BL cases [162]. By contrast, in HIV-associated cases, abnormal over-expression of wild-type RBL2 was observed [164]. This finding, in conjunction with studies indicating that the function of Rb2/p130 in the control of the G0/G1 transition can be negated by the physical interaction with the HIV encoded Tat protein [243]. This may suggest a pivotal role for HIV proteins acting synergistically with c-Myc activation in the pathogenesis of BL. HIV, by reducing the effectiveness of T-cell based immune response to oncogenic viruses can act as an indirect co-factor in the aetiology of BL [244], or by reducing the EBV-specific T-cell function, leading to proliferation of EBV infected B cells and eventual tumour formation [245]. Studies have suggested that either reducing HIV incidence, or treatment of HIV with antiretroviral drugs, may lead to a reduction of BL incidence in children [246]. Therefore, HIV infection and AIDS can also be considered a prime contributor to accelerate the pathogenesis of EBV associated BL (Fig. 10.2).

Treatment Strategy of Burkitt's Lymphoma

Over the past few years, BL research has focused on identifying more efficacious but less toxic regimens. Additionally, the rapidly growing knowledge providing molecular diagnosis of this disease has enabled the development of novel treatment options. Systemic chemotherapy is one of the treatments of choice in BL [28]. A careful patient history, physical examination and routine laboratory studies, gallium-67 scintigraphy, CAT scanning, and abdominal ultrasonography are all useful techniques for identifying tumour sites as well as follow-up examination in response to therapy [247]. The gallium concentrates preferentially in tumour nodules and is the most sensitive of the three studies [248]. The CAT scan and ultrasonogram are important for localization of the tumours in the abdomen and is also important in preparing for surgical removal [249]. In addition, the serum lactate dehydrogenase level also reflects the tumour burden and hence becomes a sensitive indicator of tumour regression and relapse [250]. BL was known as one of the few B-cell malignancies in which the treatment regimen for adults has been modeled on the basis of

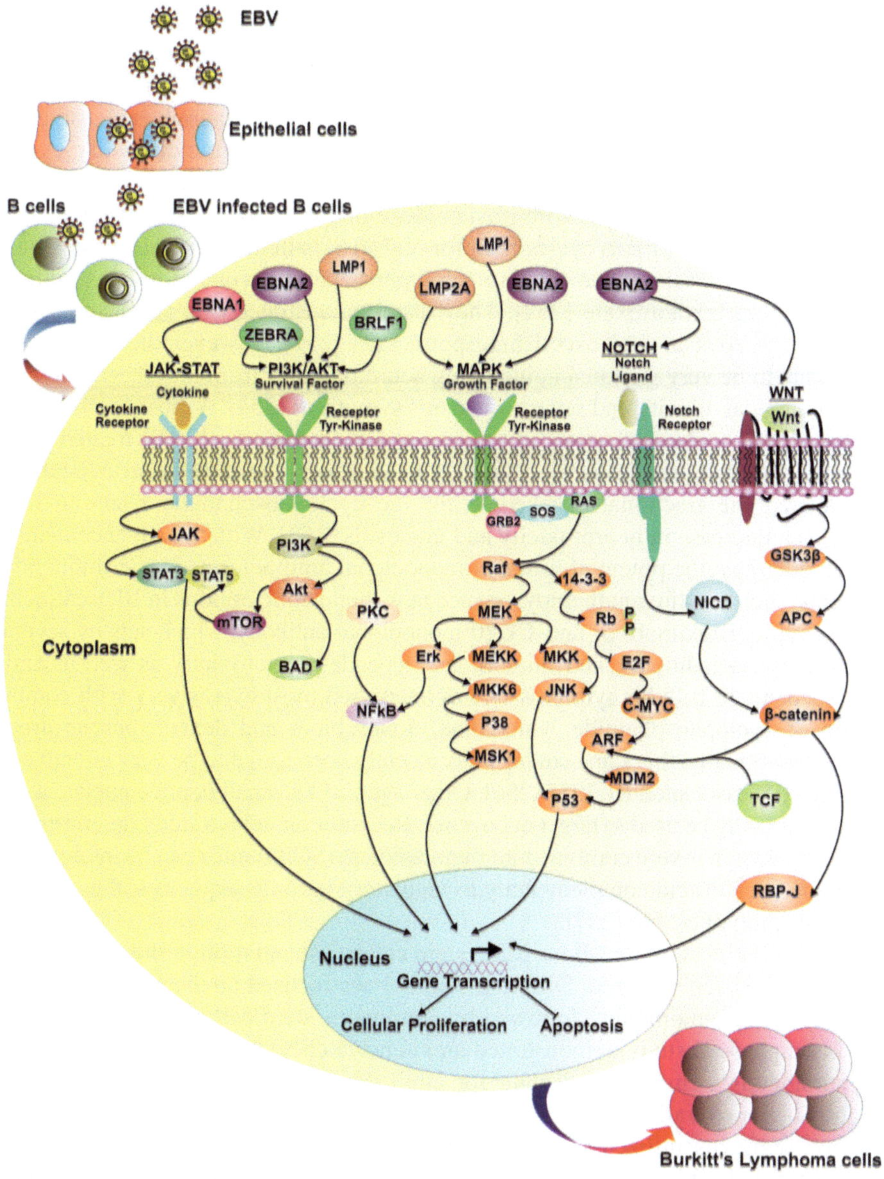

Fig. 10.2 EBV infection contributes to Burkitt's lymphoma progression by deregulation of a range of cellular processes which lead to uncontrolled proliferation of infected B-cells. After infection of the oropharyngeal epithelial cells EBV infects B-cells to establish latency. This phenomenon contributes to aberrant cell-cycle progression, genomic instability, higher angiogenic rate, abnormal cellular metastasis, and inhibition of programmed cell death [234]. Additional factors such as Malaria and HIV infection can also accelerate the oncogenic process

paediatric regimens. BL was associated with poor outcomes before the advent of high intense chemotherapy due to its high proliferative rate [251]. The prognosis for many patients with BL has changed significantly with the introduction of short, intensive chemotherapeutic regimens [251]. This advancement has significantly improved clinical outcomes for the BL patients. A report by Magrath et al., suggests that in cases of high-grade B-cell lymphomas, chemotherapeutic drugs like-cyclophosphamide, vincristine, doxorubicin, high-dose methotrexate and intrathecal therapy should be alternated with ifosfamide, etoposide, high-dose cytarabine and intrathecal therapy for two cycles each for high-risk patients, whereas those with a low risk should receive three cycles of cyclophosphamide, vincristine, doxorubicin and high-dose methotrexate [252]. They also demonstrated that short courses of intensive therapy can elicit excellent response rates [251]. However, the toxicity rate was found to be very significant, including neurotoxicities from intrathecal therapy, haematological toxicity and severe mucositis symptoms [251]. A recent report demonstrated that a phase II study utilizing a modified regimen [252], treated adult patients with reduced doses of systemic methotrexate and intrathecal cytarabine, and altered the fractionated schedule for the cyclophosphamide resulting in a significant decrease in neurotoxicity and mucositis [253]. With the advancement of immunotherapy, the potential usage of monoclonal antibodies and other biological reagents, such as adjuvant therapy, opened new therapeutic options in BL treatment. For example, rituximab, or anti-CD20 monoclonal antibody, which acts by several mechanisms including the activation of cell-dependent cytotoxicity as well as antibody-dependent cellular cytotoxicity, has been used most extensively with combination of cyclophosphamide, vincristine, doxorubicin and dexamethasone drugs [254]. Additionally, this same strategy has recently been found to be very effective in treating HIV-associated BL [255, 256]. Other agents like, small peptide nucleic acids can theoretically be used to target oncogenes. Recently, an in vivo study demonstrated that BL grown in severe combined immunodeficient (SCID) mice can be inhibited by a peptide nucleic acid complementary to regulatory intronic sequences, thus inhibiting production of c-Myc [257].

Several therapeutic strategies using stem cell transplantation in the treatment of BL have also been explored. Different studies have focused on the potential benefit of high-dose chemotherapy followed by autologous stem cell transplant. A recent report on phase II study demonstrated an intensive chemotherapy course followed by autologous stem cell transplant for adult patients resulted in comparable or slightly better overall survival rate for those with BL compared with current chemotherapy regimens utilized for comparable-aged patients [258]. Some additional reports were also found providing retrospective evaluations of allogeneic transplantation for BL. The reports demonstrated lower relapse rates for allogeneic transplant patients compared with autologous transplant recipients, but unfortunately, the mortality rate was found to be higher in allogeneic transplant patients [259]. Anti-viral therapy is also a very useful approach for treatment of viral positive BL. Latently infected BL cells with EBV remained unaffected by conventional anti-viral drugs like, acyclovir and ganciclovir [260]. They lack the expression of the viral thymidine kinase (TK) necessary to convert nucleoside analogues to their monophosphate form [261]. Moreover, it was observed that exposure to arginine butyrate can induce expression of EBV TK and sensitize the EBV-infected cells to these drugs [262]. Other drugs like cidofovir may also target expression of EBV latent genes, as some studies have demonstrated that cidofovir can down-regulate LMP1 expression and also decrease Bcl-2 expression levels in BL cells [262]. Further studies into the use of viral specific therapies for use against EBV-associated BL would provide another avenue for development as well as increased specificity and efficacy important for future targeted therapies.

Future Perspective

BL was first described as a common African childhood tumour. This exceptional tumour would quickly become an important paradigm in the field of cancer research. Since the geographical distribution pattern of BL coincided with the distribution of hyperendemic and holoendemic malaria, it was strongly suggested that malaria or other infectious agents carried by mosquitoes were likely responsible for the onset of BL [263]. The following, discovery of Epstein–Barr virus (EBV) in BL cells led to studies linking EBV infection and BL pathogenesis [264]. Extensive studies are ongoing in the field of BL research. However, to date the molecular contribution of EBV to the pathogenesis of BL remains a paradox. The functional aspects of EBV-mediated BL pathogenesis are yet to be unveiled. It is necessary also to elucidate the function of the viral microRNAs expressed in BL cells [265], and how they relate to the cellular and viral expressed genes. Further studies are required to understand the oncogenic potential of EBV antigens using transgenic models. Upon EBV infection, cellular proteins involved in regulation of multiple cellular processes like, apoptosis, differentiation, proliferation, ubiquitination, cell-cycle progression, autophagy and migration may be deregulated by viral antigens. These functional dysregulations are likely contributors to the uncontrolled cellular proliferation of infected B-cells thus facilitating the EBV-mediated progression of BL.

References

1. Epstein MA, Achong BG, Barr YM (1964) Virus Particles in Cultured Lymphoblasts from Burkitt's Lymphoma. Lancet 1:702–703
2. Burkitt D (1958) A sarcoma involving the jaws in African children. Br J Surg 46:218–223
3. Burkitt DP (1983) The discovery of Burkitt's lymphoma. Cancer 51:1777–1786
4. Bornkamm GW (2009) Epstein-Barr virus and the pathogenesis of Burkitt's lymphoma: more questions than answers. Int J Cancer 124:1745–1755
5. Burkitt D (1962) A children's cancer dependent on climatic factors. Nature 194:232–234
6. Burkitt D (1962) A "tumour safari" in East and Central Africa. Br J Cancer 16:379–386
7. van den Bosch CA (2004) Is endemic Burkitt's lymphoma an alliance between three infections and a tumour promoter? Lancet Oncol 5:738–746

8. Henle G, Henle W (1966) Immunofluorescence in cells derived from Burkitt's lymphoma. J Bacteriol 91:1248–1256
9. Henle G et al (1969) Antibodies to Epstein-Barr virus in Burkitt's lymphoma and control groups. J Natl Cancer Inst 43:1147–1157
10. Henle G, Henle W, Diehl V (1968) Relation of Burkitt's tumor-associated herpes-type virus to infectious mononucleosis. Proc Natl Acad Sci USA 59:94–101
11. Henle W, Diehl V, Kohn G, Zur Hausen H, Henle G (1967) Herpes-type virus and chromosome marker in normal leukocytes after growth with irradiated Burkitt cells. Science 157:1064–1065
12. Pope JH, Horne MK, Scott W (1968) Transformation of foetal human keukocytes in vitro by filtrates of a human leukaemic cell line containing herpes-like virus. Int J Cancer 3:857–866
13. Counter CM, Botelho FM, Wang P, Harley CB, Bacchetti S (1994) Stabilization of short telomeres and telomerase activity accompany immortalization of Epstein-Barr virus-transformed human B lymphocytes. J Virol 68:3410–3414
14. zur Hausen H et al (1970) EBV DNA in biopsies of Burkitt tumours and anaplastic carcinomas of the nasopharynx. Nature 228:1056–1058
15. Hassan R et al (2008) Clinical and demographic characteristics of Epstein-Barr virus-associated childhood Burkitt's lymphoma in Southeastern Brazil: epidemiological insights from an intermediate risk region. Haematologica 93:780–783
16. Molyneux EM et al (2012) Burkitt's lymphoma. Lancet 379(9822):1234–1244
17. Lenoir G OCG, Olweny CLM (1985) de Thé G. Epstein-Barr virus and Burkitt's lymphoma worldwide: the causal relationship revisited. IARC, Lyon
18. Parkin DMKE, Draper GJ, Masuyer E, Michaelis J, Neglia J et al (1998) International incidence of childhood cancer. IARC, Lyon
19. Makata AM, Toriyama K, Kamidigo NO, Eto H, Itakura H (1996) The pattern of pediatric solid malignant tumors in western Kenya, east Africa, 1979–1994: an analysis based on histopathologic study. Am J Trop Med Hyg 54:343–347
20. Parkin DM, Sohier R, O'Conor GT (1985) Geographic distribution of Burkitt's lymphoma. IARC Sci Publ 155–164
21. Stiller CA, Parkin DM (1990) International variations in the incidence of childhood lymphomas. Paediatr Perinat Epidemiol 4:303–324
22. Evens AM, Gordon LI (2002) Burkitt's and Burkitt-like lymphoma. Curr Treat Options Oncol 3:291–305
23. Jensen OM, Knudsen JB, McLaughlin JK, Sorensen BL (1988) The Copenhagen case–control study of renal pelvis and ureter cancer: role of smoking and occupational exposures. Int J Cancer 41:557–561
24. Parkin DM, Stiller CA, Draper GJ, Bieber CA (1988) The international incidence of childhood cancer. Int J Cancer 42:511–520
25. Abbasoglu L, Gun F, Salman FT, Celik A, Unuvar A, Gorgun O (2003) The role of surgery in intraabdominal Burkitt's lymphoma in children. Eur J Pediatr Surg 13:236–239
26. Chabner BA, Fisher RI, Young RC, DeVita VT (1980) Staging of non-Hodgkin's lymphoma. Semin Oncol 7:285–291
27. Murphy SB (1980) Classification, staging and end results of treatment of childhood non-Hodgkin's lymphomas: dissimilarities from lymphomas in adults. Semin Oncol 7:332–339
28. Ziegler JL (1981) Burkitt's lymphoma. N Engl J Med 305:735–745
29. Ziegler JL (1977) Treatment results of 54 American patients with Burkitt's lymphoma are similar to the African experience. N Engl J Med 297:75–80
30. Kelly GL, Rickinson AB (2007) Burkitt lymphoma: revisiting the pathogenesis of a virus-associated malignancy. Hematol Am Soc Hematol Educ Program 277–284
31. Diebold J (2001) Phenotype–genotype–correlation in ovarian neoplasia. Verh Dtsch Ges Pathol 85:153–160
32. Young NA, Al-Saleem T (1999) Diagnosis of lymphoma by fine-needle aspiration cytology using the revised European-American classification of lymphoid neoplasms. Cancer 87:325–345

33. McClure RF et al (2005) Adult B-cell lymphomas with Burkitt-like morphology are phenotypically and genotypically heterogeneous with aggressive clinical behavior. Am J Surg Pathol 29:1652–1660
34. Burmeister T et al (2005) Molecular heterogeneity of sporadic adult Burkitt-type leukemia/lymphoma as revealed by PCR and cytogenetics: correlation with morphology, immunology and clinical features. Leukemia 19:1391–1398
35. Gong JZ et al (2003) Burkitt lymphoma arising in organ transplant recipients: a clinicopathologic study of five cases. Am J Surg Pathol 27:818–827
36. Das DK, Gupta SK, Pathak IC, Sharma SC, Datta BN (1987) Burkitt-type lymphoma. Diagnosis by fine needle aspiration cytology. Acta Cytol 31:1–7
37. Stastny JF, Almeida MM, Wakely PE Jr, Kornstein MJ, Frable WJ (1995) Fine-needle aspiration biopsy and imprint cytology of small non-cleaved cell (Burkitt's) lymphoma. Diagn Cytopathol 12:201–207
38. Niedobitek G (1995) Patterns of Epstein-Barr virus infection in non-Hodgkin's lymphomas. J Pathol 175:259–261
39. Gregory CD, Rowe M, Rickinson AB (1990) Different Epstein-Barr virus-B cell interactions in phenotypically distinct clones of a Burkitt's lymphoma cell line. J Gen Virol 71(Pt 7):1481–1495
40. Humme S et al (2003) The EBV nuclear antigen 1 (EBNA1) enhances B cell immortalization several thousandfold. Proc Natl Acad Sci USA 100:10989–10994
41. Kennedy G, Komano J, Sugden B (2003) Epstein-Barr virus provides a survival factor to Burkitt's lymphomas. Proc Natl Acad Sci USA 100:14269–14274
42. Minsky N, Shema E, Field Y, Schuster M, Segal E, Oren M (2008) Monoubiquitinated H2B is associated with the transcribed region of highly expressed genes in human cells. Nat Cell Biol 10:483–488
43. Purwanto I, Kurnianda J, Hutajulu SH, Widayati K, Rizki M (2006) Epstein-Barr nuclear antigen-1 (EBNA-1) in diffuse large B-cell lymphoma and its relationship to the bcl-2 protein. Acta Med Indones 38:77–80
44. Sarkari F, Sanchez-Alcaraz T, Wang S, Holowaty MN, Sheng Y, Frappier L (2009) EBNA1-mediated recruitment of a histone H2B deubiquitylating complex to the Epstein-Barr virus latent origin of DNA replication. PLoS Pathog 5:e1000624
45. Schulz TF, Cordes S (2009) Is the Epstein-Barr virus EBNA-1 protein an oncogen? Proc Natl Acad Sci USA 106:2091–2092
46. Calender A, Billaud M, Aubry JP, Banchereau J, Vuillaume M, Lenoir GM (1987) Epstein-Barr virus (EBV) induces expression of B-cell activation markers on in vitro infection of EBV-negative B-lymphoma cells. Proc Natl Acad Sci USA 84:8060–8064
47. Cordier M et al (1990) Stable transfection of Epstein-Barr virus (EBV) nuclear antigen 2 in lymphoma cells containing the EBV P3HR1 genome induces expression of B-cell activation molecules CD21 and CD23. J Virol 64:1002–1013
48. Grossman SR, Johannsen E, Tong X, Yalamanchili R, Kieff E (1994) The Epstein-Barr virus nuclear antigen 2 transactivator is directed to response elements by the J kappa recombination signal binding protein. Proc Natl Acad Sci USA 91:7568–7572
49. Harada S, Yalamanchili R, Kieff E (2001) Epstein-Barr virus nuclear protein 2 has at least two N-terminal domains that mediate self-association. J Virol 75:2482–2487
50. Henkel T, Ling PD, Hayward SD, Peterson MG (1994) Mediation of Epstein-Barr virus EBNA2 transactivation by recombination signal-binding protein J kappa. Science 265:92–95
51. Lerner MR, Andrews NC, Miller G, Steitz JA (1981) Two small RNAs encoded by Epstein-Barr virus and complexed with protein are precipitated by antibodies from patients with systemic lupus erythematosus. Proc Natl Acad Sci USA 78:805–809
52. Niller HH et al (2003) The in vivo binding site for oncoprotein c-Myc in the promoter for Epstein-Barr virus (EBV) encoding RNA (EBER) 1 suggests a specific role for EBV in lymphomagenesis. Med Sci Monit 9:HY1–9
53. Toczyski DP, Steitz JA (1991) EAP, a highly conserved cellular protein associated with Epstein-Barr virus small RNAs (EBERs). EMBO J 10:459–466

54. Barth S et al (2008) Epstein-Barr virus-encoded microRNA miR-BART2 down-regulates the viral DNA polymerase BALF5. Nucleic Acids Res 36:666–675
55. Choy EY et al (2008) An Epstein-Barr virus-encoded microRNA targets PUMA to promote host cell survival. J Exp Med 205:2551–2560
56. Hemann MT, Zilfou JT, Zhao Z, Burgess DJ, Hannon GJ, Lowe SW (2004) Suppression of tumorigenesis by the p53 target PUMA. Proc Natl Acad Sci USA 101:9333–9338
57. Anderton E, Yee J, Smith P, Crook T, White RE, Allday MJ (2008) Two Epstein-Barr virus (EBV) oncoproteins cooperate to repress expression of the proapoptotic tumour-suppressor Bim: clues to the pathogenesis of Burkitt's lymphoma. Oncogene 27:421–433
58. Dawson CW, Tramountanis G, Eliopoulos AG, Young LS (2003) Epstein-Barr virus latent membrane protein 1 (LMP1) activates the phosphatidylinositol 3-kinase/Akt pathway to promote cell survival and induce actin filament remodeling. J Biol Chem 278:3694–3704
59. Eliopoulos AG, Young LS (1998) Activation of the cJun N-terminal kinase (JNK) pathway by the Epstein-Barr virus-encoded latent membrane protein 1 (LMP1). Oncogene 16:1 731–1742
60. Izumi KM, Kieff ED (1997) The Epstein-Barr virus oncogene product latent membrane protein 1 engages the tumor necrosis factor receptor-associated death domain protein to mediate B lymphocyte growth transformation and activate NF-kappaB. Proc Natl Acad Sci USA 94:12592–12597
61. Anderson LJ, Longnecker R (2009) Epstein-Barr virus latent membrane protein 2A exploits Notch1 to alter B-cell identity in vivo. Blood 113:108–116
62. Brinkmann MM, Schulz TF (2006) Regulation of intracellular signalling by the terminal membrane proteins of members of the gammaherpesvirinae. J Gen Virol 87:1047–1074
63. Caldwell RG, Wilson JB, Anderson SJ, Longnecker R (1998) Epstein-Barr virus LMP2A drives B cell development and survival in the absence of normal B cell receptor signals. Immunity 9:405–411
64. Swanson-Mungerson M, Bultema R, Longnecker R (2010) Epstein-Barr virus LMP2A imposes sensitivity to apoptosis. J Gen Virol 91:2197–2202
65. Hochberg D, Middeldorp JM, Catalina M, Sullivan JL, Luzuriaga K, Thorley-Lawson DA (2004) Demonstration of the Burkitt's lymphoma Epstein-Barr virus phenotype in dividing latently infected memory cells in vivo. Proc Natl Acad Sci USA 101:239–244
66. Klein U, Klein G, Ehlin-Henriksson B, Rajewsky K, Kuppers R (1995) Burkitt's lymphoma is a malignancy of mature B cells expressing somatically mutated V region genes. Mol Med 1:495–505
67. Babcock GJ, Decker LL, Volk M, Thorley-Lawson DA (1998) EBV persistence in memory B cells in vivo. Immunity 9:395–404
68. Joseph AM, Babcock GJ, Thorley-Lawson DA (2000) EBV persistence involves strict selection of latently infected B cells. J Immunol 165:2975–2981
69. Yates JL, Warren N, Sugden B (1985) Stable replication of plasmids derived from Epstein-Barr virus in various mammalian cells. Nature 313:812–815
70. Schaefer BC, Strominger JL, Speck SH (1995) Redefining the Epstein-Barr virus-encoded nuclear antigen EBNA-1 gene promoter and transcription initiation site in group I Burkitt lymphoma cell lines. Proc Natl Acad Sci USA 92:10565–10569
71. Kitagawa N et al (2000) Epstein-Barr virus-encoded poly(A)(–) RNA supports Burkitt's lymphoma growth through interleukin-10 induction. EMBO J 19:6742–6750
72. Nanbo A, Inoue K, Adachi-Takasawa K, Takada K (2002) Epstein-Barr virus RNA confers resistance to interferon-alpha-induced apoptosis in Burkitt's lymphoma. EMBO J 21:954–965
73. Jochner N, Eick D, Zimber-Strobl U, Pawlita M, Bornkamm GW, Kempkes B (1996) Epstein-Barr virus nuclear antigen 2 is a transcriptional suppressor of the immunoglobulin mu gene: implications for the expression of the translocated c-myc gene in Burkitt's lymphoma cells. EMBO J 15:375–382
74. Rickinson ABKE (2007) Epstein-Barr virus. Lippincott-Raven, Philadelphia
75. Zimber U et al (1986) Geographical prevalence of two types of Epstein-Barr virus. Virology 154:56–66

76. Alfieri C, Birkenbach M, Kieff E (1991) Early events in Epstein-Barr virus infection of human B lymphocytes. Virology 181:595–608
77. Abbot SD et al (1990) Epstein-Barr virus nuclear antigen 2 induces expression of the virus-encoded latent membrane protein. J Virol 64:2126–2134
78. Fahraeus R, Jansson A, Ricksten A, Sjoblom A, Rymo L (1990) Epstein-Barr virus-encoded nuclear antigen 2 activates the viral latent membrane protein promoter by modulating the activity of a negative regulatory element. Proc Natl Acad Sci USA 87:7390–7394
79. Ghosh D, Kieff E (1990) Cis-acting regulatory elements near the Epstein-Barr virus latent-infection membrane protein transcriptional start site. J Virol 64:1855–1858
80. Jin XW, Speck SH (1992) Identification of critical cis elements involved in mediating Epstein-Barr virus nuclear antigen 2-dependent activity of an enhancer located upstream of the viral BamHI C promoter. J Virol 66:2846–2852
81. Knutson JC (1990) The level of c-fgr RNA is increased by EBNA-2, an Epstein-Barr virus gene required for B-cell immortalization. J Virol 64:2530–2536
82. Laux G, Adam B, Strobl LJ, Moreau-Gachelin F (1994) The Spi-1/PU.1 and Spi-B ets family transcription factors and the recombination signal binding protein RBP-J kappa interact with an Epstein-Barr virus nuclear antigen 2 responsive cis-element. EMBO J 13:5624–5632
83. Ling PD, Rawlins DR, Hayward SD (1993) The Epstein-Barr virus immortalizing protein EBNA-2 is targeted to DNA by a cellular enhancer-binding protein. Proc Natl Acad Sci USA 90:9237–9241
84. Meitinger C, Strobl LJ, Marschall G, Bornkamm GW, Zimber-Strobl U (1994) Crucial sequences within the Epstein-Barr virus TP1 promoter for EBNA2-mediated transactivation and interaction of EBNA2 with its responsive element. J Virol 68:7497–7506
85. Sung NS, Kenney S, Gutsch D, Pagano JS (1991) EBNA-2 transactivates a lymphoid-specific enhancer in the BamHI C promoter of Epstein-Barr virus. J Virol 65:2164–2169
86. Wang F et al (1987) Epstein-Barr virus nuclear antigen 2 specifically induces expression of the B-cell activation antigen CD23. Proc Natl Acad Sci USA 84:3452–3456
87. Woisetschlaeger M, Jin XW, Yandava CN, Furmanski LA, Strominger JL, Speck SH (1991) Role for the Epstein-Barr virus nuclear antigen 2 in viral promoter switching during initial stages of infection. Proc Natl Acad Sci USA 88:3942–3946
88. Waltzer L, Logeat F, Brou C, Israel A, Sergeant A, Manet E (1994) The human J kappa recombination signal sequence binding protein (RBP-J kappa) targets the Epstein-Barr virus EBNA2 protein to its DNA responsive elements. EMBO J 13:5633–5638
89. Zimber-Strobl U et al (1994) Epstein-Barr virus nuclear antigen 2 exerts its transactivating function through interaction with recombination signal binding protein RBP-J kappa, the homologue of Drosophila Suppressor of Hairless. EMBO J 13:4973–4982
90. Johannsen E, Koh E, Mosialos G, Tong X, Kieff E, Grossman SR (1995) Epstein-Barr virus nuclear protein 2 transactivation of the latent membrane protein 1 promoter is mediated by J kappa and PU.1. J Virol 69:253–262
91. Cohen JI, Wang F, Mannick J, Kieff E (1989) Epstein-Barr virus nuclear protein 2 is a key determinant of lymphocyte transformation. Proc Natl Acad Sci USA 86:9558–9562
92. Kempkes B et al (1995) B-cell proliferation and induction of early G1-regulating proteins by Epstein-Barr virus mutants conditional for EBNA2. EMBO J 14:88–96
93. Rowe DT, Rowe M, Evan GI, Wallace LE, Farrell PJ, Rickinson AB (1986) Restricted expression of EBV latent genes and T-lymphocyte-detected membrane antigen in Burkitt's lymphoma cells. EMBO J 5:2599–2607
94. Kelly GL, Milner AE, Baldwin GS, Bell AI, Rickinson AB (2006) Three restricted forms of Epstein-Barr virus latency counteracting apoptosis in c-myc-expressing Burkitt lymphoma cells. Proc Natl Acad Sci USA 103:14935–14940
95. Owen TJ et al (2010) Epstein-Barr virus-encoded EBNA1 enhances RNA polymerase III-dependent EBER expression through induction of EBER-associated cellular transcription factors. Mol Cancer 9:241
96. Swaminathan S (2008) Noncoding RNAs produced by oncogenic human herpesviruses. J Cell Physiol 216:321–326

97. Bornkamm GW (2009) Epstein-Barr virus and its role in the pathogenesis of Burkitt's lymphoma: an unresolved issue. Semin Cancer Biol 19:351–365
98. Komano J, Maruo S, Kurozumi K, Oda T, Takada K (1999) Oncogenic role of Epstein-Barr virus-encoded RNAs in Burkitt's lymphoma cell line Akata. J Virol 73:9827–9831
99. Niller HH, Salamon D, Banati F, Schwarzmann F, Wolf H, Minarovits J (2004) The LCR of EBV makes Burkitt's lymphoma endemic. Trends Microbiol 12:495–499
100. Wu Y, Maruo S, Yajima M, Kanda T, Takada K (2007) Epstein-Barr virus (EBV)-encoded RNA 2 (EBER2) but not EBER1 plays a critical role in EBV-induced B-cell growth transformation. J Virol 81:11236–11245
101. Bell AI et al (2006) Analysis of Epstein-Barr virus latent gene expression in endemic Burkitt's lymphoma and nasopharyngeal carcinoma tumour cells by using quantitative real-time PCR assays. J Gen Virol 87:2885–2890
102. Tao Q, Robertson KD, Manns A, Hildesheim A, Ambinder RF (1998) Epstein-Barr virus (EBV) in endemic Burkitt's lymphoma: molecular analysis of primary tumor tissue. Blood 91:1373–1381
103. Kelly GL et al (2009) An Epstein-Barr virus anti-apoptotic protein constitutively expressed in transformed cells and implicated in Burkitt lymphomagenesis: the Wp/BHRF1 link. PLoS Pathog 5:e1000341
104. Austin PJ, Flemington E, Yandava CN, Strominger JL, Speck SH (1988) Complex transcription of the Epstein-Barr virus BamHI fragment H rightward open reading frame 1 (BHRF1) in latently and lytically infected B lymphocytes. Proc Natl Acad Sci USA 85:3678–3682
105. Pratt ZL, Kuzembayeva M, Sengupta S, Sugden B (2009) The microRNAs of Epstein-Barr Virus are expressed at dramatically differing levels among cell lines. Virology 386:387–397
106. Godshalk SE, Bhaduri-McIntosh S, Slack FJ (2008) Epstein-Barr virus-mediated dysregulation of human microRNA expression. Cell Cycle 7:3595–3600
107. Gatto G, Rossi A, Rossi D, Kroening S, Bonatti S, Mallardo M (2008) Epstein-Barr virus latent membrane protein 1 trans-activates miR-155 transcription through the NF-kappaB pathway. Nucleic Acids Res 36:6608–6619
108. Hemann MT et al (2005) Evasion of the p53 tumour surveillance network by tumour-derived MYC mutants. Nature 436:807–811
109. Kelly GL et al (2005) Epstein-Barr virus nuclear antigen 2 (EBNA2) gene deletion is consistently linked with EBNA3A, -3B, and -3C expression in Burkitt's lymphoma cells and with increased resistance to apoptosis. J Virol 79:10709–10717
110. Skalska L, White RE, Franz M, Ruhmann M, Allday MJ (2010) Epigenetic repression of p16(INK4A) by latent Epstein-Barr virus requires the interaction of EBNA3A and EBNA3C with CtBP. PLoS Pathog 6:e1000951
111. Leao M, Anderton E, Wade M, Meekings K, Allday MJ (2007) Epstein-Barr virus-induced resistance to drugs that activate the mitotic spindle assembly checkpoint in Burkitt's lymphoma cells. J Virol 81:248–260
112. Tomkinson B, Robertson E, Kieff E (1993) Epstein-Barr virus nuclear proteins EBNA-3A and EBNA-3C are essential for B-lymphocyte growth transformation. J Virol 67:2014–2025
113. Kilger E, Kieser A, Baumann M, Hammerschmidt W (1998) Epstein-Barr virus-mediated B-cell proliferation is dependent upon latent membrane protein 1, which simulates an activated CD40 receptor. EMBO J 17:1700–1709
114. Kaye KM, Izumi KM, Kieff E (1993) Epstein-Barr virus latent membrane protein 1 is essential for B-lymphocyte growth transformation. Proc Natl Acad Sci USA 90:9150–9154
115. Ahsan N, Kanda T, Nagashima K, Takada K (2005) Epstein-Barr virus transforming protein LMP1 plays a critical role in virus production. J Virol 79:4415–4424
116. Young LS, Murray PG (2003) Epstein-Barr virus and oncogenesis: from latent genes to tumours. Oncogene 22:5108–5121
117. Huen DS, Henderson SA, Croom-Carter D, Rowe M (1995) The Epstein-Barr virus latent membrane protein-1 (LMP1) mediates activation of NF-kappa B and cell surface phenotype via two effector regions in its carboxy-terminal cytoplasmic domain. Oncogene 10:549–560
118. Izumi KM, Cahir McFarland ED, Ting AT, Riley EA, Seed B, Kieff ED (1999) The Epstein-Barr virus oncoprotein latent membrane protein 1 engages the tumor necrosis factor receptor-

associated proteins TRADD and receptor-interacting protein (RIP) but does not induce apoptosis or require RIP for NF-kappaB activation. Mol Cell Biol 19:5759–5767
119. Mainou BA, Everly DN Jr, Raab-Traub N (2007) Unique signaling properties of CTAR1 in LMP1-mediated transformation. J Virol 81:9680–9692
120. Kieser A, Kilger E, Gires O, Ueffing M, Kolch W, Hammerschmidt W (1997) Epstein-Barr virus latent membrane protein-1 triggers AP-1 activity via the c-Jun N-terminal kinase cascade. EMBO J 16:6478–6485
121. D'souza B, Rowe M, Walls D (2000) The bfl-1 gene is transcriptionally upregulated by the Epstein-Barr virus LMP1, and its expression promotes the survival of a Burkitt's lymphoma cell line. J Virol 74:6652–6658
122. D'souza BN et al (2004) Nuclear factor kappa B-dependent activation of the antiapoptotic bfl-1 gene by the Epstein-Barr virus latent membrane protein 1 and activated CD40 receptor. J Virol 78:1800–1816
123. Bieging KT, Swanson-Mungerson M, Amick AC, Longnecker R (2010) Epstein-Barr virus in Burkitt's lymphoma: a role for latent membrane protein 2A. Cell Cycle 9:901–908
124. Bieging KT, Amick AC, Longnecker R (2009) Epstein-Barr virus LMP2A bypasses p53 inactivation in a MYC model of lymphomagenesis. Proc Natl Acad Sci USA 106: 17945–17950
125. Guasparri I, Bubman D, Cesarman E (2008) EBV LMP2A affects LMP1-mediated NF-kappaB signaling and survival of lymphoma cells by regulating TRAF2 expression. Blood 111:3813–3820
126. Swart R, Ruf IK, Sample J, Longnecker R (2000) Latent membrane protein 2A-mediated effects on the phosphatidylinositol 3-kinase/Akt pathway. J Virol 74:10838–10845
127. Morrison JA, Klingelhutz AJ, Raab-Traub N (2003) Epstein-Barr virus latent membrane protein 2A activates beta-catenin signaling in epithelial cells. J Virol 77:12276–12284
128. Bates CM, Kharzai S, Erwin T, Rossant J, Parada LF (2000) Role of N-myc in the developing mouse kidney. Dev Biol 222:317–325
129. de la Cova C, Abril M, Bellosta P, Gallant P, Johnston LA (2004) Drosophila myc regulates organ size by inducing cell competition. Cell 117:107–116
130. Packham G, Cleveland JL (1995) c-Myc and apoptosis. Biochim Biophys Acta 1242:11–28
131. Brady G, MacArthur GJ, Farrell PJ (2007) Epstein-Barr virus and Burkitt lymphoma. J Clin Pathol 60:1397–1402
132. Christian SL, Sims PV, Gold MR (2002) The B cell antigen receptor regulates the transcriptional activator beta-catenin via protein kinase C-mediated inhibition of glycogen synthase kinase-3. J Immunol 169:758–769
133. Kamijo T, Weber JD, Zambetti G, Zindy F, Roussel MF, Sherr CJ (1998) Functional and physical interactions of the ARF tumor suppressor with p53 and Mdm2. Proc Natl Acad Sci USA 95:8292–8297
134. Stott FJ et al (1998) The alternative product from the human CDKN2A locus, p14(ARF), participates in a regulatory feedback loop with p53 and MDM2. EMBO J 17:5001–5014
135. Yang CT et al (2000) Adenovirus-mediated p14(ARF) gene transfer in human mesothelioma cells. J Natl Cancer Inst 92:636–641
136. Dang CV, O'Donnell KA, Zeller KI, Nguyen T, Osthus RC, Li F (2006) The c-Myc target gene network. Semin Cancer Biol 16:253–264
137. Bishop JM (1987) The molecular genetics of cancer. Science 235:305–311
138. Klein G (1983) Specific chromosomal translocations and the genesis of B-cell-derived tumors in mice and men. Cell 32:311–315
139. Croce CM, Nowell PC (1985) Molecular basis of human B cell neoplasia. Blood 65:1–7
140. Leder P et al (1983) Translocations among antibody genes in human cancer. Science 222:765–771
141. Battey J et al (1983) The human c-myc oncogene: structural consequences of translocation into the IgH locus in Burkitt lymphoma. Cell 34:779–787
142. Dalla-Favera R, Martinotti S, Gallo RC, Erikson J, Croce CM (1983) Translocation and rearrangements of the c-myc oncogene locus in human undifferentiated B-cell lymphomas. Science 219:963–967

143. Shen-Ong GL, Keath EJ, Piccoli SP, Cole MD (1982) Novel myc oncogene RNA from abortive immunoglobulin-gene recombination in mouse plasmacytomas. Cell 31:443–452
144. Schwartz RC, Stanton LW, Riley SC, Marcu KB, Witte ON (1986) Synergism of v-myc and v-Ha-ras in the in vitro neoplastic progression of murine lymphoid cells. Mol Cell Biol 6:3221–3231
145. Langdon WY, Harris AW, Cory S, Adams JM (1986) The c-myc oncogene perturbs B lymphocyte development in E-mu-myc transgenic mice. Cell 47:11–18
146. Lombardi L, Newcomb EW, Dalla-Favera R (1987) Pathogenesis of Burkitt lymphoma: expression of an activated c-myc oncogene causes the tumorigenic conversion of EBV-infected human B lymphoblasts. Cell 49:161–170
147. Adhikary S, Eilers M (2005) Transcriptional regulation and transformation by Myc proteins. Nat Rev Mol Cell Biol 6:635–645
148. Gruhne B, Kamranvar SA, Masucci MG, Sompallae R (2009) EBV and genomic instability–a new look at the role of the virus in the pathogenesis of Burkitt's lymphoma. Semin Cancer Biol 19:394–400
149. Hofmann JJ, Iruela-Arispe ML (2007) Notch signaling in blood vessels: who is talking to whom about what? Circ Res 100:1556–1568
150. O'Connor L et al (1998) Bim: a novel member of the Bcl-2 family that promotes apoptosis. EMBO J 17:384–395
151. Clybouw C et al (2005) EBV infection of human B lymphocytes leads to down-regulation of Bim expression: relationship to resistance to apoptosis. J Immunol 175:2968–2973
152. Ionov Y et al (2003) Pim-1 protein kinase is nuclear in Burkitt's lymphoma: nuclear localization is necessary for its biologic effects. Anticancer Res 23:167–178
153. Cinti C et al (2000) Genetic alterations disrupting the nuclear localization of the retinoblastoma-related gene RB2/p130 in human tumor cell lines and primary tumors. Cancer Res 60:383–389
154. Lindstrom MS, Wiman KG (2002) Role of genetic and epigenetic changes in Burkitt lymphoma. Semin Cancer Biol 12:381–387
155. Capoulade C et al (1998) Overexpression of MDM2, due to enhanced translation, results in inactivation of wild-type p53 in Burkitt's lymphoma cells. Oncogene 16:1603–1610
156. Wilda M et al (2004) Inactivation of the ARF-MDM-2-p53 pathway in sporadic Burkitt's lymphoma in children. Leukemia 18:584–588
157. Imamura J, Miyoshi I, Koeffler HP (1994) p53 in hematologic malignancies. Blood 84:2412–2421
158. Renouf B, Hollville E, Pujals A, Tetaud C, Garibal J, Wiels J (2009) Activation of p53 by MDM2 antagonists has differential apoptotic effects on Epstein-Barr virus (EBV)-positive and EBV-negative Burkitt's lymphoma cells. Leukemia 23:1557–1563
159. Leoncini L, Bellan C, De Falco G (2006) Retinoblastoma gene family expression in lymphoid tissues. Oncogene 25:5309–5314
160. Stiegler P, Kasten M, Giordano A (1998) The RB family of cell cycle regulatory factors. J Cell Biochem Suppl 30–31:30–36
161. Hanahan D, Weinberg RA (2000) The hallmarks of cancer. Cell 100:57–70
162. Cinti C et al (2000) Genetic alterations of the retinoblastoma-related gene RB2/p130 identify different pathogenetic mechanisms in and among Burkitt's lymphoma subtypes. Am J Pathol 156:751–760
163. Hoang AT et al (1995) A link between increased transforming activity of lymphoma-derived MYC mutant alleles, their defective regulation by p107, and altered phosphorylation of the c-Myc transactivation domain. Mol Cell Biol 15:4031–4042
164. Lazzi S et al (2002) Expression of RB2/p130 tumor-suppressor gene in AIDS-related non-Hodgkin's lymphomas: implications for disease pathogenesis. Hum Pathol 33:723–731
165. Soni V, Cahir-McFarland E, Kieff E (2007) LMP1 TRAFficking activates growth and survival pathways. Adv Exp Med Biol 597:173–187
166. Saha A, Robertson ES (2011) Epstein-Barr virus-associated B-cell lymphomas: pathogenesis and clinical outcomes. Clin Cancer Res 17:3056–3063

167. Young LS, Dawson CW, Eliopoulos AG (2000) The expression and function of Epstein-Barr virus encoded latent genes. Mol Pathol 53:238–247
168. Fennewald S, van Santen V, Kieff E (1984) Nucleotide sequence of an mRNA transcribed in latent growth-transforming virus infection indicates that it may encode a membrane protein. J Virol 51:411–419
169. Higuchi M, Izumi KM, Kieff E (2001) Epstein-Barr virus latent-infection membrane proteins are palmitoylated and raft-associated: protein 1 binds to the cytoskeleton through TNF receptor cytoplasmic factors. Proc Natl Acad Sci USA 98:4675–4680
170. Mainou BA, Everly DN Jr, Raab-Traub N (2005) Epstein-Barr virus latent membrane protein 1 CTAR1 mediates rodent and human fibroblast transformation through activation of PI3K. Oncogene 24:6917–6924
171. Gires O et al (1999) Latent membrane protein 1 of Epstein-Barr virus interacts with JAK3 and activates STAT proteins. EMBO J 18:3064–3073
172. Mosialos G, Birkenbach M, Yalamanchili R, VanArsdale T, Ware C, Kieff E (1995) The Epstein-Barr virus transforming protein LMP1 engages signaling proteins for the tumor necrosis factor receptor family. Cell 80:389–399
173. Konforte D, Simard N, Paige CJ (2008) Interleukin-21 regulates expression of key Epstein-Barr virus oncoproteins, EBNA2 and LMP1, in infected human B cells. Virology 374:100–113
174. Zhang W, Liu HT (2002) MAPK signal pathways in the regulation of cell proliferation in mammalian cells. Cell Res 12:9–18
175. Haimovitz-Friedman A, Kolesnick RN, Fuks Z (1997) Ceramide signaling in apoptosis. Br Med Bull 53:539–553
176. Basu S, Kolesnick R (1998) Stress signals for apoptosis: ceramide and c-Jun kinase. Oncogene 17:3277–3285
177. Chen YR, Tan TH (2000) The c-Jun N-terminal kinase pathway and apoptotic signaling (review). Int J Oncol 16:651–662
178. Cerimele F et al (2005) Reactive oxygen signaling and MAPK activation distinguish Epstein-Barr Virus (EBV)-positive versus EBV-negative Burkitt's lymphoma. Proc Natl Acad Sci USA 102:175–179
179. zur Hausen H, O'Neill FJ, Freese UK, Hecker E (1978) Persisting oncogenic herpesvirus induced by the tumour promotor TPA. Nature 272:373–375
180. Satoh T, Hoshikawa Y, Satoh Y, Kurata T, Sairenji T (1999) The interaction of mitogen-activated protein kinases to Epstein-Barr virus activation in Akata cells. Virus Genes 18:57–64
181. Chang L, Karin M (2001) Mammalian MAP kinase signalling cascades. Nature 410:37–40
182. Tordai A, Franklin RA, Patel H, Gardner AM, Johnson GL, Gelfand EW (1994) Cross-linking of surface IgM stimulates the Ras/Raf-1/MEK/MAPK cascade in human B lymphocytes. J Biol Chem 269:7538–7543
183. Roberts ML, Cooper NR (1998) Activation of a ras-MAPK-dependent pathway by Epstein-Barr virus latent membrane protein 1 is essential for cellular transformation. Virology 240:93–99
184. Kim D, Chung J (2002) Akt: versatile mediator of cell survival and beyond. J Biochem Mol Biol 35:106–115
185. Burgering BM, Coffer PJ (1995) Protein kinase B (c-Akt) in phosphatidylinositol-3-OH kinase signal transduction. Nature 376:599–602
186. Datta SR et al (1997) Akt phosphorylation of BAD couples survival signals to the cell-intrinsic death machinery. Cell 91:231–241
187. Franke TF, Hornik CP, Segev L, Shostak GA, Sugimoto C (2003) PI3K/Akt and apoptosis: size matters. Oncogene 22:8983–8998
188. Brennan P, Mehl AM, Jones M, Rowe M (2002) Phosphatidylinositol 3-kinase is essential for the proliferation of lymphoblastoid cells. Oncogene 21:1263–1271
189. Fukuda M, Longnecker R (2004) Latent membrane protein 2A inhibits transforming growth factor-beta 1-induced apoptosis through the phosphatidylinositol 3-kinase/Akt pathway. J Virol 78:1697–1705

190. Iwakiri D, Takada K (2004) Phosphatidylinositol 3-kinase is a determinant of responsiveness to B cell antigen receptor-mediated Epstein-Barr virus activation. J Immunol 172:1561–1566
191. Baron M (2003) An overview of the Notch signalling pathway. Semin Cell Dev Biol 14:113–119
192. Kolev V et al (2005) The intracellular domain of Notch ligand Delta1 induces cell growth arrest. FEBS Lett 579:5798–5802
193. Singson A, Mercer KB, L'Hernault SW (1998) The C. elegans spe-9 gene encodes a sperm transmembrane protein that contains EGF-like repeats and is required for fertilization. Cell 93:71–79
194. Jarriault S, Brou C, Logeat F, Schroeter EH, Kopan R, Israel A (1995) Signalling downstream of activated mammalian Notch. Nature 377:355–358
195. He F et al (2009) Notch and BCR signaling synergistically promote the proliferation of Raji B-lymphoma cells. Leuk Res 33:798–802
196. Radtke F, Wilson A, MacDonald HR (2004) Notch signaling in T- and B-cell development. Curr Opin Immunol 16:174–179
197. Kuroda K et al (2003) Regulation of marginal zone B cell development by MINT, a suppressor of Notch/RBP-J signaling pathway. Immunity 18:301–312
198. Aster JC, Blacklow SC, Pear WS (2011) Notch signalling in T-cell lymphoblastic leukaemia/lymphoma and other haematological malignancies. J Pathol 223:262–273
199. Zimber-Strobl U, Strobl LJ (2001) EBNA2 and Notch signalling in Epstein-Barr virus mediated immortalization of B lymphocytes. Semin Cancer Biol 11:423–434
200. Strobl LJ, Hofelmayr H, Marschall G, Brielmeier M, Bornkamm GW, Zimber-Strobl U (2000) Activated Notch1 modulates gene expression in B cells similarly to Epstein-Barr viral nuclear antigen 2. J Virol 74:1727–1735
201. Hofelmayr H, Strobl LJ, Marschall G, Bornkamm GW, Zimber-Strobl U (2001) Activated Notch1 can transiently substitute for EBNA2 in the maintenance of proliferation of LMP1-expressing immortalized B cells. J Virol 75:2033–2040
202. Portal D, Zhao B, Calderwood MA, Sommermann T, Johannsen E, Kieff E (2011) EBV nuclear antigen EBNALP dismisses transcription repressors NCoR and RBPJ from enhancers and EBNA2 increases NCoR-deficient RBPJ DNA binding. Proc Natl Acad Sci USA 108:7808–7813
203. He Y, Pear WS (2003) Notch signalling in B cells. Semin Cell Dev Biol 14:135–142
204. Miller JR, Hocking AM, Brown JD, Moon RT (1999) Mechanism and function of signal transduction by the Wnt/beta-catenin and Wnt/Ca2+ pathways. Oncogene 18:7860–7872
205. Akiyama T (2000) Wnt/beta-catenin signaling. Cytokine Growth Factor Rev 11:273–282
206. Park JI et al (2005) Kaiso/p120-catenin and TCF/beta-catenin complexes coordinately regulate canonical Wnt gene targets. Dev Cell 8:843–854
207. Crawford HC et al (1999) The metalloproteinase matrilysin is a target of beta-catenin transactivation in intestinal tumors. Oncogene 18:2883–2891
208. Koh TJ, Bulitta CJ, Fleming JV, Dockray GJ, Varro A, Wang TC (2000) Gastrin is a target of the beta-catenin/TCF-4 growth-signaling pathway in a model of intestinal polyposis. J Clin Invest 106:533–539
209. Shackelford J, Maier C, Pagano JS (2003) Epstein-Barr virus activates beta-catenin in type III latently infected B lymphocyte lines: association with deubiquitinating enzymes. Proc Natl Acad Sci USA 100:15572–15576
210. Pennica D et al (1998) WISP genes are members of the connective tissue growth factor family that are up-regulated in wnt-1-transformed cells and aberrantly expressed in human colon tumors. Proc Natl Acad Sci USA 95:14717–14722
211. Hay-Koren A, Caspi M, Zilberberg A, Rosin-Arbesfeld R (2011) The EDD E3 ubiquitin ligase ubiquitinates and up-regulates beta-catenin. Mol Biol Cell 22:399–411
212. Portis T, Ikeda M, Longnecker R (2004) Epstein-Barr virus LMP2A: regulating cellular ubiquitination processes for maintenance of viral latency? Trends Immunol 25:422–426
213. Chung EJ et al (2002) Regulation of leukemic cell adhesion, proliferation, and survival by beta-catenin. Blood 100:982–990

214. Portis T, Longnecker R (2003) Epstein-Barr virus LMP2A interferes with global transcription factor regulation when expressed during B-lymphocyte development. J Virol 77:105–114
215. Raptis S, Bapat B (2006) Genetic instability in human tumors. EXS 96:303–320
216. Schmutte C, Fishel R (1999) Genomic instability: first step to carcinogenesis. Anticancer Res 19:4665–4696
217. Honma M (2005) Generation of loss of heterozygosity and its dependency on p53 status in human lymphoblastoid cells. Environ Mol Mutagen 45:162–176
218. Modrich P (1994) Mismatch repair, genetic stability, and cancer. Science 266:1959–1960
219. Kamranvar SA, Gruhne B, Szeles A, Masucci MG (2007) Epstein-Barr virus promotes genomic instability in Burkitt's lymphoma. Oncogene 26:5115–5123
220. Dorfman JR et al (2005) B cell memory to 3 Plasmodium falciparum blood-stage antigens in a malaria-endemic area. J Infect Dis 191:1623–1630
221. Whittle HC, Brown J, Marsh K, Blackman M, Jobe O, Shenton F (1990) The effects of Plasmodium falciparum malaria on immune control of B lymphocytes in Gambian children. Clin Exp Immunol 80:213–218
222. Whittle HC et al (1984) T-cell control of Epstein-Barr virus-infected B cells is lost during P. falciparum malaria. Nature 312:449–450
223. Magrath I (1990) The pathogenesis of Burkitt's lymphoma. Adv Cancer Res 55:133–270
224. Rochford R, Cannon MJ, Moormann AM (2005) Endemic Burkitt's lymphoma: a polymicrobial disease? Nat Rev Microbiol 3:182–187
225. Moss DJ et al (1983) A comparison of Epstein-Barr virus-specific T-cell immunity in malaria-endemic and -nonendemic regions of Papua New Guinea. Int J Cancer 31:727–732
226. Moormann AM et al (2005) Exposure to holoendemic malaria results in elevated Epstein-Barr virus loads in children. J Infect Dis 191:1233–1238
227. Yone CL, Kube D, Kremsner PG, Luty AJ (2006) Persistent Epstein-Barr viral reactivation in young African children with a history of severe Plasmodium falciparum malaria. Trans R Soc Trop Med Hyg 100:669–676
228. Morrow RH Jr (1985) Epidemiological evidence for the role of falciparum malaria in the pathogenesis of Burkitt's lymphoma. IARC Sci Publ 177–186
229. Donati D et al (2006) Increased B cell survival and preferential activation of the memory compartment by a malaria polyclonal B cell activator. J Immunol 177:3035–3044
230. Thorley-Lawson DA, Chess L, Strominger JL (1977) Suppression of in vitro Epstein-Barr virus infection. A new role for adult human T lymphocytes. J Exp Med 146:495–508
231. Sitki-Green DL, Edwards RH, Covington MM, Raab-Traub N (2004) Biology of Epstein-Barr virus during infectious mononucleosis. J Infect Dis 189:483–492
232. Arama C et al (2011) Interethnic differences in antigen-presenting cell activation and TLR responses in Malian children during Plasmodium falciparum malaria. PLoS One 6:e18319
233. Kataaha PK, Facer CA, Holborow EJ (1984) Plasmodium falciparum products enhance human lymphocyte transformation by Epstein-Barr virus. Clin Exp Immunol 56:371–376
234. Saha A, Kaul R, Murakami M, Robertson ES (2010) Tumor viruses and cancer biology: Modulating signaling pathways for therapeutic intervention. Cancer Biol Ther 10:961–978
235. Blum KA, Lozanski G, Byrd JC (2004) Adult Burkitt leukemia and lymphoma. Blood 104:3009–3020
236. Spina M et al (1998) Burkitt's lymphoma in adults with and without human immunodeficiency virus infection: a single-institution clinicopathologic study of 75 patients. Cancer 82:766–774
237. Grogg KL, Miller RF, Dogan A (2007) HIV infection and lymphoma. J Clin Pathol 60:1365–1372
238. Jaffe EHN, Stein H, Vardiman J, Raphael M, Borisch B, Jaffe E (2001) Lymphomas associated with infection by the human immune deficiency virus (HIV). IARC, Lyon
239. Gold JE, Castella A, Zalusky R (1989) B-cell acute lymphocytic leukemia in HIV-antibody-positive patients. Am J Hematol 32:200–204

240. Raphael MBB, Jaffe E (2001) Lymphomas associated with infection by the human immune deficiency virus (HIV). IARC, Lyon
241. Emmanuel B et al (2011) African Burkitt lymphoma: age-specific risk and correlations with malaria biomarkers. Am J Trop Med Hyg 84:397–401
242. Bower M (1992) The biology of HIV-associated lymphomas. Br J Cancer 66:421–423
243. Bibas M, Antinori A (2009) EBV and HIV-Related Lymphoma. Mediterr J Hematol Infect Dis 1:e2009032
244. Hecht JL, Aster JC (2000) Molecular biology of Burkitt's lymphoma. J Clin Oncol 18:3707–3721
245. Douek DC (2003) Disrupting T-cell homeostasis: how HIV-1 infection causes disease. AIDS Rev 5:172–177
246. Cohen JI (2000) Epstein-Barr virus infection. N Engl J Med 343:481–492
247. Glass RB, Fernbach SK, Conway JJ, Shkolnik A (1985) Gallium scintigraphy in American Burkitt lymphoma: accurate assessment of tumor load and prognosis. Am J Roentgenol 145:671–676
248. Richman SD, Appelbaum F, Levenson SM, Johnston GS, Ziegler JL (1975) 67 Ga radionuclide imaging in Burkitt's lymphoma. Radiology 117:639–645
249. Krudy AG, Dunnick NR, Magrath IT, Shawker TH, Doppman JL, Spiegel R (1981) CT of American Burkitt lymphoma. Am J Roentgenol 136:747–754
250. Silverman BA, Rubinstein A (1985) Serum lactate dehydrogenase levels in adults and children with acquired immune deficiency syndrome (AIDS) and AIDS-related complex: possible indicator of B cell lymphoproliferation and disease activity. Effect of intravenous gammaglobulin on enzyme levels. Am J Med 78:728–736
251. Pagano L, Caira M, Valentini CG, Fianchi L (2009) Clinical aspects and therapy of sporadic burkitt lymphoma. Mediterr J Hematol Infect Dis 1:e2009030
252. Magrath I et al (1996) Adults and children with small non-cleaved-cell lymphoma have a similar excellent outcome when treated with the same chemotherapy regimen. J Clin Oncol 14:925–934
253. Lacasce A et al (2004) Modified magrath regimens for adults with Burkitt and Burkitt-like lymphomas: preserved efficacy with decreased toxicity. Leuk Lymphoma 45:761–767
254. Thomas DA et al (2006) Chemoimmunotherapy with hyper-CVAD plus rituximab for the treatment of adult Burkitt and Burkitt-type lymphoma or acute lymphoblastic leukemia. Cancer 106:1569–1580
255. Kaplan LD et al (1989) AIDS-associated non-Hodgkin's lymphoma in San Francisco. JAMA 261:719–724
256. Levine AM et al (1991) Low-dose chemotherapy with central nervous system prophylaxis and zidovudine maintenance in AIDS-related lymphoma. A prospective multi-institutional trial. JAMA 266:84–88
257. Boffa LC et al (2007) Inhibition of Burkitt's lymphoma cells growth in SCID mice by a PNA specific for a regulatory sequence of the translocated c-myc. Cancer Gene Ther 14:220–226
258. van Imhoff GW et al (2005) Short intensive sequential therapy followed by autologous stem cell transplantation in adult Burkitt, Burkitt-like and lymphoblastic lymphoma. Leukemia 19:945–952
259. Peniket AJ et al (2003) An EBMT registry matched study of allogeneic stem cell transplants for lymphoma: allogeneic transplantation is associated with a lower relapse rate but a higher procedure-related mortality rate than autologous transplantation. Bone Marrow Transplant 31:667–678
260. Mentzer SJ, Fingeroth J, Reilly JJ, Perrine SP, Faller DV (1998) Arginine butyrate-induced susceptibility to ganciclovir in an Epstein-Barr-virus-associated lymphoma. Blood Cells Mol Dis 24:114–123
261. Littler E et al (1986) Identification of an Epstein-Barr virus-coded thymidine kinase. EMBO J 5:1959–1966

262. Abdulkarim B et al (2003) Antiviral agent cidofovir decreases Epstein-Barr virus (EBV) oncoproteins and enhances the radiosensitivity in EBV-related malignancies. Oncogene 22:2260–2271
263. Geser A, Brubaker G, Draper CC (1989) Effect of a malaria suppression program on the incidence of African Burkitt's lymphoma. Am J Epidemiol 129:740–752
264. Geser A, de The G, Lenoir G, Day NE, Williams EH (1982) Final case reporting from the Ugandan prospective study of the relationship between EBV and Burkitt's lymphoma. Int J Cancer 29:397–400
265. Cai X et al (2006) Epstein-Barr virus microRNAs are evolutionarily conserved and differentially expressed. PLoS Pathog 2:e23

Chapter 11
Molecular Biology of Burkitt Lymphoma

Lisa Giulino-Roth and Ethel Cesarman

Introduction

Burkitt lymphoma (BL) was first described by Dennis Burkitt in 1958 as a unique sarcoma involving the jaw in African children [1]. He spent the next few years visiting hospitals in East and Southern Africa and found that this tumor had a geographical distribution that overlapped with areas hyperendemic and holoendemic for malaria, suggesting a potential link to an insect vector [2]. Shortly after, a newly discovered herpes virus, now known as EBV, was isolated from BL tumors [3]. Further studies confirmed the presence of EBV in almost 100% of Burkitt lymphoma cases in Africa.

We now recognize three epidemiologic subtypes of BL: endemic, sporadic, and HIV-associated. The endemic type, as described by Burkitt, presents as an abdominal or jaw mass in children in equatorial Africa and Papa New Guinea, areas with high transmission rates of *Plasmodium falciparum* malaria. In these cases >95% of tumors are found to have EBV. The sporadic type, seen in the USA and Europe, often presents as lymph node enlargement and is associated with EBV in approximately 20% of cases. HIV-associated BL is seen worldwide and is associated with EBV in approximately 30% of cases. The unifying characteristic of all three epidemiologic subtypes is the translocation of the *MYC* proto-oncogene to one of the three immunoglobulin chains. This essentially puts *MYC* translation under the control of the immunoglobulin locus and leads to constitutive Myc activation.

L. Giulino-Roth
Department of Pediatrics, Memorial Sloan-Kettering Cancer Center, New York, NY, USA

Department of Pediatrics, Division of Pediatric Hematology and Oncology, Weill Cornell Medical Center, New York, NY, USA

E. Cesarman (✉)
Department of Pathology and Laboratory Medicine, Weill Cornell Medical College, New York, NY, USA
e-mail: ecesarm@med.cornell.edu

E.S. Robertson (ed.), *Burkitt's Lymphoma*, Current Cancer Research,
DOI 10.1007/978-1-4614-4313-1_11,

Burkitt lymphoma has an important role in history being the first human cancer to be linked to an oncogenic virus, EBV, and a cellular proto-oncogene, *MYC*. In more than 50 years since its discovery this tumor has continued to fascinate scientists due to the complex interplay between cellular genetics, infectious agents, and host immunity. In this chapter we will focus on the molecular characteristics of Burkitt lymphoma, and the complexities of Myc activation in conjunction with other cellular genetic or functional alterations that provide insights into the pathobiology of this highly aggressive malignancy.

Pathologic Diagnosis of BL

Morphology and Immunophenotype

The characteristic histologic appearance of BL is that of medium-sized monomorphic cells with round nuclei and basophilic cytoplasm. Infiltrating macrophages that have ingested apoptotic tumor cells give the classic starry sky appearance. When evaluated by immunohistochemistry BL tumor cells express common B-cell antigens (CD19, CD20, CD22, CD79a, PAX5) as well as germinal center B-cell specific markers (CD10, BCL6). They typically do not express BCL2. The proliferation index as measured by Ki67 is exceedingly high, approaching 100%.

The immunophenotype of BL is similar to that of germinal center (GC) B-cells, and this has been proposed to be the cell of origin of BL. GC B-cells represent the stage in B-cell maturation where immunoglobulin chains develop through somatic hypermutation and class switch recombination. A recent study used gene expression profiling to compare BL tumor cells to normal GC B-cells, memory B-cells, and naïve B-cells. The BL gene signature was most closely related to GC B-cells further supporting the hypothesis that GC B-cells are the normal counterpart of BL [4].

BL Karyotype

Nearly all BLs contain a translocation of the *MYC* locus (8q24). The most common partner is IgH on chromosome 14q32; however, rearrangements with the κ (22q11) or λ (2p12) light chains are also seen. There are infrequent cases of BL that lack any detectable MYC translocation as determined by cytogenetics or molecular testing [5]. While studies in adults report a simple karyotype with rare additional cytogenetic abnormalities [6], complex karyotypes are frequently seen in pediatric cases [7–10]. The most common alterations are gains in 1q, 7q, and 12q and losses in 6q, 13q, and 17p [11]. In particular, loss of 13q has been associated with inferior outcome in two retrospective pediatric studies and may have a role in risk stratification [10, 11].

The Role of Myc in BL

Myc Function

The *MYC* gene encodes for the transcription factor Myc (c-myc), which was first discovered as the cellular homologue of a retroviral oncogene encoded by the avian myelocytomatosis virus (v-myc) [12]. It is part of a family that includes N-Myc and L-Myc. Myc is a nuclear phosphoprotein with gene activating and repressing capabilities that is involved in many cellular processes including growth (increase in cell size), proliferation (DNA replication and cell cycle control), metabolism, and apoptosis. The N-terminus contains conserved regions known as Myc Box I, II, and III which play important roles in Myc stabilization and interaction with target genes. The C-terminus contains a helix-loop-helix domain, which allows Myc to form a heterodimer with the constitutively expressed protein MAX [13]. The MYC-MAX complex binds to CACGTG DNA sequences known as E boxes and activates transcription via recruitment of TRRAP-associated histone acetylation complexes and the INI1-associated chromatin modulating proteins [14]. Myc is implicated in the transcription of approximately 15% of all known genes and is one of the most commonly activated oncogenes in human cancers [15]. It has also been shown to act as a transcription repressor, one mechanism involving binding and inhibition of the transcriptional-activating protein Miz-1 [16]. A recent study by Rahl et al. also suggested a role for Myc in RNA polymerase II pause release (Rahl et al, Cell 141, 432-445 April 30, 2010). Promoter-proximal pausing is a post-initiation regulatory step that is known to play a crucial role in the control of gene expression. In this study, the authors present evidence that Myc may be responsible for the release of paused polymerase in specific genes. Large-scale gene expression profiling and chromatim immunoprecipitation studies to search for direct Myc targets have shown that thousands of genes are affected by Myc, and these genes are involved in a wide range of functions. Many are involved in cell growth, and include those in ribosome biogenesis, protein synthesis, and metabolism.

The function of Myc in normal cells is complex and nuanced, but it appears to play a central orchestrating role in differentiation as well as generation and maintenance of stem cells and their pluripotency [17]. In fact, *MYC* is among a handful of genes that in combination can induce reversion of differentiated cells into multipotent stem cells [18, 19].

Myc is activated in response to mitogenic signals and transcribes genes that are important in cellular proliferation. In the absence of apoptotic inhibiting signals, however, Myc is also responsible for initiating apoptosis. Myc drives cells into the cell cycle by inducing transcription of genes that encode for cyclins D and E and by downregulating the cyclin inhibitor p27. This drives cells from G0/G1 to the S phase of the cell cycle. An additional non-transcriptional role for Myc in DNA replication has also been documented, induced by increased replication origin activity with resulting DNA damage and checkpoint activation [20]. In addition, Myc can increase reactive oxygen species production and contribute to chromosomal instability. As a result of all of these effects, overexpression of Myc will ultimately lead to apoptosis in otherwise normal cells. There are multiple pathways by which Myc expression modulates apoptosis. Myc activates the p53 program through the nuclear tumor suppressor *ARF*. It also activates the proapoptotic protein Bim and inhibits anti-apoptotic proteins such as BCLX1 and BCL2. Myc-induced lymphomagenesis can likely only take place in the setting of inhibition of the Myc-induced apoptotic signals.

Concordantly with its role in cell growth, a role for Myc in metabolism and ribosome biogenesis has recently been appreciated [21]. In Drosophila, a hypomorphic allele of dMYC results in flies with a "Minute" phenotype that resemble those that result from loss of function in genes involved in ribosome biogenesis, so it has been postulated that this may be the primordial function of Myc [21]. In addition to numerous genes involved in glucose and glutamine metabolism (which are transcribed by RNA polymerase II), Myc stimulates genes transcribed by RNA Polymenrase II (E.G. tRNA and 5S rRNA genes) [22], and RNA polymerase I, which transcribes genes encoding ribosomal RNA [23]. Myc also is thought to integrate proliferation with glucose metablolism (promoting both oxidative phosphorylation and glycolysis) and glutamine catabolism [24].

Molecular Mechanisms of Myc Deregulation in BL

In the case of BL, Myc becomes deregulated as a result of a reciprocal translocation between the *MYC* gene and one of the three immunoglobulin chains. The most common translocation, seen in approximately 80% of BL cases, is between *MYC* and the IgH gene (t(8;14)) (Fig. 11.1) [25, 26]. In the remainder of cases *MYC* is

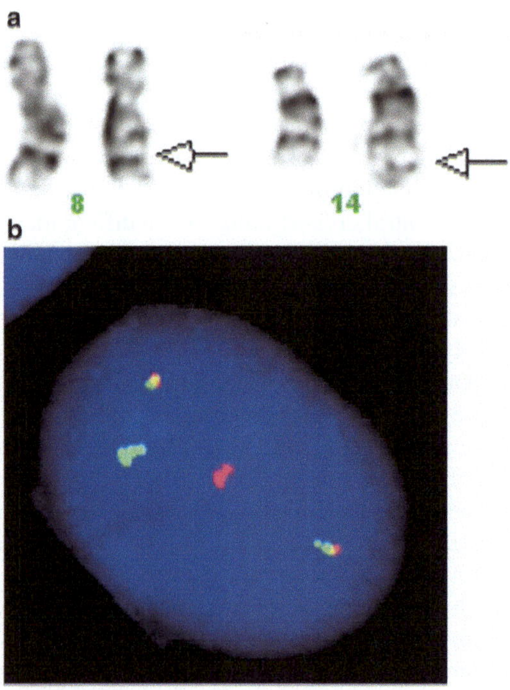

Fig. 11.1 Cytogenetic analysis of a case of Burkitt lymphoma. (**a**) Metaphase spread shows a conventional t(8;14)(q24;q32) chromosomal translocation. (**b**) Interphase FISH shows a balanced translocation involving the MYC and IgH loci. The chromosome 8 centromere is labeled with spectrum aqua, MYC probe is labeled in spectrum *orange* and IGH is labeled with spectrum *green*. Two fusion signals are seen, as well as one *red* and one *green* representing the normal chromosomes. Images courtesy of Susan Mathew

translocated to the IgL κ (t(8;22)) or λ (t(2;8)) genes. This places *MYC* under the control of the immunoglobulin locus resulting in constitutive activation.

Activation-Induced Cytidine Deaminase

MYC translocation is mediated by the enzyme activation-induced cytidine deaminase (AID). AID is highly expressed in germinal center B-cells and is responsible for both class switch recombination (CSR) and somatic hypermutation (SHM) [27]. Expression of AID leads to deamination of cytidine residues on the DNA of Ig variable or switch regions, which results in a U:G mismatch. This mismatch is repaired by endonuclease cleavage generating a DNA double strand break. In a transgenic murine model AID has been shown to induce Ig-MYC translocations that are similar to those seen in BL [28, 29].

A new method, called translocation-capture sequencing, has been used to search the entire genome for genomic rearrangements, and estimate the frequency of *c-myc/IgH* translocations in primary mouse B-cells expressing AID, which occur in approximately 1 of 17,000 cells [30, 31]. This confirms that in germinal center B-cells AID-mediated translocation between Ig and MYC occurs with relative frequency, and, in the absence of other genetic events, is of no pathologic consequence.

Variations in Myc-IgH Breakpoint

Interestingly, the breakpoint in t(8;14) varies by epidemiologic subtype [32]. In the endemic form of disease the Myc breakpoint is >100 kb upstream of the first coding region. The IgH breakpoint occurs more frequently in the joining region as a result of aberrant VDJ joining and SHM. In contrast, in the sporadic and HIV-associated forms of BL, the *MYC* breakpoint occurs immediately 5′ of *MYC* or within the first exon of *MYC*, which is non-coding. In these cases the breakpoint in IgH occurs on the switch region and is thought to be a result of aberrant CSR. The consequences and significance of these different breakpoints are not well understood.

Mutations in Non-coding Regions of Myc and P1/P2 Utilization

In the endemic form of BL, where the Ig regulatory elements are at a great distance, mutations in the first exon of MYC have been found that lead to a release in a block of transcriptional regulation, contributing to deregulated expression [33]. However, the regulatory elements of the *MYC* gene are complex, and still incompletely characterized. Two major promoters in the MYC gene have been described: P1 and P2. While both are used in normal cells, a shift to the upstream P1 was shown to occur in BL [34, 35]. There seems to be relationship between the block of transcriptional elongation and promoter utilization. The P1-initiated c-myc transcripts were not found to terminate at discrete sites near the 3′ end of exon 1 where this block is located, whereas P2-initiated transcripts either terminate or read through the transcription block signals. This led to the conclusion that over-expression from the P1 promoter of MYC may contribute to readthrough transcription in Burkitt lymphoma cells and eventually abnormal levels of Myc protein [36].

Mutations in Myc Coding Regions

Point mutations in the coding region of Myc are frequent in many B-cell lymphomas including BL [37–40]. The conserved Myc box I region has multiple mutational hotspots, the most common of which is a missense mutation affecting threonine 58 (T58). Phosphorylation of T58 by GSK-3β targets Myc for degradation by the proteosome. Point mutations affecting T58 inhibit Myc degradation resulting in stabilization of the protein and enhanced transforming activity [41]. The second most common mutation interferes with Pro57 and likely has the same effect due to the fact that Pro57 is required for T58 phosphorylation. These mutations allow Myc, which normally has a short half-life of <30 min, to escape degradation in BL cells.

microRNA Expression in BL Cases Lacking a Myc Translocation

A small subset (<10%) of both endemic and sporadic BL lack the Myc translocation. Examination of these cases demonstrates elevated expression of Myc at levels equivalent to that seen in cases of BL with Myc translocation [42]. There is evidence that micro-RNAs (miRNAs) are responsible for Myc overexpression in translocation-negative cases. MiRNAs are small non-coding RNA strands that bind to mRNA and regulate gene expression by mRNA cleavage or translational inhibition [43].

Downregulation of hsa-miR-34b and hsa-miR-9 has been implicated as mechanisms of translocation independent upregulation of Myc [42, 44]. Leucci et al. investigated the miRNA expression pattern in BL cases with and without a Myc translocation. They found downregulation of hsa-miR-34b, a miRNA predicted to target Myc, in translocation-negative cases but not in translocation-positive cases. The role of hsa-miR-34b in Myc expression is supported by in vitro studies showing a dose-dependent inverse relationship between hsa-miR-34b and Myc. Lymphoblastoid cell lines (LCLs) transfected with synthetic hsa-miR-34b showed a dose-dependent decrease in Myc expression. Conversely, transfection with a hsa-miR-34b-inhibitor resulted in increased in Myc expression [42].

A more recent study evaluating miRNAs in BL found that downregulation of hsa-miR-9 may also be responsible for Myc upregulation in BL cases lacking a Myc translocation [44]. Hsa-miR-9 expression was found to be decreased in translocation-negative cases when compared with translocation-positive cases. These cases were found to have heavy methylation of the hsa-miR-9 gene. Has-miR-9 modulates E2F1, a transcription factor that upregulates Myc expression. E2F1 was found to be upregulated only in BL cases that lacked a Myc translocation. LCLs transfected with a hsa-miR-9-inhibitor showed increased Myc expression, implicating the role for hsa-miR-9 in lymphomagenesis in BL cases lacking a Myc translocation. Data from these two studies imply that two distinct mechanisms may be responsible for Myc overexpression in BL: translocation of Myc to an immunoglobulin locus or downregulation of miRNAs which modulate Myc expression.

Consequence of Myc Overexpression in BL

The mechanism by which Myc overexpression drives BL tumor development has been evaluated using in vitro and in vivo models. Myc overexpression in LCLs results in EBV independent cell growth [45] and upregulation of germinal center markers such as CD10 and CD38 which are hallmarks of BL [46, 47]. It also results in decreased in cellular immunogenicity, which is typical of BL tumor cells. LCLs with Myc overexpression have decreased HLA expression and decreased expression of components of the antigen-processing pathway [48, 49]. This implies that Myc overexpression may contribute to the ability of BL to evade the host immune response.

Murine models have been developed to evaluate the effect of the Myc-immunoglobulin translocation. Fusion of WT MYC to an IgH enhancer in transgenic mice results in tumors, but they are of pre-B-cell origin unlike the GC phenotype seen in BL [50]. In contrast, mice transgenic for a mutated MYC derived from BL cells translocated to the IgL locus develop tumors that more closely resemble BL [51]. This implies that mutations seen in Myc may contribute to BL oncogenesis.

Additional Pathway Alterations in BL

In addition to Myc overexpression, many cases of BL demonstrate alterations in p53, RB, and Bim pathways, which likely contribute to lymphomagenesis.

p53 Deregulation

Approximately 30% of endemic BL and 55% of sporadic BL cases have alterations in the p53 pathway, either due to p53 mutation or overexpression of MDM2, a negative regulator of p53 [52–55]. P53 is a known tumor suppressor gene that is altered in almost half of all human tumors. Mutations in p53 that are seen in BL cluster around the core DNA binding and activation domain and have been shown to functionally affect p-53-mediated apoptosis and cell cycle arrest [56]. Cases with WT p53 have been found to have other alterations that affect the p53 pathway including MDM2 overexpression or less frequently, homozygous deletion in p14ARF, a protein which stabilizes p53 [57]. Promoter methylation of INK4a, a component of the RB tumor suppressor pathway, has also been documented in WT p53 BL cases implying that alterations in both the p53 and RB pathways exist in BL [58]. These alterations likely complement Myc activation by inhibiting Myc-mediated apoptosis.

RBL2 Mutations in Endemic BL

RBL2/p130 is one of the three members of the retinoblastoma family of genes along with pRb and p107 [59]. The pocket region, which is homologous in all three family members, mediates interactions with E2F/DP members and viral oncoproteins. Loss of genes in this pathway may confer growth advantage or resistance to apoptosis in BL. While the pRB pathway is intact in BL, RBL2/p130 is mutated in most cases of endemic BL and some cases of sporadic BL. These mutations interfere with the nuclear localization of the protein product [60, 61]. HIV-associated BL (HIV-BL), in contrast, does not harbor mutations in RBL2/p130. Another mechanism of RBL2/p130 inactivation, specifically in HIV-BL may be via interactions between the HIV-1 TAT protein and RBL2/p130 [62, 63]. However, HIV does not directly infect BL cells, so this process would have to be a result of entry of Tat protein into BL cells at sufficiently high concentrations, after release from infected T cells or macrophages, which has not been experimentally documented to occur in vivo.

The importance of RBL2/p130 downregulation in complementing Myc has been demonstrated in vitro and in vivo [4]. Introduction of WT RBL2/p130 into BL cell lines with RBL2/p130 mutation results in cell cycle arrest via a G0-G1 phase block. These cells also have altered expression genes important in apoptosis, B-cell activation, and cell proliferation [64]. Overexpression of Myc and silencing of RBL2/p130 in EBV-positive B-cell lines accelerates cell proliferation and decreases apoptosis. This effect is greater than either alterations in Myc or RBL2/p130 alone. In vivo xenograft murine models that are transfected to overexpress Myc and silence RBL2/p130 demonstrate development of B-cell lymphomas. In conclusion, RBL2/p130 signaling is deregulated in endemic and some sporadic BL and may cooperate with Myc to mediate lymphomagenesis.

Role of Bim in Evasion of Apoptosis

Another mechanism by which Myc mediates apoptosis is by indirect upregulation of the proapoptotic protein Bim, also known as BCL-2-like protein 11. Bim initiates apoptosis by inactivating BCL2 and MCL1, both members of the BCL2 family of proteins [65, 66]. Mutant forms of Myc have been described in BL that lose the ability to stimulate Bim expression. Mutations have been described in the MYC box 1 region at residues 57 or 58 (P57S or T58A). Evidence from murine models indicates that these mutations result in the inability of Myc to stimulate Bim-mediated

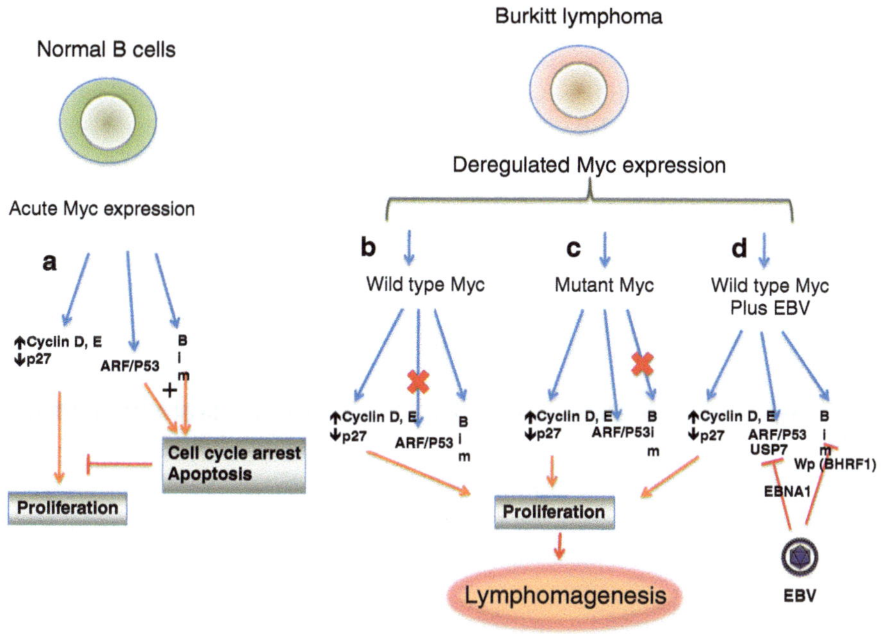

Fig. 11.2 Mechanisms for escaping c-MYC-induced apoptosis. *Panels* **a–c** are adapted from Dang et al. Cancer Cell 2005; 8:177-178 (**a**) Acute activation of Myc induces target genes involved in proliferation, but the activation of ARF, p53, and Bim (which inhibits Bcl2) leads to apoptosis or cell cycle arrest. Activation of both the ARF/p53 and Bim pathways is required for apoptosis induction (**b**) Chronic expression of wild-type Myc induces lymphomagenesis coordinately with the inactivation of ARF or p53. (**c**) Chronic expression of Myc mutants derived from Burkitt lymphoma (BL) cells fail to activate Bim and hence promote lymphomagenesis despite the presence of wild-type p53 or ARF. (**d**) In our proposed model, EBV in a Wp-restricted form of latency downregulates Bim in BL cells and thus contributes to lymphomagenesis. Adapted from Rickinson, PhD; Alfred Reiter, MD; and John T. Sandlund, MD, Hematology 2007

apoptosis [67]. Irradiated mice that are immune reconstituted with hematopoietic stem cells containing mutated Myc develop tumors at a faster rate than mice reconstituted with WT Myc. Tumors as a result of mutated Myc do not have alterations in the p53 pathway but demonstrate decreased expression of Bim. These studies are validated with work in BL tumor samples that shows that BL cases with WT Myc are more likely to have p53 mutations and cases with mutated Myc are more likely to have decreased Bim expression [67].

It is therefore likely that there are multiple mechanisms by which BL cells can evade Myc-mediated apoptosis (Fig. 11.2). For tumors with WT Myc, apoptosis is inhibited via alterations in the AFR/p53 pathway. In cases of Myc mutations, the p53 pathway remains intact but apoptosis is inhibited via decreased expression of Bim.

Anti-apoptotic Function of EBV in BL

EBV may represent another mechanism by which BL cells are able to avert Myc-mediated apoptosis. EBV is present in almost all endemic BL and a subset of sporadic and HIV-associated BL. EBV is a γ-herpes virus that can exist in lytic and latent states. The majority of adults have been infected with EBV and carry the latent virus in 1 of every 10^5 to 10^6 circulating memory B-cells. In EBV-positive BL, EBV is found in every tumor cell, implying a role for the virus in generation of a malignant clone. While EBV is known to have growth-transforming capacity in B-cells this may not be its role in BL as the majority of EBV-transforming proteins are not expressed in BL. In the case of BL, EBV exists in a latency I pattern where only Epstein Barr nuclear antigen-1 (EBNA1), and non-coding EBV-encoded RNAs (EBERs) are expressed. There is mounting evidence that the role of EBV in BL may not be to transform B-cells but to counteract Myc-induced apoptosis. Two EBV encoded proteins have been suggested to have an anti-apoptotic role.

EBNA1

EBNA1 is essential for EBV episome replication and is expressed in all EBV-associated malignancies. Overexpression of a dominant-negative EBNA1 mutant in EBV-positive BL cell lines is associated with increased cell death [68]. Similarly, downregulation of EBNA1 in BL cell lines by RNA interference results in moderately decreased cell proliferation [69, 70]. One proposed mechanism by which EBNA1 inhibits apoptosis is by interfering with WT p53 [68, 71]. EBNA1 binds the deubiquitinizing enzyme HAUSP/USP7. This enzyme is known to bind to p53 leading to p53 stabilization. EBNA1 competes with p53 for binding to USP7 and is thought to reduce p53 stability. The importance of EBNA1 in evading apoptosis in BL, however, has been debated. Studies in LCLs treated with DNA cross linking agents have shown that latent EBV does not result in alterations in p53 levels or p53 phosphorylation [72]. A recent study suggested that an alternative mechanism of by which EBNA1 may counteract apoptosis is via upregulation of survivin, an anti-apoptotic protein [73].

BHRF1

Expression of BHRF1, a viral homologue of BCL2, has been described in a subset of endemic BL and is shown to have a more dramatic anti-apoptoic effect than EBNA1 expression alone. BHRF1 is expressed as part of an alternative EBV transcriptional program known as "Wp-restricted latency" which has been described in approximately 15% of endemic BL [74]. Wp-restricted BL cell lines are known to be particularly resistant to apoptosis [75]. In this latency pattern, EBNA transcripts are derived from the Wp promoter; however, a deletion removes EBNA2 resulting in transcription of EBNA1, EBNA 3A, 3B, and 3C, and a truncated form of EBNA-LP. Deletion of EBNA2 puts BHRF1 in close proximity to the active BamH1 W promoter resulting in expression of this protein, which is usually only seen in lytic replication. BHRF1 is known to protect B-cells from programmed cell death including Myc-mediated apoptosis [76, 77]. BHRF1 expression in latency I BL cell lines protects cells from apoptosis [78]. Additionally, knockdown of BHRF1 by RNA interference in Wp-restricted BL cells results in increased cell death [79]. These results support the role of EBV in the evasion of Myc-inducted apoptosis in BL.

mRNA and miRNA Profiling in BL

Microarray technology has been used to provide additional insights into the molecular pathways relevant in BL. Gene expression data has identified a genetic signature that can distinguish BL from DLBCL. Similar technology has been used to evaluate differences between the BL epidemiologic subtypes.

It is occasionally difficult to reliably differentiate BL from DLBCL using morphology, immunophenotype, and standard molecular testing, and descriptors such as BL-like or atypical BL have been used to describe these cases. The current WHO classification schema now recognizes a separate diagnostic category of B-cell lymphoma unclassifiable with features intermediate between BL and DLBCL (BCL, U) [80]. Differentiating BL from DLBCL is clinically relevant as the optimal therapy varies between the two.

Gene expression profiling (GEP) has identified a BL that is unique from DLBCL [6, 81]. These studies, which included cases of sporadic BL, compared BL to DLBCL and found the BL signature to be enriched in Myc targets and GC B-cell genes. MHC class I and NF-κB target genes were downregulated in BL [81]. Importantly, tumors with the "molecular BL" signature included not only cases that were pathologically diagnosed as BL but also cases of BCL, U and some cases of DLCBL. Patients with tumors molecularly classified as BL had a superior outcome when treated with intensive BL-type therapy than those treated as DLCBL [81]. These studies highlight the difficulty in diagnosing BL by standard methods and identify a sporadic BL-specific signature that can be obtained by molecular profiling.

More recently GEP profiling has been performed on all three epidemiologic subtypes of BL [4]. Unsupervised clustering shows that the BL subtypes cluster together apart from other aggressive lymphomas. While the epidemiologic subtypes were relatively homogeneous, some modest differences were reported. Endemic and HIV-associated BL cluster together apart from sporadic BL. Differences between endemic BL and sporadic BL include genes important in B-cell receptor signaling, TNF-α/NF-κB pathways and IL-dependent signaling cascades. It has been postulated that differences may be related to chronic antigenic stimulation in the context of endemic BL.

Microarrays evaluating miRNA profiles in BL have found similar patterns [82, 83]. The miRNA signature of BL differs from that of DLCBL in Myc-regulated and in NF-κB pathway-associated miRNA. Only minimal differences were noted between endemic and sporadic BL.

Conclusions

The hallmark genetic alteration of BL is a translocation that leads to deregulation of Myc. While we have known this for over 30 years, Myc is an extremely complex protein, in terms of its both regulation and function [84]. Its expression seems to be tightly controlled, and subtle changes in this control, rather than simple upregulation, may be involved in the pathogenesis of BL. Functionally, Myc affects many essential cellular functions that include growth, metabolism, and differentiation, and is thought to play the role of integrator of these functions. Myc is an obvious therapeutic target in BL, but so far, no Myc inhibitors have been developed in spite of serious efforts. A variety of approaches have been proposed that target specific Myc-mediated effects. A recent example is the discovery of a selectively small molecule bromodomain inhibitor that suppresses the transcriptional effects of Myc by BET bromodomain proteins that serve as transcriptional coactivators [85]. Understanding of the molecular pathogenesis of BL has led to the understanding of the complexities of Myc that has been extrapolated to numerous other malignancies and is likely to lead to significant new targeted therapies.

References

1. Burkitt D (1958) A sarcoma involving the jaws in African children. Br J Surg 46:218–223
2. Hutt MS, Burkitt D (1965) Geographical distribution of cancer in East Africa: a new clinicopathological approach. Br Med J 2:719–722
3. Epstein MA, Achong BG, Barr YM (1964) Virus particles in cultured lymphoblasts from Burkitt's lymphoma. Lancet 1:702–703
4. Piccaluga PP, De Falco G, Kustagi M et al (2011) Gene expression analysis uncovers similarity and differences among Burkitt lymphoma subtypes. Blood 117:3596–3608
5. Haralambieva E, Schuuring E, Rosati S et al (2004) Interphase fluorescence in situ hybridization for detection of 8q24/MYC breakpoints on routine histologic sections: validation in Burkitt lymphomas from three geographic regions. Genes Chromosomes Cancer 40:10–18
6. Hummel M, Bentink S, Berger H et al (2006) A biologic definition of Burkitt's lymphoma from transcriptional and genomic profiling. N Engl J Med 354:2419–2430
7. Lai JL, Fenaux P, Zandecki M, Nelken B, Huart JJ, Deminatti M (1989) Cytogenetic studies in 30 patients with Burkitt's lymphoma or L3 acute lymphoblastic leukemia with special reference to additional chromosome abnormalities. Ann Genet 32:26–32
8. Lones MA, Sanger WG, Le Beau MM et al (2004) Chromosome abnormalities may correlate with prognosis in Burkitt/Burkitt-like lymphomas of children and adolescents: a report from Children's Cancer Group Study CCG-E08. J Pediatr Hematol Oncol 26:169–178
9. Onciu M, Schlette E, Zhou Y et al (2006) Secondary chromosomal abnormalities predict outcome in pediatric and adult high-stage Burkitt lymphoma. Cancer 107:1084–1092

10. Poirel HA, Cairo MS, Heerema NA et al (2009) Specific cytogenetic abnormalities are associated with a significantly inferior outcome in children and adolescents with mature B-cell non-Hodgkin's lymphoma: results of the FAB/LMB 96 international study. Leukemia 23:323–331
11. Nelson M, Perkins SL, Dave BJ et al (2010) An increased frequency of 13q deletions detected by fluorescence in situ hybridization and its impact on survival in children and adolescents with Burkitt lymphoma: results from the Children's Oncology Group study CCG-5961. Br J Haematol 148:600–610
12. Vennstrom B, Sheiness D, Zabielski J, Bishop JM (1982) Isolation and characterization of c-myc, a cellular homolog of the oncogene (v-myc) of avian myelocytomatosis virus strain 29. J Virol 42:773–779
13. Blackwood EM, Eisenman RN (1991) Max: a helix-loop-helix zipper protein that forms a sequence-specific DNA-binding complex with Myc. Science 251:1211–1217
14. McMahon SB, Wood MA, Cole MD (2000) The essential cofactor TRRAP recruits the histone acetyltransferase hGCN5 to c-Myc. Mol Cell Biol 20:556–562
15. God JM, Haque A (2010) Burkitt lymphoma: pathogenesis and immune evasion. J Oncol 2010. pii 516047
16. Peukert K, Staller P, Schneider A, Carmichael G, Hanel F, Eilers M (1997) An alternative pathway for gene regulation by Myc. EMBO J 16:5672–5686
17. Smith K, Dalton S (2010) Myc transcription factors: key regulators behind establishment and maintenance of pluripotency. Regen Med 5:947–959
18. Takahashi K, Yamanaka S (2006) Induction of pluripotent stem cells from mouse embryonic and adult fibroblast cultures by defined factors. Cell 126:663–676
19. Wernig M, Meissner A, Foreman R et al (2007) In vitro reprogramming of fibroblasts into a pluripotent ES-cell-like state. Nature 448:318–324
20. Dominguez-Sola D, Ying CY, Grandori C et al (2007) Non-transcriptional control of DNA replication by c-Myc. Nature 448:445–451
21. Dang CV, Enigmatic MYC (2010) Conducts MYC conducts an unfolding systems biology symphony. Genes Cancer 1:526–531
22. Gomez-Roman N, Grandori C, Eisenman RN, White RJ (2003) Direct activation of RNA polymerase III transcription by c-Myc. Nature 421:290–294
23. Arabi A, Wu S, Ridderstrale K et al (2005) c-Myc associates with ribosomal DNA and activates RNA polymerase I transcription. Nat Cell Biol 7:303–310
24. Dang CV (2010) Rethinking the Warburg effect with Myc micromanaging glutamine metabolism. Cancer Res 70:859–862
25. Dalla-Favera R, Bregni M, Erikson J, Patterson D, Gallo RC, Croce CM (1982) Human c-myc onc gene is located on the region of chromosome 8 that is translocated in Burkitt lymphoma cells. Proc Natl Acad Sci USA 79:7824–7827
26. Taub R, Kirsch I, Morton C et al (1982) Translocation of the c-myc gene into the immunoglobulin heavy chain locus in human Burkitt lymphoma and murine plasmacytoma cells. Proc Natl Acad Sci USA 79:7837–7841
27. Muramatsu M, Kinoshita K, Fagarasan S, Yamada S, Shinkai Y, Honjo T (2000) Class switch recombination and hypermutation require activation-induced cytidine deaminase (AID), a potential RNA editing enzyme. Cell 102:553–563
28. Ramiro AR, Jankovic M, Eisenreich T et al (2004) AID is required for c-myc/IgH chromosome translocations in vivo. Cell 118:431–438
29. Robbiani DF, Bothmer A, Callen E et al (2008) AID is required for the chromosomal breaks in c-myc that lead to c-myc/IgH translocations. Cell 135:1028–1038
30. Oliveira TY, Resch W, Jankovic M, Casellas R, Nussenzweig MC, Klein IA (2012) Translocation capture sequencing: a method for high throughput mapping of chromosomal rearrangements. J Immunol Methods 375(1–2):176–181
31. Klein IA, Resch W, Jankovic M et al (2011) Translocation-capture sequencing reveals the extent and nature of chromosomal rearrangements in B lymphocytes. Cell 147:95–106
32. Shiramizu B, Barriga F, Neequaye J et al (1991) Patterns of chromosomal breakpoint locations in Burkitt's lymphoma: relevance to geography and Epstein-Barr virus association. Blood 77:1516–1526

33. Cesarman E, Dalla-Favera R, Bentley D, Groudine M (1987) Mutations in the first exon are associated with altered transcription of c-myc in Burkitt lymphoma. Science 238:1272–1275
34. Siebenlist U, Hennighausen L, Battey J, Leder P (1984) Chromatin structure and protein binding in the putative regulatory region of the c-myc gene in Burkitt lymphoma. Cell 37:381–391
35. Taub R, Moulding C, Battey J et al (1984) Activation and somatic mutation of the translocated c-myc gene in burkitt lymphoma cells. Cell 36:339–348
36. Spencer CA, LeStrange RC, Novak U, Hayward WS, Groudine M (1990) The block to transcription elongation is promoter dependent in normal and Burkitt's lymphoma c-myc alleles. Genes Dev 4:75–88
37. Rabbitts TH, Hamlyn PH, Baer R (1983) Altered nucleotide sequences of a translocated c-myc gene in Burkitt lymphoma. Nature 306:760–765
38. Showe LC, Ballantine M, Nishikura K, Erikson J, Kaji H, Croce CM (1985) Cloning and sequencing of a c-myc oncogene in a Burkitt's lymphoma cell line that is translocated to a germ line alpha switch region. Mol Cell Biol 5:501–509
39. Bhatia K, Huppi K, Spangler G, Siwarski D, Iyer R, Magrath I (1993) Point mutations in the c-Myc transactivation domain are common in Burkitt's lymphoma and mouse plasmacytomas. Nat Genet 5:56–61
40. Yano T, Sander CA, Clark HM, Dolezal MV, Jaffe ES, Raffeld M (1993) Clustered mutations in the second exon of the MYC gene in sporadic Burkitt's lymphoma. Oncogene 8:2741–2748
41. Bahram F, von der Lehr N, Cetinkaya C, Larsson LG (2000) c-Myc hot spot mutations in lymphomas result in inefficient ubiquitination and decreased proteasome-mediated turnover. Blood 95:2104–2110
42. Leucci E, Cocco M, Onnis A et al (2008) MYC translocation-negative classical Burkitt lymphoma cases: an alternative pathogenetic mechanism involving miRNA deregulation. J Pathol 216:440–450
43. Ambros V (2004) The functions of animal microRNAs. Nature 431:350–355
44. Onnis A, De Falco G, Antonicelli G et al (2010) Alteration of microRNAs regulated by c-Myc in Burkitt lymphoma. PLoS One 5(9). pii: e12960
45. Lombardi L, Newcomb EW, Dalla-Favera R (1987) Pathogenesis of Burkitt lymphoma: expression of an activated c-myc oncogene causes the tumorigenic conversion of EBV-infected human B lymphoblasts. Cell 49:161–170
46. Polack A, Hortnagel K, Pajic A et al (1996) c-myc activation renders proliferation of Epstein-Barr virus (EBV)-transformed cells independent of EBV nuclear antigen 2 and latent membrane protein 1. Proc Natl Acad Sci USA 93:10411–10416
47. Pajic A, Staege MS, Dudziak D et al (2001) Antagonistic effects of c-myc and Epstein-Barr virus latent genes on the phenotype of human B cells. Int J Cancer 93:810–816
48. Schlee M, Holzel M, Bernard S et al (2007) C-myc activation impairs the NF-kappaB and the interferon response: implications for the pathogenesis of Burkitt's lymphoma. Int J Cancer 120:1387–1395
49. Staege MS, Lee SP, Frisan T et al (2002) MYC overexpression imposes a nonimmunogenic phenotype on Epstein-Barr virus-infected B cells. Proc Natl Acad Sci USA 99:4550–4555
50. Adams JM, Harris AW, Pinkert CA et al (1985) The c-myc oncogene driven by immunoglobulin enhancers induces lymphoid malignancy in transgenic mice. Nature 318:533–538
51. Kovalchuk AL, Qi CF, Torrey TA et al (2000) Burkitt lymphoma in the mouse. J Exp Med 192:1183–1190
52. Wilda M, Bruch J, Harder L et al (2004) Inactivation of the ARF-MDM-2-p53 pathway in sporadic Burkitt's lymphoma in children. Leukemia 18:584–588
53. Bhatia KG, Gutierrez MI, Huppi K, Siwarski D, Magrath IT (1992) The pattern of p53 mutations in Burkitt's lymphoma differs from that of solid tumors. Cancer Res 52:4273–4276
54. Capoulade C, Bressac-de paillerets B, lefrere I et al (1998) Overexpression of MDM2, due to enhanced translation, results in inactivation of wild-type p53 in Burkitt's lymphoma cells. Oncogene 16:1603–1610
55. Cherney BW, Bhatia KG, Sgadari C et al (1997) Role of the p53 tumor suppressor gene in the tumorigenicity of Burkitt's lymphoma cells. Cancer Res 57:2508–2515

56. Vousden KH, Crook T, Farrell PJ (1993) Biological activities of p53 mutants in Burkitt's lymphoma cells. J Gen Virol 74(Pt 5):803–810
57. Lindstrom MS, Klangby U, Wiman KG (2001) p14ARF homozygous deletion or MDM2 overexpression in Burkitt lymphoma lines carrying wild type p53. Oncogene 20:2171–2177
58. Klangby U, Okan I, Magnusson KP, Wendland M, Lind P, Wiman KG (1998) p16/INK4a and p15/INK4b gene methylation and absence of p16/INK4a mRNA and protein expression in Burkitt's lymphoma. Blood 91:1680–1687
59. Stiegler P, Giordano A (1998) Big brothers are watching: the retinoblastoma family and growth control. Prog Mol Subcell Biol 20:25–42
60. Cinti C, Claudio PP, Howard CM et al (2000) Genetic alterations disrupting the nuclear localization of the retinoblastoma-related gene RB2/p130 in human tumor cell lines and primary tumors. Cancer Res 60:383–389
61. Cinti C, Leoncini L, Nyongo A et al (2000) Genetic alterations of the retinoblastoma-related gene RB2/p130 identify different pathogenetic mechanisms in and among Burkitt's lymphoma subtypes. Am J Pathol 156:751–760
62. De Falco G, Bellan C, Lazzi S et al (2003) Interaction between HIV-1 Tat and pRb2/p130: a possible mechanism in the pathogenesis of AIDS-related neoplasms. Oncogene 22:6214–6219
63. Lazzi S, Bellan C, De Falco G et al (2002) Expression of RB2/p130 tumor-suppressor gene in AIDS-related non-Hodgkin's lymphomas: implications for disease pathogenesis. Hum Pathol 33:723–731
64. De Falco G, Leucci E, Lenze D et al (2007) Gene-expression analysis identifies novel RBL2/p130 target genes in endemic Burkitt lymphoma cell lines and primary tumors. Blood 110:1301–1307
65. Egle A, Harris AW, Bouillet P, Cory S (2004) Bim is a suppressor of Myc-induced mouse B cell leukemia. Proc Natl Acad Sci USA 101:6164–6169
66. Strasser A (2005) The role of BH3-only proteins in the immune system. Nat Rev Immunol 5:189–200
67. Hemann MT, Bric A, Teruya-Feldstein J et al (2005) Evasion of the p53 tumour surveillance network by tumour-derived MYC mutants. Nature 436:807–811
68. Kennedy G, Komano J, Sugden B (2003) Epstein-Barr virus provides a survival factor to Burkitt's lymphomas. Proc Natl Acad Sci USA 100:14269–14274
69. Hong M, Murai Y, Kutsuna T et al (2006) Suppression of Epstein-Barr nuclear antigen 1 (EBNA1) by RNA interference inhibits proliferation of EBV-positive Burkitt's lymphoma cells. J Cancer Res Clin Oncol 132:1–8
70. Yin Q, Flemington EK (2006) siRNAs against the Epstein Barr virus latency replication factor, EBNA1, inhibit its function and growth of EBV-dependent tumor cells. Virology 346:385–393
71. Saridakis V, Sheng Y, Sarkari F et al (2005) Structure of the p53 binding domain of HAUSP/USP7 bound to Epstein-Barr nuclear antigen 1 implications for EBV-mediated immortalization. Mol Cell 18:25–36
72. O'Nions J, Turner A, Craig R, Allday MJ (2006) Epstein-Barr virus selectively deregulates DNA damage responses in normal B cells but has no detectable effect on regulation of the tumor suppressor p53. J Virol 80:12408–12413
73. Lu J, Murakami M, Verma SC et al (2011) Epstein-Barr virus nuclear antigen 1 (EBNA1) confers resistance to apoptosis in EBV-positive B-lymphoma cells through up-regulation of survivin. Virology 410:64–75
74. Kelly G, Bell A, Rickinson A (2002) Epstein-Barr virus-associated Burkitt lymphomagenesis selects for downregulation of the nuclear antigen EBNA2. Nat Med 8:1098–1104
75. Kelly GL, Milner AE, Tierney RJ et al (2005) Epstein-Barr virus nuclear antigen 2 (EBNA2) gene deletion is consistently linked with EBNA3A, -3B, and -3C expression in Burkitt's lymphoma cells and with increased resistance to apoptosis. J Virol 79:10709–10717
76. Henderson S, Huen D, Rowe M, Dawson C, Johnson G, Rickinson A (1993) Epstein-Barr virus-coded BHRF1 protein, a viral homologue of Bcl-2, protects human B cells from programmed cell death. Proc Natl Acad Sci USA 90:8479–8483

77. Fanidi A, Hancock DC, Littlewood TD (1998) Suppression of c-Myc-induced apoptosis by the Epstein-Barr virus gene product BHRF1. J Virol 72:8392–8395
78. Kelly GL, Long HM, Stylianou J et al (2009) An Epstein-Barr virus anti-apoptotic protein constitutively expressed in transformed cells and implicated in burkitt lymphomagenesis: the Wp/BHRF1 link. PLoS Pathog 5:e1000341
79. Watanabe A, Maruo S, Ito T, Ito M, Katsumura KR, Takada K (2010) Epstein-Barr virus-encoded Bcl-2 homologue functions as a survival factor in Wp-restricted Burkitt lymphoma cell line P3HR-1. J Virol 84:2893–2901
80. Swerdlow SH, Campo E, Harris NL et al (2008) WHO classification of tumours of haematopoietic and lymphoid tissues, 4th edn. IARC Press, Lyon
81. Dave SS, Fu K, Wright GW et al (2006) Molecular diagnosis of Burkitt's lymphoma. N Engl J Med 354:2431–2442
82. Lenze D, Leoncini L, Hummel M et al (2011) The different epidemiologic subtypes of Burkitt lymphoma share a homogenous micro RNA profile distinct from diffuse large B-cell lymphoma. Leukemia 25(12):1869–1876
83. Robertus JL, Kluiver J, Weggemans C et al (2010) MiRNA profiling in B non-Hodgkin lymphoma: a MYC-related miRNA profile characterizes Burkitt lymphoma. Br J Haematol 149:896–899
84. Meyer N, Penn LZ (2008) Reflecting on 25 years with MYC. Nat Rev Cancer 8:976–990
85. Delmore JE, Issa GC, Lemieux ME et al (2011) BET bromodomain inhibition as a therapeutic strategy to target c-Myc. Cell 146:904–917

Chapter 12
Immune Responses to Burkitt's Lymphoma

Ann Moormann and Christian Münz

Introduction

Epstein Barr virus (EBV) is a common human γ-herpesvirus that infects more than 90% of the human adult population [1]. After transmission via saliva exchange, EBV primarily infects and establishes persistence in human B cells. Depending on the differentiation stage of the infected B cell, EBV infection leads to the expression of latency programs, consisting of eight proteins in naïve B cells, three proteins in germinal center B cells, and zero or transient single protein expression in memory B cells (latencies III, II and I, respectively) [2]. These latency proteins (six nuclear antigens or EBNAs and two membrane proteins or LMPs) are thought to drive infected B cells into memory B-cell differentiation for long-term persistence in this cellular compartment and reactivation of virus producing, lytic infection after B-cell receptor cross-linking on EBV infected memory B cells [3, 4]. Accordingly, most EBV-associated tumors that are thought to emerge from these B cell differentiation stages are B cell lymphomas and express different sets of EBV latent proteins. Post-transplant lymphoproliferative disease carries latency III, Hodgkin's lymphoma latency II, and Burkitt's lymphoma latency I. In addition, EBV associated T and NK cell lymphomas, as well as carcinomas of epithelial cell origin exist, but their etiology remains poorly defined [5].

EBV-associated Burkitt's lymphoma (BL) develops primarily during coinfection with the immunomodulatory pathogens *Plasmodium falciparum* malaria and human immunodeficiency virus [6], resulting in endemic BL (95% EBV associated) and

A. Moormann
Department of Pediatrics, University of Massachusetts Medical School,
Worcester, MA 01605, USA
e-mail: ann.moormann@umass.med.edu

C. Münz (✉)
Viral Immunobiology, Institute of Experimental Immunology, University of Zürich,
Winterthurerstrasse 190, 8057 Zürich, Switzerland
e-mail: christian.muenz@uzh.ch

E.S. Robertson (ed.), *Burkitt's Lymphoma*, Current Cancer Research,
DOI 10.1007/978-1-4614-4313-1_12,

HIV-associated BL (40% EBV associated), respectively. These coinfections are known to compromise adaptive antiviral and stimulate humoral immune responses which could weaken immune control and enhance production of BL cells, respectively. Since EBV latency I tumors like BL are the least immunogenic of all EBV-associated malignancies, due to the expression of a sole EBV antigen at the protein level, even a slight weakening of EBV-associated immune control could lead to BL development. Accordingly, we will focus on three aspects of immune responses to BL in this chapter. We will discuss innate and adaptive immunity to EBV latency I, intrinsic immune escape mechanisms that protect BL cells, and changes that the BL predisposing coinfections HIV and malaria cause in the immune system, which could explain failing immune control over EBV.

Innate Immune Responses to Burkitt's Lymphoma

Since overexpression of the oncogene c-myc, due to either the translocation into the immunoglobulin loci or down-regulation of c-myc targeting miRNAs, drives BL proliferation [7], these tumor cells express only few viral products which are thought to block apoptosis of proliferating cells [8]. In fact most BL tumors express only the nuclear antigen 1 of EBV (EBNA1) at the protein level and non-translated EBV-encoded RNAs (EBERs) from the viral episomes that they harbor. And thus leave the immune system few clues by which to detect BL cells. Innate immune activation involves lymphocytes and antigen presenting cells, such as dendritic cells (DCs) that detect pathogens via germ-line encoded receptors for pathogen-associated molecular patterns recognized by toll-like receptors (TLRs), or for stress-induced ligands that activate natural killer (NK) cell [9, 10]. These innate leukocytes then interact with each other before priming adaptive lymphocytes [11]. While the innate immune response was originally thought to limit pathogen burden prior to immune control by adaptive immunity, it has recently become clear that innate lymphocytes also contribute to immune control of persistent infections [11]. Nevertheless, pathogen detection by the innate immune system is required to initiate adaptive immunity to EBV.

Of the few viral components that are expressed in BL cells, viral DNA has been reported to stimulate plasmacytoid DCs [12, 13]. These type I IFN producing cells were able to detect viral episomes via TLR9 (Fig. 12.1). This recognition limited EBV infection in a human peripheral blood mononuclear cell (PBMC) xenotransplant model of NOD-SCID mice. However, type I IFN only prevented B-cell transformation by EBV within the first 24 h after infection [14]. While plasmacytoid DCs are, however, innate effector cells in antiviral immune responses, their capacity to present antigen for the priming of adaptive immune responses is not their primary function [15]. Thus, activation of conventional DCs should accompany plasmacytoid DC stimulation in order to initiate adaptive immune responses. Along these lines, EBERs have recently been proposed to stimulate conventional human DCs [16]. It was found that EBERs by intramolecular base pairing from stem-loop structures

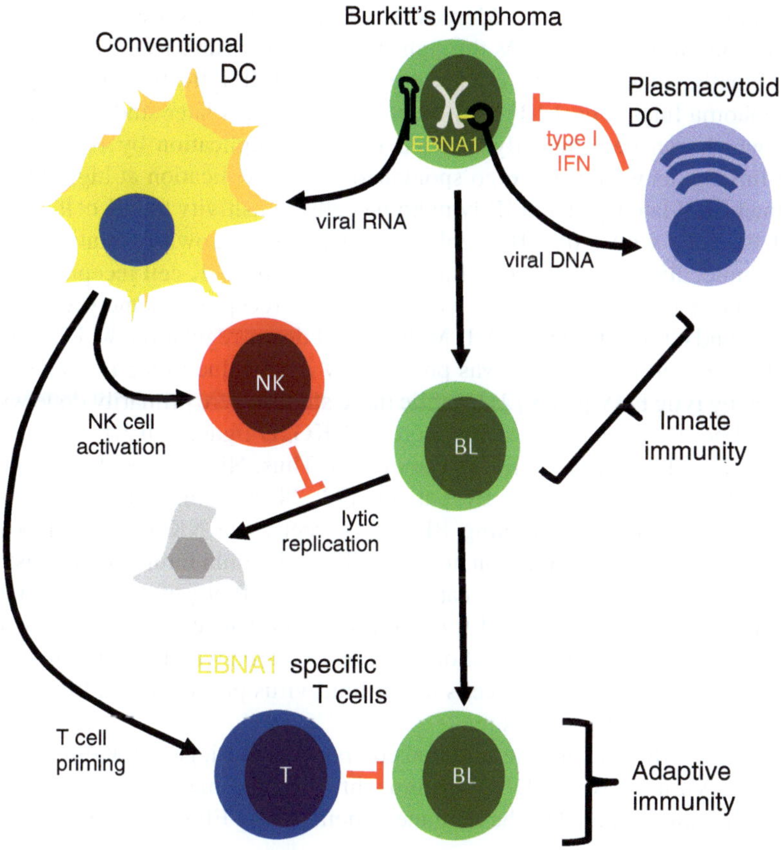

Fig. 12.1 Innate and adaptive immune responses to EBV components in Burkitt's lymphoma. Viral DNA was suggested to stimulate plasmacytoid DCs via TLR9 to produce type I IFN, which blocks B-cell transformation by EBV only in the first 24 h. Viral RNA, especially the small non-translated RNAs called EBERs, stimulate conventional DCs via TLR3. These antigen presenting cells then mature, allowing them to efficiently activate NK cells and prime EBV-specific T cells. The activated NK cells can efficiently target infected B cells undergoing lytic replication via cytotoxicity, and restrict B-cell transformation by EBV via IFN-γ. Among the primed EBV-specific T cells, EBNA1-specific $CD4^+$ T-cell responses can target BL cells. However, cell intrinsic immune escape mechanisms and immunosuppressive coinfections like HIV infection and malaria can compromise these

stimulated the double-stranded (ds) RNA receptor TLR3 and EBER-matured DCs were in turn able to stimulate T-cell responses. Thus BL cells could provide EBV DNA and RNA for plasmacytoid and conventional DC stimulation in order to activate innate and prime adaptive lymphocytes in tandem.

Although innate NK cells have been suggested to restrict EBV infection, they appear dispensable in the mouse γ-herpesvirus 68 model [17]. For human γ-herpesvirus EBV, however, NK cell depletion rendered PBMC xenografted mice more susceptible to infection [18]. Moreover, tonsillar NK cells were able to restrict B-cell transformation by EBV through their superior capacity to produce IFN-γ [19]. Finally, cytolytic NK cells were able to kill lytically EBV replicating B-lymphoma lines (Fig. 12.1) [20]. Interestingly, in this later study BL cells were used, which can be efficiently induced into lytic replication by B-cell receptor cross-linking, as well as undergo spontaneous lytic replication at higher frequencies than EBV latency II and III lymphoma cells. Sensitivity to NK cell cytotoxicity of BL cells with lytic EBV replication was due to down-regulation of MHC class I molecules, which serve as ligands for inhibitory NK cell receptors, and up-regulation of two ligands for activating NK cell receptors, namely ULBP-1 for NKG2D and CD112 for DNAM-1. MHC class I down-regulation, which sensitizes cells for NK cell recognition, was presumably in part due to the immune evasins encoded by lytic EBV genes [21]. While these studies were primarily done with the BL cell line Akata and derivatives thereof, NKG2D ligand (ULBP-1) expression was also found on the BL cell line Daudi [22]. Thus, NK cells could theoretically restrict elevated EBV titers in BL patients [23, 24] by eliminating lytically EBV replicating B cells, and targeting BL cells directly via NKG2D and DNAM-1-mediated recognition. In addition, tonsillar NK cells could limit B-cell transformation by EBV [19]. Their superior capacity to produce IFN-γ after activation allows delayed establishment of B-cell transforming EBV latency. In contrast to type I IFN, this blocking of transformation by IFN-γ is effective during the first 3 days after infection. Therefore, NK cells might limit virus production and B-cell transformation during EBV infection.

Altogether, BL contains the essential components to trigger EBV directed innate immunity. Viral RNA and DNA are thought to be the main pathogen associated molecular patterns that alert the immune system during EBV infection.

Adaptive Immune Responses to Burkitt's Lymphoma

In addition to innate immune recognition, EBV is targeted by adaptive T- and B-cell responses. While the abundant humoral immune responses against EBNA1 and antigens in the viral particle are used to diagnose symptomatic EBV infections, they are generally considered non-protective against tumor cells that only harbor latent antigens. In contrast, T-cell responses are thought to protect healthy virus carriers from EBV-associated malignancies [25, 26]. Indeed immunosuppressive treatments or immune compromising coinfections that inhibit T-cell responses result in increased incidence of EBV-associated malignancies, such as post-transplant lymphoproliferative disease (PTLD) and HIV-associated lymphomas [5]. Some of these, primarily documented for PTLDs, can be treated by adoptive transfer of EBV specific T-cell lines [27]. These T-cell lines, which are expanded by stimulation with EBV transformed lymphoblastoid cell lines (LCLs), and EBV-specific T-cell responses of healthy virus carriers are able to recognize EBV gene products following a distinct hierarchy [25]. While cytotoxic $CD8^+$ T cells mainly recognize EBNA3A,

3B and 3C, as well as early lytic antigens (i.e., the immediate early transactivators BZLF1 and BRLF1) helper CD4⁺ T cells are specific for EBNA1, 2 and 3C, as well as late viral antigens. Within this hierarchy in EBV antigen recognition only a small proportion of T cells would have the capacity to mediate immune control over BL cells.

In fact, the majority of BL cells express only EBNA1 as the sole viral antigen, and only a subset (around 15%) additionally express EBNA3A, -3B, -3C, -LP, and BHRF1 [8, 28, 29]. Both EBNA1 and BHRF1 are targeted by $CD4^+$ T cells, some of which have been shown to recognize BL cells (Fig. 12.1) [30–32]. In contrast, EBV-specific $CD8^+$ T cells are unable to detect viral antigens in BL cells even when they are ectopically expressed [33–35]. Therefore, $CD4^+$ T cells exert the majority of immune control over BL cells. Indeed, it has been shown that EBNA1 is the most consistently recognized $CD4^+$ T-cell antigen among the latent EBV gene products [36, 37]. Moreover, Th1 polarized EBNA1-specific $CD4^+$ T cells are cytotoxic for EBV transformed B cells [38], and EBNA1-specific $CD4^+$ T cell clones can kill transformed B cells of all EBV latencies [31], as well as restrict B-cell transformation by EBV in vitro [39]. EBNA1 transfected mouse B-cell lymphoma cells with c-myc translocations are controlled by EBNA1-specific $CD4^+$ T cells in vivo [40]. $CD4^+$ T-cell recognition of EBNA1-positive EBV transformed B-cell lines is in part due to antigen processing for MHC class II presentation via macroautophagy, a catabolic pathway that delivers cytoplasmic constituents for lysosomal degradation [41, 42]. Although BL cells display lower constitutive macroautophagy levels than EBV transformed B cells of other latencies ([43] and Münz, unpublished observations), the very same pathway might sensitize BL cells for killing by $CD4^+$ T cells. Thus, since antigen presentation by MHC class I molecules is blocked in BL cells, MHC class II restricted $CD4^+$ T-cell responses might be the only adaptive immune control over BL tumor cells.

Immune Escape by Burkitt's Lymphoma Cells

In addition to the limited number of EBV protein antigens that are expressed in BL cells and targeted by the adaptive immune system, immune escape mechanisms are also employed by this tumor, which affect antigen processing for MHC class I presentation in general, limit antigen presentation of EBNA1 and condition the tumor microenvironment for immune suppression [29, 44]. Along these lines, c-myc overexpression, which is caused by translocation of this oncogene into the immunoglobulin loci in BL cells, has been linked to deficient MHC class I antigen presentation to $CD8^+$ T cells [45]. C-myc down-regulates proteasomal activity, which generates most MHC class I ligands, and activates other intracellular proteolysis pathways, like the subtilisin-like protease tripeptidylpeptidase II (TPPII), which might destroy MHC class I ligands by generating peptides, which are too short for MHC class I presentation [46]. These mechanisms have been suggested to be responsible for low MHC class I antigen presentation by BL cells. Indeed, TPPII can compensate for proteasome function to ensure cell survival of proteasome inhibitor treated cells [47], and might allow survival of BL cells with decreased proteasomal activity. In addition to proteasomal inhibition, BL cells also seem to have decreased expression of the transporter associated with antigen processing (TAP), which imports proteasomal products into the endoplasmic reticulum for loading onto MHC class I molecules in this organelle [34]. Interestingly, while c-myc overexpression seems to induce these effects, viral LMP1 is able to restore efficient antigen processing for MHC class I presentation. Thus, EBV latency I and the c-myc translocation seem to cooperate in reducing immunogenicity of BL cells for CD8$^+$ T-cell recognition.

In addition to this reduced antigen processing and presentation function on MHC class I molecules of BL cells, the sole EBV antigen that is expressed in most BL cells, namely EBNA1, also limits its antigen processing in cis. EBNA1 carries a glycine-alanine (GA) repeat domain that inhibits its translation and proteasomal degradation. EBNA1 compromises its translation by the high purine content of its messenger RNA and inhibition of ribosome assembly by the nascent GA repeat [48–50]. This reduced translation decreases defective ribosomal product (DRiP) formation, which constitutes the major source for EBNA1-derived CD8$^+$ T-cell epitopes [51–53]. In addition, the GA repeat also inhibits proteasomal degradation, in order to both limit antigen processing for MHC class I presentation from mature EBNA1 proteins and ensure that constant levels of this important viral episome maintenance protein are sustained in infected cells [54, 55]. Probably due to this evasion from proteasomal degradation, EBNA1 is alternatively turned over by macroautophagy and processed for MHC class II presentation to CD4$^+$ T cells [42]. However, its nuclear localization also limits macroautophagy of EBNA1 because this catabolic pathway degrades only cytoplasmic constituents [41]. Once nuclear import of EBNA1 is compromised, this viral antigen is more efficiently processed for MHC class II presentation via macroautophagy. Thus, the only EBV antigen expressed in most BL cells actively prevents its own presentation by MHC class I and II molecules, and thereby becomes difficult to detect by T cells.

Apart from these deficiencies in viral antigen presentation on BL cells, the tumor microenvironment might further suppress adaptive immune responses at the tumor sites. Along these lines, EBNA1 has been described to up-regulate the expression of the chemokine CCL20, which attracts regulatory T cells (Tregs) [56]. Indeed, EBNA1-specific Tregs have been isolated from virus carriers [57]. However, the primary leukocyte infiltrate of BL are macrophages, which gives the tumor a "starry sky" appearance [58]. These macrophages both nurture the lymphoma cells and suppress immune responses via IL-10 production [59]. One of these suppressed responses might be EBNA1-specific T-cell recognition. Indeed, decreased T-cell responses against EBNA1 have been found in Kenyan children with BL [60]. Thus, BL seems to utilize both immune suppressive T cells and macrophages to escape immune detection in its tumor microenvironment, and systemic defects in EBNA1-specific T-cell immunity may in addition play a role in BL ontogeny.

Influence of Malaria Coinfection on Immune Responses to Burkitt's Lymphoma

Plasmodium falciparum malaria was geographically associated with BL incidence in Africa soon after it was first described by Denis Burkitt [61, 62]; however, the precise mechanisms by which malaria coinfections modulate viral persistence and EBV-specific T-cell immunity in the etiology of BL have only recently begun to be elucidated [63, 64]. Malaria parasites can stimulate host immune responses as well as suppress them exerting their influence on both innate and adaptive immune systems with differing effects depending on malaria transmission intensity and age of infection [65]. What is unclear is if malaria coinfections continue to contribute to pathogenesis and BL cell tropism after tumorigenesis has been initiated in the B cell. B cells with c-myc translocations have been found in peripheral blood of normal individuals [66], suggesting that successive oncogenic steps are required before a malignancy is established. Children in Africa are infected with EBV before the age of 3 years [67], yet BL does not present in children residing in high malaria transmission areas until they are on average 5–9 years of age, in contrast to BL patients from low malaria transmission areas who do not develop BL until they become adolescents [68, 69]. In addition, younger patients tend to present with tumors of the jaw whereas older patients and those with sporadic BL (which is 30–40% associated with EBV) tend to have abdominal tumors. Moreover, studies conducted in Kenya over the past 8 years serendipitously coinciding with malaria control efforts that have significantly decreased parasite transmission intensity with subsequent reductions in malaria-associated morbidity and mortality [70] allude to an increasing proportion of BL patients diagnosed with abdominal tumors and fewer with jaw tumors independent of age (Moormann, unpublished observations). It is possible that increased cancer awareness and improved diagnosis of abdominal tumors may account for this shift in clinical presentation for endemic BL, but it is also possible that lower malaria transmission intensity allows the persistence of less severe, chronic malaria infections (as experienced by older children and adults who have developed premonition to malaria) that may influence where BL cells migrate in the body.

Along these lines host genetic susceptibility to severe malaria infections might also influence the risk for BL development. A point mutation in the hemoglobin beta gene (AS heterozygosity or sickle cell trait) decreases parasite density and malaria disease severity [71], thus begging the question, if this mutation also confers a decreased risk for BL. Studies addressing this question are few and have yielded inconclusive results due to small sample size and appropriateness of controls selected for allele frequency comparisons [72–74]. In our BL study population ($n=608$), we found an intermediate frequency of AS heterozygosity compared to the general population ([75] and Moormann, unpublished observation). This suggests that perhaps the host's ability to become repeatedly infected with malaria yet not succumb to malaria-associated mortality, which is accompanied by an unregulated pro-inflammatory response, is a more important risk factor for developing BL than severe malaria, thus emphasizing the need for longitudinal studies to understand the role of malaria coinfections in BL pathology.

We know that children diagnosed with BL at some point become selectively deficient in their Th1 polarized (IFN-γ producing) cell immunity to EBNA1 [60], yet we have not determined whether EBNA1-specific T cell immunity is restored during remission and is associated with long-term survival, nor if its deficiency predisposes for BL development. However, it has been proposed that blood stage malaria infection is controlled by Th2 polarized immunity [76], which could compromise the simultaneous priming of protective Th1 immunity against EBV. Moreover, the *Plasmodium falciparum* erythrocyte membrane protein (PfEMP1) has been shown to inhibit early IFN-γ production [77], which could also divert EBV specific T-cell immunity from Th1. Finally, *Plasmodium* infected erythrocytes were found to inhibit dendritic cell function [78], which could compromise priming of efficient EBV-specific immune control. Indeed this immune control was found to be compromised by malaria infection [79] and loss of EBNA1-specific T-cell responses was observed in BL patients [60].

In addition to this immunomodulatory function of malaria, which could impair EBV-specific immune control, *Plasmodium* infection might also predispose for BL development via B-cell stimulation. Malaria parasite-derived TLR ligands have been shown to signal innate immune responses via TLR4 [80] and TLR9 [81]. Thus, it is curious to note that c-myc translocations, the hallmark of BL cells, are created by activation-induced cytidine deaminase (AID) during antibody class switching or somatic hypermutation [82] and that expression of AID may be mediated by TLR9 in cooperation with IL-10 signaling [83]. Furthermore, *Plasmodium* antigen driven B-cell activation, by the polyclonal B-cell activator PfEMP1 [84], could also drive more EBV-infected B cells into germinal center reactions, which could favor AID mediated c-myc translocation. It is speculation at this point if repeated malaria infections continue to exacerbate this dynamic and thereby increase the risk of BL relapse. Nevertheless, malaria-driven immune modulation and B-cell activation could both favor BL development.

Immunomodulation by HIV Infection During Burkitt's Lymphoma

EBV is found in 40–60% of HIV-associated BL cases [85, 86] and often occurs as the first sign of the acquired immunodeficiency syndrome (AIDS) [87]. Interestingly, an altered viral set-point for EBV infection in HIV carrying individuals does not correlate with the development of EBV-associated lymphomas during the progression to AIDS [88], suggesting that selective loss of EBV immune control contributes to the development of HIV-associated BL. While other EBV-associated lymphomas, like diffuse large B-cell lymphomas (DLBCL) occur later in the progression of AIDS and have been found to be responsive to highly active anti-retroviral treatment (HAART) [89, 90], BL frequencies and outcome have not been significantly influenced by HAART. This suggests that selective defects in EBV-specific immune control, affecting the limited repertoire of immune responses that can target this tumor, are not easily reinstated by HAART, while those that target DLBCL might be more readily recovered.

Along these lines, EBNA1-specific T-cell responses were found selectively decreased prior to lymphoma development in HIV-infected individuals with non-Hodgkin lymphoma [91]. Not only $CD4^+$ T-cell responses to EBNA1 were most severely affected, but also $CD8^+$ T-cell responses against this viral protein were diminished. In contrast, $CD4^+$ T-cell responses against the immediate early lytic EBV antigen BZLF-1 were preserved in HIV-infected individuals progressing to AIDS with the development of EBV-positive lymphomas. Prior to this study the same group had suggested a protective effect of $CD4^+$ T cells in EBV-specific immune control, because EBV-specific $CD4^+$, but not $CD8^+$ T-cell frequencies were inversely correlated with EBV viral loads in HIV-infected individuals [92]. Moreover, HAART seems to restore EBNA1-specific T-cell responses, but the slow kinetics of this restoration (5 years) might not be able to efficiently counteract HIV-associated BL development [88]. Confirming a selective loss of EBV-specific $CD4^+$ T-cell responses during HIV associated lymphoma development, it was found that patients with primary CNS lymphomas lacked EBV specific $CD4^+$ T-cell responses, irrespective of total $CD4^+$ T-cell count [93]. Thus, it is tempting to speculate that $CD4^+$ T cells, activated by persistent EBV infection, might be preferentially depleted by HIV infection. This depletion, followed by functional exhaustion of EBV-specific $CD8^+$ T-cell responses [94], could predispose for HIV-associated lymphoma development. Among EBV-specific $CD4^+$ T cells EBNA1-specific responses might become diminished first due to the ubiquitous expression of this antigen in all latency stages, thereby compromising BL-specific immune control that can target only EBNA1.

Conclusions

The restricted EBV gene expression pattern of endemic BL makes these tumors difficult to detect for the human immune system. While viral DNA and RNA, harbored also in BL cells, can activate plasmacytoid and conventional dendritic cells, respectively, only one EBV antigen is expressed at the protein level in most BL cells and can be recognized by the adaptive immune system. Besides being the only EBV antigen expressed in BL cells, EBNA1 down-modulates its processing onto MHC class I for $CD8^+$ T-cell recognition and the BL-characteristic c-myc overexpression by translocation compromises further MHC class I antigen processing. Only EBNA1-specific $CD4^+$ T-cell responses show a limited reactivity against BL cells. But the $CD4^+$ T-cell compartment and particularly Th1 polarized $CD4^+$ T cells, which orchestrate cell-mediated immunity, are compromised by HIV and *Plasmodium falciparum* coinfections. Thus, strengthening of this immune response by vaccination during antiretroviral therapy and malaria containing treatment should be explored to prevent BL development.

Acknowledgments Work in the Münz laboratory is in part supported by the National Cancer Institute (R01CA108609), Cancer Research Switzerland (KFS-02652-08-2010), the Association for International Cancer Research (11–0516), the Sassella Foundation (10/02), the Vontobel Foundation, the Baugarten Foundation, Novartis and the Swiss National Science Foundation (310030_126995). Work in the Moormann laboratory is in part supported by the National Cancer Institute (CA134051), The Worcester Foundation ARF Grant, and the University of Massachusetts Medical School Dean's Challenge Award.

References

1. Young LS, Rickinson AB (2004) Epstein-Barr virus: 40 years on. Nat Rev Cancer 4:757–768
2. Babcock JG, Hochberg D, Thorley-Lawson AD (2000) The expression pattern of Epstein-Barr virus latent genes in vivo is dependent upon the differentiation stage of the infected B cell. Immunity 13:497–506
3. Babcock JG, Decker LL, Volk M, Thorley-Lawson DA (1998) EBV persistence in memory B cells in vivo. Immunity 9:395–404
4. Laichalk LL, Thorley-Lawson DA (2005) Terminal differentiation into plasma cells initiates the replicative cycle of Epstein-Barr virus in vivo. J Virol 79:1296–1307
5. Kutok JL, Wang F (2006) Spectrum of Epstein-Barr virus-associated diseases. Annu Rev Pathol 1:375–404
6. Thorley-Lawson DA, Allday MJ (2008) The curious case of the tumour virus: 50 years of Burkitt's lymphoma. Nat Rev Microbiol 6:913–924
7. Leucci E, Cocco M, Onnis A, De Falco G, van Cleef P, Bellan C, van Rijk A, Nyagol J, Byakika B, Lazzi S, Tosi P, van Krieken H, Leoncini L (2008) MYC translocation-negative classical Burkitt lymphoma cases: an alternative pathogenetic mechanism involving miRNA deregulation. J Pathol 216:440–450
8. Kelly GL, Milner AE, Baldwin GS, Bell AI, Rickinson AB (2006) Three restricted forms of Epstein-Barr virus latency counteracting apoptosis in c-myc-expressing Burkitt lymphoma cells. Proc Natl Acad Sci USA 103:14935–14940
9. Iwasaki A, Medzhitov R (2004) Toll-like receptor control of the adaptive immune responses. Nat Immunol 5:987–995
10. Münz C, Steinman RM, Fujii S (2005) Dendritic cell maturation by innate lymphocytes: coordinated stimulation of innate and adaptive immunity. J Exp Med 202:203–207
11. Chijioke O, Münz C (2011) Interactions of human myeloid cells with natural killer cell subsets in vitro and in vivo. J Biomed Biotechnol 2011:251679
12. Fiola S, Gosselin D, Takada K, Gosselin J (2010) TLR9 contributes to the recognition of EBV by primary monocytes and plasmacytoid dendritic cells. J Immunol 185:3620–3631
13. Lim WH, Kireta S, Russ GR, Coates PT (2006) Human plasmacytoid dendritic cells regulate immune responses to Epstein-Barr virus (EBV) infection and delay EBV-related mortality in humanized NOD-SCID mice. Blood 109:1043–1050
14. Lotz M, Tsoukas CD, Fong S, Carson DA, Vaughan JH (1985) Regulation of Epstein-Barr virus infection by recombinant interferons. Selected sensitivity to interferon-gamma. Eur J Immunol 15:520–525
15. Gilliet M, Cao W, Liu YJ (2008) Plasmacytoid dendritic cells: sensing nucleic acids in viral infection and autoimmune diseases. Nat Rev Immunol 8:594–606
16. Iwakiri D, Zhou L, Samanta M, Matsumoto M, Ebihara T, Seya T, Imai S, Fujieda M, Kawa K, Takada K (2009) Epstein-Barr virus (EBV)-encoded small RNA is released from EBV-infected cells and activates signaling from Toll-like receptor 3. J Exp Med 206:2091–2099
17. Usherwood EJ, Meadows SK, Crist SG, Bellfy SC, Sentman CL (2005) Control of murine gammaherpesvirus infection is independent of NK cells. Eur J Immunol 35:2956–2961
18. Baiocchi RA, Ward JS, Carrodeguas L, Eisenbeis CF, Peng F, Roychowdhury S, Vourganti S, Sekula T, O'Brien M, Moeschberger M, Caligiuri MA (2001) GM-CSF and IL-2 induce

specific cellular immunity and provide protection against Epstein-Barr virus lymphoproliferative disorder. J Clin Invest 108:887–894
19. Strowig T, Brilot F, Arrey F, Bougras G, Thomas D, Muller WA, Münz C (2008) Tonsilar natural killer cells restrict B cell transformation by the Epstein Barr virus via IFN-γ. PLoS Pathog 4:e27
20. Pappworth IY, Wang EC, Rowe M (2007) The switch from latent to productive infection in epstein-barr virus-infected B cells is associated with sensitization to NK cell killing. J Virol 81:474–482
21. Ressing ME, Horst D, Griffin BD, Tellam J, Zuo J, Khanna R, Rowe M, Wiertz EJ (2008) Epstein-Barr virus evasion of CD8+ and CD4+ T cell immunity via concerted actions of multiple gene products. Scmin Cancer Biol 18:397–408
22. Pende D, Rivera P, Marcenaro S, Chang CC, Biassoni R, Conte R, Kubin M, Cosman M, Ferrone S, Moretta L, Moretta A (2002) Major histocompatibility complex class I-related chain a and UL16-binding protein expression on tumor cell lines of different histotypes: analysis of tumor susceptibility to NKG2D-dependent natural killer cell cytotoxicity. Cancer Res 62:6178–6186
23. Moormann AM, Chelimo K, Sumba OP, Lutzke ML, Ploutz-Snyder R, Newton D, Kazura J, Rochford R (2005) Exposure to holoendemic malaria results in elevated Epstein-Barr virus loads in children. J Infect Dis 191:1233–1238
24. Njie R, Bell AI, Jia H, Croom-Carter D, Chaganti S, Hislop AD, Whittle H, Rickinson AB (2009) The effects of acute malaria on Epstein-Barr virus (EBV) load and EBV-specific T cell immunity in Gambian children. J Infect Dis 199:31–38
25. Hislop AD, Taylor GS, Sauce D, Rickinson AB (2007) Cellular responses to viral infection in humans: lessons from epstein-barr virus. Annu Rev Immunol 25:587–617
26. Long HM, Taylor GS, Rickinson AB (2011) Immune defence against EBV and EBV-associated disease. Curr Opin Immunol 23:258–264
27. Gottschalk S, Rooney CM, Heslop HE (2005) Post-transplant lymphoproliferative disorders. Annu Rev Med 56:29–44
28. Kelly G, Bell A, Rickinson AB (2002) Epstein-Barr virus-associated Burkitt lymphomagenesis selects for downregulation of the nuclear antigen EBNA2. Nat Med 8:1098–1104
29. Taylor GS, Blackbourn DJ (2011) Infectious agents in human cancers: lessons in immunity and immunomodulation from gammaherpesviruses EBV and KSHV. Cancer Lett 305: 263–278
30. Khanna R, Burrows SR, Thomson SA, Moss DJ, Cresswell P, Poulsen LM, Cooper L (1997) Class I processing-defective Burkitt's lymphoma cells are recognized efficiently by CD4+ EBV-specific CTLs. J Immunol 158:3619–3625
31. Paludan C, Bickham K, Nikiforow S, Tsang ML, Goodman K, Hanekom WA, Fonteneau JF, Stevanovic S, Münz C (2002) EBNA1 specific CD4+ Th1 cells kill Burkitt's lymphoma cells. J Immunol 169:1593–1603
32. Voo KS, Fu T, Heslop HE, Brenner MK, Rooney CM, Wang RF (2002) Identification of HLA-DP3-restricted peptides from EBNA1 recognized by CD4+ T cells. Cancer Res 62:7195–7199
33. Rooney CM, Rowe M, Wallace LE, Rickinson AB (1985) Epstein-Barr virus-positive Burkitt's lymphoma cells not recognized by virus-specific T-cell surveillance. Nature 317:629–631
34. Rowe M, Khanna R, Jacob CA, Argaet V, Kelly A, Powis S, Belich M, Croom-Carter D, Lee S, Burrows SR, Trowsdale J, Moss DJ, Rickinson AB (1995) Restoration of endogenous antigen processing in Burkitt's lymphoma cells by Epstein-Barr virus latent membrane protein-1: coordinate up-regulation of peptide transporters and HLA-class I antigen expression. Eur J Immunol 25:1374–1384
35. Torsteinsdottir S, Masucci MG, Ehlin-Henriksson B, Brautbar C, Ben Bassat H, Klein G, Klein E (1986) Differentiation-dependent sensitivity of human B-cell-derived lines to major histocompatibility complex-restricted T-cell cytotoxicity. Proc Natl Acad Sci USA 83:5620–5624
36. Leen A, Meij P, Redchenko I, Middeldorp J, Bloemena E, Rickinson AB, Blake NW (2001) Differential immunogenicity of Epstein-Barr virus latent-cycle proteins for human CD4+ T-helper 1 responses. J Virol 75:8649–8659

37. Münz C, Bickham KL, Subklewe M, Tsang ML, Chahroudi A, Kurilla MG, Zhang D, O'Donnell M, Steinman RM (2000) Human CD4+ T lymphocytes consistently respond to the latent Epstein-Barr virus nuclear antigen EBNA1. J Exp Med 191:1649–1660
38. Bickham K, Münz C, Tsang ML, Larsson M, Fonteneau JF, Bhardwaj N, Steinman RM (2001) EBNA1-specific CD4+ T cells in healthy carriers of Epstein-Barr virus are primarily Th1 in function. J Clin Invest 107:121–130
39. Nikiforow S, Bottomly K, Miller G, Münz C (2003) Cytolytic CD4+-T-cell clones reactive to EBNA1 inhibit Epstein-Barr virus-induced B-cell proliferation. J Virol 77:12088–12104
40. Fu T, Voo KS, Wang RF (2004) Critical role of EBNA1-specific CD4+ T cells in the control of mouse Burkitt lymphoma in vivo. J Clin Invest 114:542–550
41. Leung CS, Haigh TA, Mackay LK, Rickinson AB, Taylor GS (2010) Nuclear location of an endogenously expressed antigen, EBNA1, restricts access to macroautophagy and the range of CD4 epitope display. Proc Natl Acad Sci USA 107:2165–2170
42. Paludan C, Schmid D, Landthaler M, Vockerodt M, Kube D, Tuschl T, Münz C (2005) Endogenous MHC class II processing of a viral nuclear antigen after autophagy. Science 307:593–596
43. Schmid D, Pypaert M, Münz C (2007) MHC class II antigen loading compartments continuously receive input from autophagosomes. Immunity 26:79–92
44. Münz C, Moormann A (2008) Immune escape by Epstein-Barr virus associated malignancies. Semin Cancer Biol 18:381–387
45. Staege MS, Lee SP, Frisan T, Mautner J, Scholz S, Pajic A, Rickinson AB, Masucci MG, Polack A, Bornkamm GW (2002) MYC overexpression imposes a nonimmunogenic phenotype on Epstein-Barr virus-infected B cells. Proc Natl Acad Sci USA 99:4550–4555
46. Gavioli R, Frisan T, Vertuani S, Bornkamm GW, Masucci MG (2001) c-myc overexpression activates alternative pathways for intracellular proteolysis in lymphoma cells. Nat Cell Biol 3:283–288
47. Wang EW, Kessler BM, Borodovsky A, Cravatt BF, Bogyo M, Ploegh HL, Glas R (2000) Integration of the ubiquitin-proteasome pathway with a cytosolic oligopeptidase activity. Proc Natl Acad Sci USA 97:9990–9995
48. Apcher S, Komarova A, Daskalogianni C, Yin Y, Malbert-Colas L, Fahraeus R (2009) MRNA translation regulation by the Gly-Ala repeat of Epstein-Barr virus nuclear antigen 1. J Virol 83:1289–1298
49. Tellam J, Smith C, Rist M, Webb N, Cooper L, Vuocolo T, Connolly G, Tscharke DC, Devoy MP, Khanna R (2008) Regulation of protein translation through mRNA structure influences MHC class I loading and T cell recognition. Proc Natl Acad Sci USA 105:9319–9324
50. Yin Y, Manoury B, Fahraeus R (2003) Self-inhibition of synthesis and antigen presentation by Epstein-Barr virus-encoded EBNA1. Science 301:1371–1374
51. Lee SP, Brooks JM, Al-Jarrah H, Thomas WA, Haigh TA, Taylor GS, Humme S, Schepers A, Hammerschmidt W, Yates JL, Rickinson AB, Blake NW (2004) CD8 T cell recognition of endogenously expressed Epstein-Barr virus nuclear antigen 1. J Exp Med 199:1409–1420
52. Tellam J, Connolly G, Green KJ, Miles JJ, Moss DJ, Burrows SR, Khanna R (2004) Endogenous presentation of CD8+ T cell epitopes from Epstein-Barr virus nuclear antigen 1. J Exp Med 199:1421–1431
53. Voo KS, Fu T, Wang HY, Tellam J, Heslop HE, Brenner MK, Rooney CM, Wang RF (2004) Evidence for the presentation of major histocompatibility complex class I-restricted Epstein-Barr virus nuclear antigen 1 peptides to CD8+ T lymphocytes. J Exp Med 199:459–470
54. Levitskaya J, Coram M, Levitsky V, Imreh S, Steigerwald-Mullen PM, Klein G, Kurilla MG, Masucci MG (1995) Inhibition of antigen processing by the internal repeat region of the Epstein-Barr virus nuclear antigen-1. Nature 375:685–688
55. Levitskaya J, Sharipo A, Leonchiks A, Ciechanover A, Masucci MG (1997) Inhibition of ubiquitin/proteasome-dependent protein degradation by the Gly-Ala repeat domain of the Epstein-Barr virus nuclear antigen 1. Proc Natl Acad Sci USA 94:12616–12621
56. Baumforth KR, Birgersdotter A, Reynolds GM, Wei W, Kapatai G, Flavell JR, Kalk E, Piper K, Lee L, Machado L, Hadley K, Sundblad A, Sjoberg J, Bjorkholm M, Porwit AA, Yap LF,

Teo S, Grundy SG, Young LS, Ernberg I, Woodman CB, Murray PG (2008) Expression of the Epstein-Barr virus-encoded Epstein-Barr virus nuclear antigen 1 in Hodgkin's lymphoma cells mediates Up-regulation of CCL20 and the migration of regulatory T cells. Am J Pathol 173:195–204

57. Voo KS, Peng G, Guo Z, Fu T, Li Y, Frappier L, Wang RF (2005) Functional characterization of EBV-encoded nuclear antigen 1-specific CD4+ helper and regulatory T cells elicited by in vitro peptide stimulation. Cancer Res 65:1577–1586
58. Bedoya V, Grimley PM, Rabson AS (1969) Ultrastructural evidence to in vitro interaction among Burkitt lymphoma cells: possible relevance of the "phagocytic" activity of starry sky histiocytes in vivo. Cancer Res 29:753–762
59. Ogden CA, Pound JD, Batth BK, Owens S, Johannessen I, Wood K, Gregory CD (2005) Enhanced apoptotic cell clearance capacity and B cell survival factor production by IL-10-activated macrophages: implications for Burkitt's lymphoma. J Immunol 174:3015–3023
60. Moormann AM, Heller KN, Chelimo K, Embury P, Ploutz-Snyder R, Otieno JA, Oduor M, Münz C, Rochford R (2009) Children with endemic Burkitt lymphoma are deficient in EBNA1-specific IFN-gamma T cell responses. Int J Cancer 124:1721–1726
61. Burkitt D (1958) A sarcoma involving the jaws in African children. Br J Surg 46:218–223
62. Dalldorf G, Bergamini F (1964) Unidentified, filtrable agents isolated from African children with malignant lymphomas. Proc Natl Acad Sci USA 51:263–265
63. Moormann AM, Snider CJ, Chelimo K (2011) The company malaria keeps: how co-infection with Epstein-Barr virus leads to endemic Burkitt lymphoma. Curr Opin Infect Dis 24:435–441
64. Rochford R, Cannon MJ, Moormann AM (2005) Endemic Burkitt's lymphoma: a polymicrobial disease? Nat Rev Microbiol 3:182–187
65. Moormann AM (2009) How might infant and paediatric immune responses influence malaria vaccine efficacy? Parasite Immunol 31:547–559
66. Limpens J, Stad R, Vos C, de Vlaam C, de Jong D, van Ommen GJ, Schuuring E, Kluin PM (1995) Lymphoma-associated translocation t(14;18) in blood B cells of normal individuals. Blood 85:2528–2536
67. Biggar RJ, Henle W, Fleisher G, Bocker J, Lennette ET, Henle G (1978) Primary Epstein-Barr virus infections in African infants. I. Decline of maternal antibodies and time of infection. Int J Cancer 22:239–243
68. Burkitt D, Wright D (1966) Geographical and tribal distribution of the African lymphoma in Uganda. Br Med J 1:569–573
69. Moormann AM, Snider CJ, Chelimo K (2011) The company malaria keeps: how co-infection with Epstein Barr virus leads to Burkitt lymphoma. Curr Opin Infect Dis 24(5):435–441
70. Okiro EA, Alegana VA, Noor AM, Snow RW (2010) Changing malaria intervention coverage, transmission and hospitalization in Kenya. Malar J 9:285
71. Beutler E, Dern RG, Flanagan CL (1955) Effect of sickle-cell trait on resistance to malaria. Br Med J 1:1189–1191
72. Nkrumah FK, Perkins IV (1976) Sickle cell trait, hemoglobin C trait, and Burkitt's lymphoma. Am J Trop Med Hyg 25:633–636
73. Pike MC, Morrow RH, Kisuule A, Mafigiri J (1970) Burkitt's lymphoma and sickle cell trait. Br J Prev Soc Med 24:39–41
74. Williams AO (1966) Haemoglobin genotypes, ABO blood groups, and Burkitt's tumour. J Med Genet 3:177–179
75. Moormann AM, Embury PE, Opondo J, Sumba OP, Ouma JH, Kazura JW, John CC (2003) Frequencies of sickle cell trait and glucose-6-phosphate dehydrogenase deficiency differ in highland and nearby lowland malaria-endemic areas of Kenya. Trans R Soc Trop Med Hyg 97:513–514
76. Langhorne J, Cross C, Seixas S, Li C, von der Weid T (1998) A role for B cells in the development of T cell helper function in a malaria infection in mice. Proc Natl Acad Sci USA 95:1730–1734

77. D'Ombrain MC, Voss TS, Maier AG, Pearce JA, Hansen DS, Cowman AF, Schofield L (2007) Plasmodium falciparum erythrocyte membrane protein-1 specifically suppresses early production of host interferon-gamma. Cell Host Microbe 2:130–138
78. Urban BC, Ferguson DJ, Pain A, Willcox N, Plebanski M, Austyn JM, Roberts DJ (1999) Plasmodium falciparum-infected erythrocytes modulate the maturation of dendritic cells. Nature 400:73–77
79. Whittle HC, Brown J, Marsh K, Greenwood BM, Seidelin P, Tighe H, Wedderburn L (1984) T-cell control of Epstein-Barr virus-infected B cells is lost during P. falciparum malaria. Nature 312:449–450
80. Corr SC, O'Neill LA (2009) Genetic variation in Toll-like receptor signalling and the risk of inflammatory and immune diseases. J Innate Immun 1:350–357
81. Parroche P, Lauw FN, Goutagny N, Latz E, Monks BG, Visintin A, Halmen KA, Lamphier M, Olivier M, Bartholomeu DC, Gazzinelli RT, Golenbock DT (2007) Malaria hemozoin is immunologically inert but radically enhances innate responses by presenting malaria DNA to Toll-like receptor 9. Proc Natl Acad Sci USA 104:1919–1924
82. Ramiro AR, Jankovic M, Eisenreich T, Difilippantonio S, Chen-Kiang S, Muramatsu M, Honjo T, Nussenzweig A, Nussenzweig MC (2004) AID is required for c-myc/IgH chromosome translocations in vivo. Cell 118:431–438
83. He B, Qiao X, Cerutti A (2004) CpG DNA induces IgG class switch DNA recombination by activating human B cells through an innate pathway that requires TLR9 and cooperates with IL-10. J Immunol 173:4479–4491
84. Chene A, Donati D, Guerreiro-Cacais AO, Levitsky V, Chen Q, Falk KI, Orem J, Kironde F, Wahlgren M, Bejarano MT (2007) A molecular link between malaria and Epstein-Barr virus reactivation. PLoS Pathog 3:e80
85. Bornkamm GW (2009) Epstein-Barr virus and the pathogenesis of Burkitt's lymphoma: more questions than answers. Int J Cancer 124:1745–1755
86. Carbone A, Cesarman E, Spina M, Gloghini A, Schulz TF (2009) HIV-associated lymphomas and gamma-herpesviruses. Blood 113:1213–1224
87. Kalter SP, Riggs SA, Cabanillas F, Butler JJ, Hagemeister FB, Mansell PW, Newell GR, Velasquez WS, Salvador P, Barlogie B, Rios A, Hersh EM (1985) Aggressive non-Hodgkin's lymphomas in immunocompromised homosexual males. Blood 66:655–659
88. Piriou ER, van Dort K, Nanlohy NM, Miedema F, van Oers MH, van Baarle D (2004) Altered EBV viral load setpoint after HIV seroconversion is in accordance with lack of predictive value of EBV load for the occurrence of AIDS-related non-Hodgkin lymphoma. J Immunol 172:6931–6937
89. Lim ST, Karim R, Nathwani BN, Tulpule A, Espina B, Levine AM (2005) AIDS-related Burkitt's lymphoma versus diffuse large-cell lymphoma in the pre-highly active antiretroviral therapy (HAART) and HAART eras: significant differences in survival with standard chemotherapy. J Clin Oncol 23:4430–4438
90. Spina M, Simonelli C, Talamini R, Tirelli U (2005) Patients with HIV with Burkitt's lymphoma have a worse outcome than those with diffuse large-cell lymphoma also in the highly active antiretroviral therapy era. J Clin Oncol 23:8132–8133
91. Piriou E, van Dort K, Nanlohy NM, van Oers MH, Miedema F, van Baarle D (2005) Loss of EBNA1-specific memory $CD4^+$ and $CD8^+$ T cells in HIV-infected patients progressing to AIDS-related non-Hodgkin lymphoma. Blood 106:3166–3174
92. Piriou ER, van Dort K, Nanlohy NM, van Oers MH, Miedema F, van Baarle D (2005) Novel method for detection of virus-specific $CD41^+$ T cells indicates a decreased EBV-specific $CD4^+$ T cell response in untreated HIV-infected subjects. Eur J Immunol 35:796–805
93. Gasser O, Bihl FK, Wolbers M, Loggi E, Steffen I, Hirsch HH, Gunthard HF, Walker BD, Brander C, Battegay M, Hess C (2007) HIV patients developing primary CNS lymphoma lack EBV-specific $CD4^+$ T cell function irrespective of absolute $CD4^+$ T cell counts. PLoS Med 4:e96
94. van Baarle D, Nanlohy NM, Otto S, Plunkett FJ, Fletcher JM, Akbar AN (2008) Progressive telomere shortening of Epstein-Barr virus-specific memory T cells during HIV infection: contributor to exhaustion? J Infect Dis 198:1353–1357

Chapter 13
The Many Roles of Malaria in the Etiology of Endemic Burkitt Lymphoma

Rosemary Rochford and Amolo S. Asito

Epidemiology of Malaria and eBL

Following the first clinical description by Denis Burkitt of the lymphoma now bearing his name [1], several epidemiologic studies were done to determine the geographic distribution of this cancer. The earliest study was undertaken by Denis Burkitt who embarked on a "tumor safari" to map cases of eBL throughout Africa [2]. He generated a low-resolution map of eBL that describes a lymphoma belt across equatorial Africa. Case identification was based on response to questionnaires and personal reporting. Haddow [3] used this data to determine that eBL had a striking geographical restriction with cases occurring in a band approximately 10° north or south of the equator and within that region, not occurring in areas with altitudes greater than 1,500 m. Papua New Guinea was the only other region of the world that where cases of BL similar to the "African" lymphoma were found [4]. Based on these observations, early investigators hypothesized that an infectious agent, possibly a vectored virus such as an arbovirus, might be etiologically linked with this cancer [3, 5]. However, it quickly became evident that eBL occurred at a high incidence in regions where malaria transmission of *Plasmodium falciparum* was sustained and intense, i.e. holoendemic [6, 7].

Because of the limitations of cancer registries in Africa and availability of accurate population data, a direct correlation of eBL incidence rates with *P. falciparum*

R. Rochford (✉)
Department of Microbiology and Immunology, SUNY Upstate Medical University, Syracuse, NY, USA
e-mail: rochforr@upstate.edu

A.S. Asito
Department of Microbiology and Immunology, SUNY Upstate Medical University, Syracuse, NY, USA

Centre for Global Health Research, Kenya Medical Research Institute, Kisumu, Kenya

E.S. Robertson (ed.), *Burkitt's Lymphoma*, Current Cancer Research, DOI 10.1007/978-1-4614-4313-1_13, © Springer Science+Business Media New York 2013

parasite prevalence at a finer geographic level of analysis wasn't done for almost two decades after the original discovery of eBL [8]. More recently, a study based in Kenya reexamined the association between eBL and malaria using new ecological models of malaria transmission [9]. Consistent with the earlier studies, eBL incidence rates were greater in regions with chronic and intense malaria transmission intensity than in regions with no or sporadic malaria transmission.

The variability in eBL onset age correlates with differences in malaria exposure. For example, patients living in holoendemic malaria areas develop eBL younger than those living in sporadic or seasonal malaria areas [8]. A ten-year study in Uganda during the 1960s detected a median onset age of 12 years in areas where malaria transmission was weak or inconsistent (hypo-endemic), compared to 8 and 6 years, respectively, in areas with meso- and hyper-endemic transmission [10]. Burkitt and Wright detected an equal susceptibility, but older onset age, among persons migrating from low- to high-risk eBL areas, which is ecologically consistent with non-malarious and endemic malaria zones, respectively [11].

While the above studies firmly established an ecologic link between eBL risk and malaria endemicity, two recent case–control studies based in Uganda and Malawi have provided more direct evidence of a biologic link between malaria exposure and increased risk for eBL [12, 13]. Malaria-specific antibody titers in children with eBL and age-matched hospital-based controls were examined. Risk for eBL increased with increasing antibody titers against malaria. Cases were also more likely to have elevated antibody titers against both malaria and EBV relative to controls suggesting a synergistic linkage between these two pathogens in the etiology of eBL. Interestingly, a correlation between age when multiple *P. falciparum* genotypes were detected in the population and age of peak onset of eBL was found [14] suggesting that infection with multiple *P. falciparum* genotypes could be linked to onset of eBL. This observation is consistent with an etiologic model presented below that has the repeated infections associated with holoendemic malaria that are driving increased risk.

In sum, since eBL was first described there has been a consistent epidemiologic association with high levels of malaria transmission and increased risk for eBL. The efforts underway to reduce malaria in sub-Saharan Africa should be monitored closely to determine if eBL incidence also decreases.

P. falciparum Malaria Pathogenesis

To understand why malaria increases the risk of eBL, there are three features of *P. falciparum* pathogenesis that provide clues to this question. First is the varying transmission dynamic of *P. falciparum* malaria. As discussed in the first section, eBL is correlated with holoendemic transmission of malaria, not just a single *P. falciparum* infection. *P. falciparum* malaria only elicits protective immunity after several years of continuous exposure, during which time recurring infections and illness occur [15]. Because of this, children aged 1–5 years living in holoendemic malaria regions are at the highest risk of morbidity and mortality associated with

P. falciparum infections [16]. Of relevance to the role of malaria in the etiology of eBL, the peak in eBL incidence peaks right after this time period [9, 17]. The repeated malaria infections are thought to result in impairment of cellular immunity to malaria [18–20], to other pathogens [21–25] and to vaccines [26].

The second feature is the high antigenic burden imposed by these repeated *P. falciparum* infections. During acute clinical malaria, greater than 5,000 parasitized RBC per μl of whole blood. Even in children with asymptomatic parasitemia, there can be high levels of parasitized RBC [27]. In holoendemic regions, greater than 50 % of children are asymptomatic but parasitemic at any given time [28]. So in essence, children living in a malaria endemic region have a high systemic antigen load along with continual reinfection. Under these conditions, *Plasmodium* infection in children could be considered a chronic infection, and during this period the child's immune system is under constant stress from the repeated infections. As early as 1970, O'Conor had proposed that chronic antigenic stimulation from malaria infections might play a role in the emergence of premalignant lesions [29].

In addition to chronic antigen stimulation of the immune system, recent studies have indicated that *P. falciparum* malaria results in alterations in B-cell homeostasis [30] resulting in expansion of immature transitional (CD19+IgD+CD10+) B cells as well as the emergence of atypical memory B cells [31]. *P. falciparum* can also act as a B-cell mitogen [32, 33] and induce hyper-gammaglobulinemia [34]. How these features of malaria pathogenesis could potentially intersect with eBL etiology will be discussed below.

Interaction of Malaria with EBV-Infected B Cells

There are two pathogens linked to the etiology of eBL, *P. falciparum* and Epstein–Barr virus (EBV). For a more extensive discussion of the biology of EBV and its link to eBL pathogenesis, see Chapter 10. Relevant to the role of malaria, EBV exists as a persistent infection in B cells throughout the lifetime of the host and this infection is controlled by both $CD4^+$ and $CD8^+$ T-cell responses.

Several studies have pointed to a profound dysregulation of EBV persistence in children due to *P. falciparum* malaria [27, 35–40]. For example, increases in EBV-infected B cells were observed during single episodes of acute *P. falciparum* malaria [35, 39]. There is also evidence that malaria induces reactivation from latently infected cells both in vitro [41] and in children with acute malaria [36, 37]. Serologic evidence of ongoing EBV reactivation in children living in malaria holoendemic region has also been reported [40]. A higher EBV load set point—indicative of the frequency of latently infected cells—occurs in children from malaria endemic regions relative to children from malaria sporadic regions [27] and the viral load observed in these children more closely matches levels seen in patients with acute infectious mononucleosis [35].

Two potential but not exclusive mechanisms for these observations exist: reactivation and infection of new B cells or expansion of latently infected B cells. Because of the high antigen burden, clearance of the parasite-infected red blood cells (RBC) in the spleen—an organ rich in B cells—there is a strong likelihood that infected RBC could directly contact EBV-infected B cells. The *P. falciparum* antigen cysteine-rich interdomain region 1α (CIDRα) expressed on the surface of infected red blood cells can directly bind to B cells and induce lytic reactivation of EBV [32]. Reactivation of EBV would result in elevated viral loads through release of infectious virus and reinfection of naive B cells. That this pathway is essential for maintenance of EBV loads in healthy individuals was recently demonstrated by Hoshino et al. [42] who found that treatment of healthy EBV-positive individuals with valacyclovir, an antiviral drug that blocks lytic infection, resulted in the reduction in frequency of EBV-infected cells over time.

The alternative possibility for elevated viral loads is that the *P. falciparum* is driving memory B-cell expansion through interaction with TLR9 on memory B cells. *P. falciparum* has a ligand for TLR9 [43]. TLR9 is expressed on B cells and TLR9 signaling also essential for B-cell proliferation [44]. Thus, interaction of a latently infected B cell with the *P. falciparum* TLR9 ligand could drive those cells to proliferate.

A recent study found that infants living in a high malaria transmission region of Kenya were infected with EBV significantly earlier in life (7.3 months of age) compared to infants from a non-malaria endemic region (8.4 months) pointing to an additional role of malaria in modulating EBV persistence [45]. In addition, the earlier age of infection led to more frequent detection of EBV and higher EBV viral loads over time. Interestingly, these data support a model first proposed by de-Thé in 1978 who hypothesized that infection of infants with EBV early in life could result in an infection that was poorly controlled by the host and thus increased the risk for eBL [46]. What remains to be determined is why are these infants infected with EBV so early in life and whether malaria also plays a role in this.

What is the relevance of high viral loads to an increased risk for eBL? EBV latency membrane protein (LMP)-1 interacts with DNA methyltransferase and results in epigenetic modification and subsequent down-regulation of the pro-apoptotic Bim gene [47]. So latently infected memory B cells would have reduced the levels of Bim even though the LMP-1 protein is no longer expressed in these cells, i.e. this would be a consequence of them being "marked" by their primary infection with EBV when all the EBV latent proteins are expressed [48]. Thus, higher viral loads in children from malaria endemic regions would result in a greater number of circulating B cells that were resistant to apoptotic stimuli.

Interestingly, signaling through TLR was shown to induce the enzyme activation-induced cytidine deaminase (AID) in human B cells [49, 50]. AID over-expression induces IgH-c-myc translocations [51] characteristic of BL. Thus, elevated and unregulated AID expression in B cells triggered by *P. falciparum* could increase the risk for a c-myc translocation. If over-expression of c-myc occurred following an AID-mediated translocation, normal B cells would die by apoptosis. However, because of the down-regulation of Bim, the memory B cells would be resistant to apoptosis and would tolerate the c-myc translocation. Cells that escaped apoptosis and carrying the c-myc translocation would ultimately lead to the emergence of a malignant clone [52]. Escape from T-cell surveillance would also be critical and how malaria plays a role in this will be discussed next.

Interaction of Malaria with EBV-Specific T Cell Immunity

Three early studies suggested that *P. falciparum* malaria could interfere with EBV-specific cellular immune responses. Whittle et al. [24] demonstrated that peripheral blood lymphocytes isolated from adult patients with acute malaria were unable to control outgrowth of EBV-transformed cells in a standard regression assay to assess EBV-specific T-cell function. Moss et al. [53], with a similar assay, demonstrated that healthy adults living in malaria holoendemic regions of Papua New Guinea had impaired EBV-specific T-cell responses. In children experiencing an episode of acute malaria, spontaneous outgrowth of EBV-transformed B cells ex vivo occurred at even greater frequency compared to the same children following recovery from malaria [54]. Subsequent to these studies, Moormann et al. [55] found that Kenyan children from a malaria holoendemic area had significantly fewer EBV-specific IFN-γ responses compared to children from a highland area with infrequent malaria exposure. This effect was most pronounced in children 5–9 years old, coinciding with the peak incident age of eBL. Njie et al. [35] found that during an episode of acute malaria in children from the Gambia there was a transient decrease in EBV-specific CD8 T-cell immunity. In a longitudinal cohort in Kenya, following infants EBV-specific T-cell responses after prospective cohort [45], there was a significant difference in the capacity of children living in a malaria holoendemic region compared to malaria sporadic region to maintain a T-cell response to EBV lytic antigens (Asito, Piriou, Moormann, and Rochford, unpublished observation). This suggests that *P. falciparum* malaria contributes to loss of EBV-specific immunity by inducing the collapse of an antiviral IFN-γ-mediated CD8+ T-cell response. More detailed discussion of the effects of malaria on EBV T cell immunity is found in Chap. 12.

Interestingly, a potential role is also indicated for $\gamma\delta$ T cells in the etiology of eBL. *P. falciparum* infection is associated with expansion of $V\delta1^+$ T cells in peripheral blood [56, 57]. This suggests that chronic exposure to *P. falciparum* in children would affect normal $\gamma\delta$ T-cell immunity and expand $V\delta1^+$ T cells. Of interest relative to the link between *P. falciparum* and EBV in eBL etiology is the studies that show increased EBV viral load as described above and increased B-cell activation in children living in malaria holoendemic regions. One possible outcome of elevated EBV viral load and activated B cells would be an expansion of the $V\delta1^+$ T cells in these children living in a region where the malaria is holoendemic and the risk for eBL is high. Interestingly, alterations in $V\delta1^+$ T-cell activation and frequencies in children with eBL are comparable to children with acute *P. falciparum* malaria [58]. Moreover, recent studies have found that tumor derived $V\delta1^+$ cells isolated from breast cancer patients can negatively down-modulate $\alpha\beta$ T-cell responses and inhibit the capacity of $CD8^+$ T cells to kill tumor cells in an in vivo model [59] suggesting that expansion of $V\delta1^+$ T cells during *P. falciparum* infection could have the unintended consequence of losing antitumor immunity and allowing the emergence of a malignant B-cell clone. Further studies to evaluate a potential role for $\gamma\delta$ T cells in EBV immunity and risk for eBL are needed.

A Model for the Role of Malaria in the Etiology of Endemic BL

Early reviews postulating on the mechanism by which malaria increases the risk for eBL postulated either a role for inducing B-cell activation or causing T-cell suppression. However, given the chronic nature of *P. falciparum* infections, the high antigen burden, and the overall impact the holoendemic malaria has on a population, malaria likely serves many nonexclusive roles in increasing the risk for eBL. As shown in Fig. 13.1, malaria plays a role by first increasing the number of latently infected B cells via a number of potential mechanisms; second, through loss of immune control

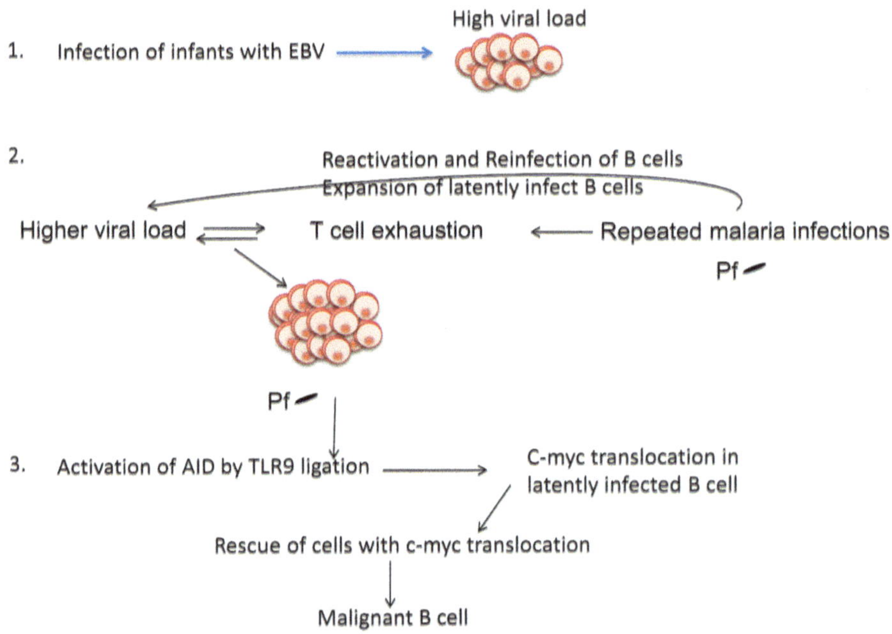

Fig. 13.1 Model for the different roles of malaria in increasing risk for eBL. In stage 1, infants are infected at less than 6 months of age, increasing the numbers of latently infected B cells. While this phenomenon is age dependent, living a malaria endemic region increases the frequency of early age of EBV infection [45]. In stage 2, repeated malaria infections during infancy and early childhood expand the numbers of latently infected B cells [27, 35–40]. The higher EBV load also results in loss of EBV-specific CD8+ T cell immunity [55] further amplifying this effect. In stage 3, the higher viral load equates to greater numbers of latently infected B cells resulting in a greater stochastic chance for a direct interaction of a TLR9 ligand derived from P. falciparum [43] to bind to TLR9 on memory B cells. This could result in activation of the enzyme AID [49, 50]. AID is required for c-myc translocations in mouse models [51], and it is postulated that aberrant AID activation results in the c-myc translocation characteristic of BL. If over-expression of c-myc occurred in a normal B cell at the wrong stage of B-cell development, regulatory mechanisms resulting in apoptotic death of the B cell would occur. However, if the B cell had been epigenetically marked by EBV, loss of expression of the pro-apoptotic protein Bim could result in a cell that could tolerate c-myc over-expression and ultimately lead to emergence of malignant clone

of latently infected B cells and finally, by inducing c-myc translocation through an AID-mediated mechanism. The combined effects of malaria infections result in increasing risk for the emergence of a malignant clone and the likelihood of a child presenting with Burkitt lymphoma.

References

1. Burkitt D (1958) A sarcoma involving the jaws in African children. Br J Surg 46:218–223
2. Burkitt D (1962) A "tumour safari" in East and Central Africa. Br J Cancer 16:379–386
3. Haddow AJ (1963) An improved map for the study of Burkitt's lymphoma syndrome in Africa. East Afr Med J 40:429–432
4. Booth K, Burkitt DP, Bassett DJ, Cooke RA, Biddulph J (1967) Burkitt lymphoma in Papua, New Guinea. Br J Cancer 21:657–664
5. Burkitt D (1962) Determining the climatic limitations of a children's cancer common in Africa. Br Med J 5311:1019–1023
6. Wright DH (1967) The epidemiology of Burkitt's tumor. Cancer Res 27:2424–2438
7. Dalldorf G (1962) Lymphomas of African children. JAMA 181:1026–1028
8. Morrow RH (1985) Epidemiological evidence for the role of faciparum malaria in the pathogenesis of Burkitt's lymphoma. In: Lenoir G, O'Connor G, Olweny C (eds) Burkitt's lymphoma: a human cancer model, vol 60. IARC Press, Lyons, pp 177–185
9. Rainey JJ, Mwanda WO, Wairiumu P, Moormann AM, Wilson ML, Rochford R (2007) Spatial distribution of Burkitt's lymphoma in Kenya and association with malaria risk. Trop Med Int Health 12:936–943
10. Morrow RH, Kisuule A, Pike MC, Smith PG (1976) Burkitt's lymphoma in the Mengo Districts of Uganda: epidemiologic features and their relationship to malaria. J Natl Cancer Inst 56:479–483
11. Burkitt D, Wright D (1966) Geographical and tribal distribution of the African lymphoma in Uganda. Br Med J 5487:569–573
12. Mutalima N, Molyneux E, Jaffe H et al (2008) Associations between Burkitt lymphoma among children in Malawi and infection with HIV, EBV and malaria: results from a case–control study. PLoS One 3:e2505
13. Carpenter LM, Newton R, Casabonne D et al (2008) Antibodies against malaria and Epstein-Barr virus in childhood Burkitt lymphoma: a case–control study in Uganda. Int J Cancer 122:1319–1323
14. Emmanuel B, Kawira E, Ogwang MD et al (2011) African Burkitt lymphoma: age-specific risk and correlations with malaria biomarkers. Am J Trop Med Hyg 84:397–401
15. Marsh K, Otoo L, Hayes RJ, Carson DC, Greenwood BM (1989) Antibodies to blood stage antigens of Plasmodium falciparum in rural Gambians and their relation to protection against infection. Trans R Soc Trop Med Hyg 83:293–303
16. Snow RW, Omumbo JA, Lowe B et al (1997) Relation between severe malaria morbidity in children and level of Plasmodium falciparum transmission in Africa. Lancet 349:1650–1654
17. Orem J, Mbidde EK, Lambert B, de Sanjose S, Weiderpass E (2007) Burkitt's lymphoma in Africa, a review of the epidemiology and etiology. Afr Health Sci 7:166–175
18. Ho M, Webster HK, Looareesuwan S et al (1986) Antigen-specific immunosuppression in human malaria due to Plasmodium falciparum. J Infect Dis 153:763–771
19. Ho M, Webster HK, Green B, Looareesuwan S, Kongchareon S, White NJ (1988) Defective production of and response to IL-2 in acute human falciparum malaria. J Immunol 141:2755–2759
20. Hviid L, Jakobsen PH, Abu-Zeid YA, Theander TG (1992) T-cell responses in malaria. APMIS 100:95–106

21. Mabey DC, Brown A, Greenwood BM (1987) Plasmodium falciparum malaria and Salmonella infections in Gambian children. J Infect Dis 155:1319–1321
22. Cook IF (1985) Herpes zoster in children following malaria. J Trop Med Hyg 88:261–264
23. Thursz MR, Kwiatkowski D, Torok ME et al (1995) Association of hepatitis B surface antigen carriage with severe malaria in Gambian children. Nat Med 1:374–375
24. Whittle HC, Brown J, Marsh K et al (1984) T-cell control of Epstein-Barr virus-infected B cells is lost during *P. falciparum* malaria. Nature 312:449–450
25. Gunapala DE, Facer CA, Davidson R, Weir WR (1990) In vitro analysis of Epstein-Barr virus: host balance in patients with acute Plasmodium falciparum malaria. I. Defective T-cell control. Parasitol Res 76:531–535
26. Williamson WA, Greenwood BM (1978) Impairment of the immune response to vaccination after acute malaria. Lancet 1:1328–1329
27. Moormann AM, Chelimo K, Sumba OP et al (2005) Exposure to holoendemic malaria results in elevated Epstein-Barr virus loads in children. J Infect Dis 191:1233–1238
28. Hogh B (1996) Clinical and parasitological studies on immunity to Plasmodium falciparum malaria in children. Scand J Infect Dis Suppl 102:1–53
29. O'Conor GT (1970) Persistent immunologic stimulation as a factor in oncogenesis with special reference to Burkitt's tumor. Am J Med 48:279–285
30. Nagaoka H, Gonzalez-Aseguinolaza G, Tsuji M, Nussenzweig MC (2000) Immunization and infection change the number of recombination activating gene (RAG)-expressing B cells in the periphery by altering immature lymphocyte production. J Exp Med 191:2113–2120
31. Weiss GE, Crompton PD, Li S et al (2009) Atypical memory B cells are greatly expanded in individuals living in a malaria-endemic area. J Immunol 183:2176–2182
32. Donati D, Zhang LP, Chen Q et al (2004) Identification of a polyclonal B-cell activator in Plasmodium falciparum. Infect Immun 72:5412–5418
33. Greenwood BM, Oduloju AJ, Platts-Mills TA (1979) Partial characterization of a malaria mitogen. Trans R Soc Trop Med Hyg 73:178–182
34. Greenwood BM (1974) Possible role of a B-cell mitogen in hypergammaglobulinaemia in malaria and trypanosomiasis. Lancet 1:435–436
35. Njie R, Bell AI, Jia H et al (2009) The effects of acute malaria on Epstein-Barr virus (EBV) load and EBV-specific T cell immunity in Gambian children. J Infect Dis 199:31–38
36. Donati D, Espmark E, Kironde F et al (2006) Clearance of circulating Epstein-Barr virus DNA in children with acute malaria after antimalaria treatment. J Infect Dis 193:971–977
37. Rasti N, Falk KI, Donati D et al (2005) Circulating Epstein-Barr virus in children living in malaria-endemic areas. Scand J Immunol 61:461–465
38. Yone CL, Kube D, Kremsner PG, Luty AJ (2006) Persistent Epstein-Barr viral reactivation in young African children with a history of severe Plasmodium falciparum malaria. Trans R Soc Trop Med Hyg 100:669–676
39. Lam KM, Syed N, Whittle H, Crawford DH (1991) Circulating Epstein-Barr virus-carrying B cells in acute malaria. Lancet 337:876–878
40. Piriou E, Kimmel R, Chelimo K et al (2009) Serological evidence for long-term Epstein-Barr virus reactivation in children living in a holoendemic malaria region of Kenya. J Med Virol 81:1088–1093
41. Chene A, Donati D, Guerreiro-Cacais AO et al (2007) A molecular link between malaria and Epstein-Barr virus reactivation. PLoS Pathog 3:e80
42. Hoshino Y, Katano H, Zou P et al (2009) Long-term administration of valacyclovir reduces the number of Epstein-Barr virus (EBV)-infected B cells but not the number of EBV DNA copies per B cell in healthy volunteers. J Virol 83:11857–11861
43. Parroche P, Lauw FN, Goutagny N et al (2007) Malaria hemozoin is immunologically inert but radically enhances innate responses by presenting malaria DNA to Toll-like receptor 9. Proc Natl Acad Sci U S A 104:1919–1924
44. Peng SL (2005) Signaling in B cells via Toll-like receptors. Curr Opin Immunol 17:230–236
45. Piriou E, Asito AS, Sumba OP et al (2012) Early age of primary EBV infection results in poorly controlled viral infection in infants from Western Kenya: clues to the etiology of endemic Burkitt lymphoma. J Infect Dis 205(6):906–913

46. de-The G (1977) Is Burkitt's lymphoma related to perinatal infection by Epstein-Barr virus? Lancet 1:335–338
47. Paschos K, Smith P, Anderton E, Middeldorp JM, White RE, Allday MJ (2009) Epstein-Barr virus latency in B cells leads to epigenetic repression and CpG methylation of the tumour suppressor gene Bim. PLoS Pathog 5:e1000492
48. Babcock GJ, Thorley-Lawson DA (2000) Tonsillar memory B cells, latently infected with Epstein-Barr virus, express the restricted pattern of latent genes previously found only in Epstein-Barr virus-associated tumors. Proc Natl Acad Sci U S A 97:12250–12255
49. Capolunghi F, Cascioli S, Giorda E et al (2008) CpG drives human transitional B cells to terminal differentiation and production of natural antibodies. J Immunol 180:800–808
50. Potup P, Kumsiri R, Kano S et al (2009) Blood stage Plasmodium falciparum antigens induce immunoglobulin class switching in human enriched B cell culture. Southeast Asian J Trop Med Public Health 40:651–664
51. Ramiro AR, Jankovic M, Callen E et al (2006) Role of genomic instability and p53 in AID-induced c-myc-Igh translocations. Nature 440:105–109
52. Brady G, MacArthur GJ, Farrell PJ (2007) Epstein-Barr virus and Burkitt lymphoma. J Clin Pathol 60:1397–1402
53. Moss DJ, Burrows SR, Castelino DJ et al (1983) A comparison of Epstein-Barr virus-specific T-cell immunity in malaria- endemic and -nonendemic regions of Papua New Guinea. Int J Cancer 31:727–732
54. Whittle HC, Brown J, Marsh K, Blackman M, Jobe O, Shenton F (1990) The effects of Plasmodium falciparum malaria on immune control of B lymphocytes in Gambian children. Clin Exp Immunol 80:213–218
55. Moormann AM, Chelimo K, Sumba PO, Tisch DJ, Rochford R, Kazura JW (2007) Exposure to holoendemic malaria results in suppression of Epstein-Barr virus-specific T cell immunosurveillance in Kenyan children. J Infect Dis 195:799–808
56. Hviid L, Kurtzhals JA, Adabayeri V et al (2001) Perturbation and proinflammatory type activation of V delta 1(+) gamma delta T cells in African children with Plasmodium falciparum malaria. Infect Immun 69:3190–3196
57. Hviid L, Kurtzhals JA, Dodoo D et al (1996) The gamma/delta T-cell response to Plasmodium falciparum malaria in a population in which malaria is endemic. Infect Immun 64:4359–4362
58. Futagbi G, Welbeck JE, Tetteh JK, Hviid L, Akanmori BD (2007) Selective activation of TCR-gammadelta+ cells in endemic Burkitt's lymphoma. Malar J 6:69
59. Peng G, Wang HY, Peng W, Kiniwa Y, Seo KH, Wang RF (2007) Tumor-infiltrating gammadelta T cells suppress T and dendritic cell function via mechanisms controlled by a unique toll-like receptor signaling pathway. Immunity 27:334–348

Chapter 14
Therapeutic Approaches to Burkitt's Lymphoma

James Armitage and Donald W. Coulter

History

The treatment of Burkitt lymphoma has evolved over the last 50 years, and that progression has been contingent upon understanding the biological characteristics of the disease, such as the rapid doubling time of the tumor, the propensity for extranodal sites, high chemosensitivity, and the potential for CNS relapses [1]. The combined efforts of multiple consortiums, including the BFM, SFOP, CCG, and UKCCG, have advanced treatment since Dr. Denis Burkitt's first description of events in Uganda in 1958 [2]. Although Dr. Burkitt lost his right eye at age 11, the result of a thrown stone during a school-yard fight, his keen observation skills remained unaffected [3].

> Let me take you back 30 years to a morning that I was surgeon on duty at the teaching hospital in Uganda. I was called in consultation by the physician on duty, Dr. Hugh Trowell, to see a patient who had some sort of lesion involving all four quadrants of the jaws. I could not make out what it was. It did not fit in with a tumor…it did not fit in with sepsis…it did not fit in with anything. I documented it in my mind, believing it to be an oddity you might see once in a lifetime, and did not give it any more thought.
>
> About two weeks later, while on ward rounds in another hospital 30 miles away, I looked out the window and saw another child with a swollen face. Giving up my ward round, I went out to find this child with tumors of some kind in all four quadrants of the jaws. I put the child and his mother in my car, drove them back to the hospital, and began to investigate these jaw tumors [4].

Although first described as a "round cell sarcoma," Burkitt and O'Connor defined the disease as a malignant lymphoma in 1961, including the pathological terminology of a "starry sky" background still used today [5].

J. Armitage (✉)
The Joe Shapiro Professor of Internal Medicine, University of Nebraska Medical Center
e-mail: joarmita@unmc.edu

D.W. Coulter
Assistant Professor of Pediatrics
e-mail: dwcoulter@unmc.edu

E.S. Robertson (ed.), *Burkitt's Lymphoma*, Current Cancer Research,
DOI 10.1007/978-1-4614-4313-1_14,

Pediatric Treatment History

The specific biology of Burkitt lymphoma drove early attempts at therapy. Surgery was an early accepted treatment modality until the multifocal nature of the disease was understood, making radical surgery pointless [6].

Given the rapid rate of tumor growth, the plausibility of radiotherapy as a treatment modality was evaluated. Irradiation induced rapid regression of tumors; however, as in the case of surgical resection, patients eventually succumbed to growth of multifocal untreated masses [6].

The multifocal nature of the disease made systemic chemotherapy the early treatment of choice. The earliest described monotherapy involved nitrogen mustard, either injected intravenously or intra-arterially at doses ranging from 0.2 to 2.5 mg/kg, which produced rapid improvement that often times only lasted a few weeks [5, 7].

Other early monotherapy included cyclophosphamide, either orally or intravenously, and methotrexate either infused through the external carotid artery or administered orally. The results again showed only temporary regression of the tumors.

Through the 1960s, monotherapy with many of the drugs available at the time confirmed the high degree of chemosensitivity of Burkitt lymphoma. Dr. Burkitt originally documented rapid response and sometimes durable remission to cyclophosphamide given as a one-time dose of 40 mg/kg IV [8]. This dosing regimen was chosen based on necessity, given the short hospitalization stays of African children in Uganda [9]. Agents such as cyclophosphamide, methotrexate, or vincristine usually induced rapid regression of tumor bulk, but most patients who maintained their original good response had limited disease [10–13]. The majority of patients treated in the early 1960s had long-term survival rates approaching 20% [14]. A summary of agents given as monotherapy and the resulting response rates is outlined in Table 14.1 [15].

Table 14.1 Previous monotherapy used in the treatment of Burkitt lymphoma [15]

Drug	No. of patients	CR	CR+PR	OR (%)
Cyclophosphamide	163	43	132	81
Orthomerphalan	14	?	14	100
Chlorambucil	12	3	10	83
Nitrogen mustard	61	10	44	72
Melphalan	26	8	16	61
Procarbazine	6	0	0	0
BCNU	5	0	4	80
Vincristine	21	10	17	81
Vinblastine	2	0	0	0
Methotrexate	45	11	26	58
6-Mercaptopurine	3	0	0	0
Cystosine arabinoside	3	2	2	2
Epipodophyllotoxin	2	2	2	2
Actinomycin D	4	1	4	4

Variety of doses and schedules were used, even for the same drug
CR complete response
OR overall response
PR partial response

Further chemotherapeutic advances occurred in 1967, when the Uganda Cancer Institute (UCI) of Makerere University in Kampala, Uganda and the United States National Cancer Institute (NCI) began collaborating. From July 1967 to August 1969 (Trial I), 57 patients were admitted to the Lymphoma Treatment Center in Kampala and received a single dose of cyclophosphamide at a dose of 40 mg/kg IV. Patients who achieved a complete remission to single-dose therapy were then randomized to five more doses of cyclophosphamide at 2- to 3-week intervals or no further therapy. All partial remissions following single-dose therapy were not randomized and received five more doses of cyclophosphamide at 2- to 3-week intervals. Relapses were treated with combination therapy including vincristine 1.4 mg/m2 IV on day 1, methotrexate 15 mg/m2 PO on days 1–4, and 10–14 days later cytarabine 250 mg/m2 daily for 3 days (BIKE). This combination therapy regimen was repeated for two cycles [16].

Of the 57 patients enrolled in the study, 42 had a complete response to monotherapy with cyclophosphamide. Ten patients died from advanced disease in the first week of treatment, three had partial responses, and two had no response to cyclophosphamide monotherapy [16].

Patients randomized to multiple doses of cyclophosphamide had longer remissions and fewer relapses than patients who received only a single dose. Seven patients who received single-dose cyclophosphamide relapsed and were able to achieve complete responses after multiple doses of cyclophosphamide. Ten patients relapsed after multiple doses of cyclophosphamide, and BIKE chemotherapy induced complete response in 9 patients with 8 patients remaining disease-free for up to 14 months [15].

The second trial using combination chemotherapy occurred from August 1969 to June 1971 (Trial II). Higher stage patients were randomized to receive cyclophosphamide 40 mg/kg IV in repeated doses at 2- to 3-week intervals versus cyclophosphamide 40 mg/kg IV followed by vincristine 1.4 mg/m2 IV on day 1, methotrexate 15 mg/m2 PO on days 1–4, and then 10–14 days later cytarabine 250 mg/m2 daily for 3 days (TRIKE) [17]. Initial results in the higher risk patients revealed a survival trend in favor of TRIKE therapy, although this finding was not confirmed until 1980 [18].

Given the results of Trial II indicating that upfront combination chemotherapy may be advantageous, a randomized trial comparing cyclophosphamide alone versus cyclophosphamide, vincristine and methotrexate (COM) was initiated [19]. The proportion of relapses treated with cyclophosphamide alone or with COM was similar, but the location of relapse was different. In patients treated with monotherapy, relapse was identified systemically and in the CNS, in contrast to patients treated with COM who had relapse in the CNS alone. Later follow-up identified a survival advantage for patients treated initially with COM, and this regimen was adopted by the US NCI as the backbone for subsequent therapy [15].

During these early years of treatment, the central nervous system presented a problem to investigators, both as a primary site of disease and as a location of relapse. Early investigations into craniospinal irradiation yielded poor results, both as a factor of the limited availability of the technology in equatorial Africa and the poor outcomes for patients [20]. In an effort to evaluate intrathecal chemotherapy for the almost 50% of patients who presented with CNS positive disease, treatment was given with either intrathecal methotrexate or cytarabine with comparative outcomes [21].

Thus, the stage was set for the incorporation of intrathecal chemotherapy into trials using multiagent therapy, both elements of treatment plans used today. During the 1970s, treatment studies for Burkitt lymphoma focused on combination chemotherapy, central nervous system prophylaxis, and salvage therapy for patients who experienced relapse [9]. This work resulted in an increase in overall survival from 20% to 50%. In 1977, a landmark study (CCG-551) comparing 18 months of therapy with cyclophosphamide, vincristine, methotrexate, and prednisone (COMP) to the ten-drug LSA2L2 regimen (cyclophosphamide, vincristine, prednisone, daunomycin, methotrexate, cytarabine, thioguanine, L-asparaginase, carmustine, and hydroxyurea) revealed that patients with Burkitt lymphoma fared better with four-drug therapy (57% versus 28% 2-year disease-free survival), and that patients with bone marrow or central nervous system involvement had the worst outcome (30%) [22]. These results were later verified to be stable at 5 years (50% versus 29%) [23].

The French Society of Pediatric Oncology (SFOP) completed a series of four successive Lymphome malin B (LMB) trials, which continued to increase the event-free survival for patients with Burkitt lymphoma. The LMB 0181 Pilot Study was conducted between February and October 1981, accruing 32 patients [24]. The protocol was designed to increase survival by employing treatment with chemotherapy alone (no irradiation or surgical debulking), intensifying therapy in the third and fourth months of treatment to decrease relapses, and to improve central nervous system prophylaxis without using cranial irradiation. Although the treatment proved efficacious, a high amount of toxicity was identified, requiring modification of the protocol. Subsequently, the LMB 0281 study ran from November 1981 to March 1984. Therapy included vincristine, prednisone, doxorubicin, cyclophosphamide, and methotrexate with therapeutic reinforcement using two courses based on continuous infusion of cytarabine. Maintenance therapy lasted 8 months and CNS prophylaxis included high-dose methotrexate, intrathecal methotrexate and cytarabine, continuous infusion cytarabine, and lomustine. The results showed increased survival for high-stage patients without CNS disease (75%), but an unacceptable toxic death rate (10%) [24]. The CNS relapse rate was only 1%.

A pervasive focus of subsequent therapy became decreasing treatment toxicity while keeping survival stable. From July 1984 to September 1987, the LMB 84 study compared 7-month therapy versus 4-month therapy in 216 patients without CNS disease. Therapy included an initial reductive phase of cyclophosphamide, vincristine, and prednisone (COP) with intrathecal methotrexate and hydrocortisone. The purpose of the cytoreductive phase was to solve metabolic problems, most due to acute tumor lysis, without being forced to manage the complications of intensive therapy such as aplasia and mucositis [25]. The results revealed an equivalent cure rate (78%), with a decrease in the toxic death rate (6%) [26].

Other information gleaned from these early trials included the emergence of risk factors, such as CNS involvement, no response to a cytoreductive phase, and no complete response after the third or fourth cycles [27]. In July 1989, the LMB 89 study sorted patients into one of the three therapeutic groups (A, B, or C) dependent upon their disease stage and prognostic factors. Group A patients had achieved complete resection of Stage I and abdominal Stage II tumors. Group C patients had CNS involvement or Burkitt leukemia with at least 70% blasts in the bone marrow. All remaining patients were stratified to group B. The results revealed that 90% survival could be obtained when treatment is modified for the risk factors of the patient [25].

These results lead to the FAB LMB 96 trial completed by the Societe Francaise d'Oncologie Pediatrique (SFOP), Children's Cancer Group (CCG), and the United Kingdom Children's Cancer Study Group (UKCCG). This international trial showed that treatment reduction in both cyclophosphamide and doxorubicin for early responding patients was possible [28]. Response to therapy was identified as the most significant prognostic factor, with patients showing <20% reduction of disease after prophase reduction having an event-free survival of 30% [29]. Finally, the results showed that patients presenting with CNS-positive disease received no survival benefit from craniospinal irradiation [28].

Adult Treatment History

Treatment for adults has been based on the success achieved in pediatric patients. In 1995 the results of a retrospective review of 65 adult patients treated according to the pediatric LMB 81, 84, 86, and 89 regimens revealed an 89% complete response rate with a three-year overall survival of 74% [30]. In 1996, these results were confirmed by a prospective study evaluating 72 adult patients treated according to the LMB protocol (CR rate 83%, 2 year OS 66%) [31].

A more recent prospective study of 72 adult patients treated with LMB 89 therapy revealed a 72% complete response rate with a 2-year overall survival rate of 70%. Patients with higher lactate dehydrogenase levels and advanced age tended to do worse (2-year OS rate of 84% in patients aged <33 years compared to 60% in patients aged >33 years) [31].

Other therapies used in children and adults include CODOX-M and IVAC, pioneered by Magrath [32]. This regimen utilizes three cycles of CODOX-M for patients with low-risk disease, and four cycles of alternating CODOX-M and IVAC for patients with high-risk disease. In 1996, Magrath et al. reported a 2-year event-free survival of 85% in children, and 100% in adults with a mean age of 25 years [32]. Two years later, an updated report revealed complete responses in 24 of 26 adult patients studied, with 22 patients alive and disease-free (follow-up 12–91 months) [33]. In Europe, attempts to use CODOX-M/IVAC have not produced similar results, although mean patient age may be a factor. The United Kingdom Lymphoma Group reported a 2-year event-free survival of 64.6% in a group of patients with a mean age of 35 years, with side effects of myelosuppression and mucositis [34].

HyperCVAD has been used exclusively in adults, and investigators at The University of Texas M.D. Anderson Cancer Center showed a complete response rate of 81% in 26 adult patients with a median age of 58 [35]. The addition of a monoclonal antibody against CD20 (rituximab) has improved the results of HyperCVAD with a 3-year overall survival of 89% in patients less than 60 years of age [36].

Rituximab is currently being investigated in pediatric patients when combined with intensive chemotherapy based on the French LMB–89 protocol. Results of the study are currently pending.

In the past, patients with HIV-associated Burkitt lymphoma had greater treatment-related mortality than patients with endemic or sporadic disease [37]. Early studies in the era of combination antiretroviral therapy have improved the survival for these patients, although changes are being tested to reduce the morbidity for patients [38].

After showing efficacy in untreated patients with diffuse large B-cell lymphoma [39], dose-adjusted etoposide, prednisone, vincristine, cyclophosphamide, and doxorubicin with rituximab (DA-EPOCH-R) has been evaluated in patients with Burkitt lymphoma. Twenty-nine adult patients, including 17 with Stage III/IV disease and 10 with HIV were treated with DA-EPOCH-R with event-free and overall survival of 97% and 100%, respectively, at a median follow-up of 57 months. Treatment was well tolerated, with notable toxicities including tumor lysis syndrome in one patient and febrile neutropenia in 16% of cycles [39].

Pediatric Treatment Recommendations

Patients with Burkitt lymphoma require intensive multi-agent therapy with CNS prophylaxis. Given the extremely rapid growth rate of Burkitt lymphoma, it is imperative that the time course from diagnosis and staging to initial treatment be as short as possible. The current treatment recommendations for newly diagnosed pediatric patients with Burkitt lymphoma are listed in Table 14.2 with agents listed in Table 14.3. Prior to initiating chemotherapy it is recommended that all patients be placed on cooperative study protocols if available.

Adult Treatment Recommendations

As in pediatric patients, delays in instituting therapy in adult patients can be detrimental, and all efforts should be made to have patients diagnosed and staged as rapidly as possible. Treatment options for adult patients are outlined in the most recent National Comprehensive Cancer Network practice guidelines (version 3.2012) [40]. Recommendations are made for low-risk patients (normal LDH, completely resected abdominal lesion or single extra-abdominal mass measuring <10 cm) or high-risk patients. DA-EPOCH-R and other treatment options for low-risk patients are outlined in Table 14.4. CODOX-M/IVAC with or without rituximab or HyperCVAD alternating with methotrexate plus cytarabine with or without rituximab are suggested for the high-risk patients [40]. Further suggestions for the care of high-risk patients are outlined in Table 14.5.

Table 14.2 Treatment recommendations for pediatric patients with newly diagnosed Burkitt lymphoma. Modified from the Physicians Data Query [68]

	Stratum	Disease manifestations	Treatment
FAB/LMB – 96 (COG-5961)	A	Completely resected	Two cycles of COPAD chemotherapy
	B	Multiple extra-abdominal sites Non-resected Stage I, II, III, IV Marrow < 25% Blasts No CNS disease	Prephase (COP) + four cycles of chemotherapy (reduced intensity arm)
	C	Mature B- Cell ALL (> 25% Blasts in Marrow) and/or CNS Disease	Prephase (COP) + eight cycles of chemotherapy (full intensity arm)
BFM Group	R1	Completely resected	Two cycles of chemotherapy
	R2	Non-resected Stage I/II and Stage III with LDH < 500 IU/L	Prephase (COP) + four cycles of chemotherapy (4 h methotrexate infusion)
	R3	Stage III with LDH 500–999 IU/L Stage IV, B Cell ALL (> 25% Blasts) and LDH < 1,000 IU/L No CNS Disease	Prephase (COP) + five cycles of chemotherapy (24 h methotrexate infusion)
	R4	Stage III, IV, B-Cell ALL with LDH > 1,000 IU/L Any CNS Disease	Prephase (COP) + six cycles of chemotherapy (24 h methotrexate infusion)

Table 14.3 Chemotherapeutic agents used for pediatric patients with newly diagnosed Burkitt lymphoma. Modified from the Physicians Data Query [68]

Phase	Agents
COPAD	Vincristine Prednisone Cyclophosphamide Doxorubicin
COP	Cyclophosphamide Vincristine Prednisone Intrathecal methotrexate and hydrocortisone
COPADM1	Vincristine Prednisone Methotrexate Folinic acid Cyclophosphamide Doxorubicin Intrathecal methotrexate and hydrocortisone
COPADM2	Vincristine Prednisone Methotrexate Folinic acid Cyclophosphamide Doxorubicin Intrathecal methotrexate and hydrocortisone

(continued)

Table 14.3 (continued)

Phase	Agents
CYM	Methotrexate Folinic acid Cytarabine Intrathecal methotrexate, and hydrocortisone
Maintenance	Vincristine Prednisone Cyclophosphamide Methotrexate Folinic acid Doxorubicin Intrathecal methotrexate, cytarabine and Hydrocortisone

Table 14.4 Adult low- risk regimens. Modified from NCCN [69]

Regimen	Agents
CALGB 9251	Cyclophosphamide Prednisone Ifosfamide Methotrexate Leucovorin Vincristine Dexamethasone Doxorubicin or etoposide or cytarabine Methotrexate IT Cytarabine IT Hydrocortisone IT
CODOX-M	Cyclophosphamide Doxorubicin Vincristine Methotrexate IT Cytarabine IT Methotrexate ± Rituximab
Dose adjusted EPOCH - R (Minimum three cycles with one additional cycle beyond CR)	Etoposide Prednisone Vincristine Cyclophosphamide Doxorubicin Methotrexate IT Rituximab
HyperCVAD	Cyclophosphamide Vincristine Doxorubicin Dexamethasone Methotrexate Cytarabine Rituximab

Table 14.5 Adult high-risk regimens. Modified from NCCN [69]

Regimen	Agents
CALGB9251 (with prophylactic CNS irradiation in certain patients)	Cyclophosphamide Prednisone Ifosfamide Methotrexate Leucovorin Vincristine Dexamethasone Doxorubicin or etoposide or cytarabine Methotrexate IT Cytarabine IT Hydrocortisone IT
CODOX-M alternating with IVAC	Cyclophosphamide Doxorubicin Vincristine Methotrexate IT Cytarabine IT Methotrexate Ifosfamide Cytarabine Etoposide Methotrexate IT ± Rituximab
Dose adjusted EPOCH - R	Etoposide Prednisone Vincristine Cyclophosphamide Doxorubicin Methotrexate IT Rituximab
HyperCVAD	Cyclophosphamide Vincristine Doxorubicin Dexamethasone Methotrexate Cytarabine Rituximab

Follow-up

The majority of patients who remain in remission for over 1 year can be classified as cured of their disease. For patients enrolled on clinical trials, follow-up will be determined by the recommendations of the protocol. To evaluate other patients, definitions of response have been developed by the International Working Group (IWG) and are outlined in Table 14.6 [41]. Although the recommendations list 18-Fluoro-deoxyglucose positron emission tomography (FDG-PET) as an evaluation tool, this modality has not been proven to add benefit to the workup of Burkitt

Table 14.6 IWG definitions of response in patients diagnosed with non-Hodgkins Lymphoma. Although listed, FDG or PET are not usually completed in the workup of patients with Burkitt lymphoma

Response	Definition	Nodal masses	Spleen, liver	Bone marrow
CR	Disappearance of all evidence of disease	(a) FDG-avid or PET positive prior to therapy; mass of any size permitted if PET negative (b) Variably FDG-avid or PET negative; regression to normal size on CT	Not palpable, nodules disappeared	Infiltrate cleared on repeat biopsy; if indeterminate by morphology, immunohistochemistry should be negative
PR	Regression of measurable disease and no new sites	≥50% decrease in SPD of up to 6 largest dominant masses; no increase in size of other nodes (a) FDG-avid or PET positive prior to therapy; one or more PET positive at previously involved site (b) Variably FDG-avid or PET negative; regression on CT	≥50% decrease in SPD of nodules (for single nodule in greatest transverse diameter); no increase in size of liver or spleen	Irrelevant if positive prior to therapy; cell type should be specified
SD	Failure to attain CR/PR or PD	(a) FDG-avid or PET positive prior to therapy; PET positive at prior sites of disease and no new sites on CT or PET (b) Variably FDG-avid or PET negative; no change in size of previous lesions on CT		
Relapsed disease or PD	Any new lesion or increase by ≥50% of previously involved sites from nadir	Appearance of a new lesion(s) > 1.5 cm in any axis, ≥50% increase in SPD of more than one node, or ≥50% increase in longest diameter of a previously identified node > 1 cm in short axis Lesions PET positive if FDG-avid lymphoma or PET positive prior to therapy	>50% increase from nadir in the SPD of any previous lesions	New or recurrent involvement

CR complete remission, *FDG* [^{18}F]fluorodeoxyglucose, *PET* positron emission tomography, *PR* partial remission, *SPD* sum of the product of the diameters, *SD* stable disease, *PD* progressive disease

lymphoma patients and is not routinely completed [42]. Recommendations regarding the frequency of surveillance evaluations will be dependent upon clinical judgment, but a general guideline usually includes visits at lengthening intervals for the first 5 years with yearly visits thereafter [43]. Complete history and physical exam with emphasis on previous disease sites is important. Routine labs including CBC, electrolytes, liver function tests, and LDH are also important. CT scans are also used for follow-up, but have no proven impact on outcome and should not be used superfluously given the high dose of radiation as a possible cancer risk [44–46].

There is no defined standard treatment for patients with recurrent disease, and these patients should be encouraged to participate in clinical trials. Both pediatric and adult patients usually do not benefit from autologous hematopoietic cell transplantation [47, 48].

Complications

The introduction of high intensity short duration chemotherapy regimens has significantly improved the outcome for patients with Burkitt lymphoma. Patients still face the toxic consequences of the disease, both before and after the treatment is initiated. Tumor lysis syndrome occurs frequently in Burkitt lymphoma, probably related to the extraordinary doubling time and chemosensitivity of the tumor [49]. The finding that uric acid levels were often raised in Burkitt lymphoma patients prior to receiving chemotherapy was reported in 1972, with a description of a patient who had a serum uric acid level of 54 mg per 100 ml on the day of death [50].

The syndrome is characterized by hyperuricemia, hyperkalemia, hyperphosphatemia, and hypocalcemia [51]. In 2004, a proposal was made to define tumor lysis syndrome by both laboratory (LTLS) and clinical (CTLS) criteria and use these criteria to develop a grading system [52]. More recently, some authors have suggested changes to the LTLS and CTLS definitions, specifically that two or more metabolic abnormalities be present simultaneously to denote LTLS, and a 25% change from baseline should not be considered a criterion for CTLS [53].

In 1980, Cohen et al. reported 37 patients with Burkitt lymphoma and acute tumor lysis syndrome and made recommendations for treatment including the use of hydration, allopurinol, and close monitoring of electrolytes [49]. Over the last 30 years, little has changed in the management of these patients, with the exception of urinary alkalinization, which is no longer recommended, and the availability of urate oxidase (rasburicase) [54]. A multicenter trial involving patients with advanced stage Burkitt lymphoma in France and the USA compared the use of rasburicase versus allopurinol for acute tumor lysis syndrome prevention. All patients received the same chemotherapy and aggressive hydration, with the French participants receiving rasburicase rather than allopurinol given that rasburicase was not yet approved for use in the USA. The results showed that 9% of French children developed tumor lysis syndrome versus 26% of children treated in the USA [29]. All newly diagnosed Burkitt lymphoma patients should start allopurinol immediately.

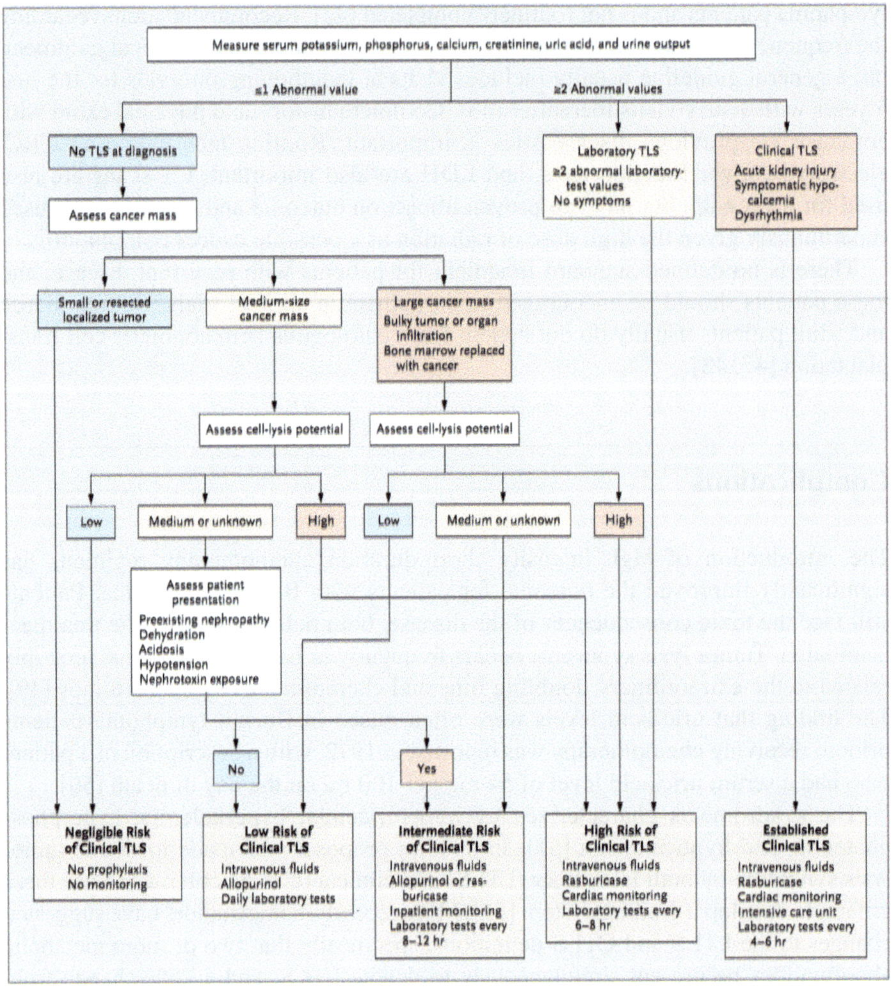

Fig. 14.1 Treatment algorithm for patients presenting with acute tumor lysis syndrome

Thereafter, the need for rasburicase administration can be evaluated. Whether to continue allopurinol in patients treated with rasburicase has not been definitively studied. The agents have different mechanisms for reducing uric acid load. Allopurinol prevents formation and rasburicase metabolizes already formed uric acid. Many clinicians will stop allopurinol when administering rasburicase and restart 24 h later for ongoing TLS while others continue allopurinol [54]. A recent review article by Howard et al. provides an excellent treatment algorithm to guide care at the time of presentation, shown in Fig. 14.1 [53].

Other toxicity experienced by patients include mucositis, cerebellar toxicity, and thrombocytopenia-related hemorrhage [55]. Over the years, reduction of doses of methotrexate and intrathecal cytarabine and altered fractionated schedule of cyclophosphamide have helped to alleviate some of these issues for contemporary patients [56]. To further minimize toxicities, many treatment regimens incorporate fungal, bacterial, and viral prophylaxis, although the value of adding such agents has never been validated by controlled studies [55]. Although no definitive data exists for the use of G-CSF in adult patients with Burkitt lymphoma, it has been shown to reduce the average time to neutrophil recovery [35].

New Directions

Despite the vast improvement noted in outcomes from Dr. Burkitt's first description in 1958 to the present day, further understanding regarding mechanisms of treatment failures and novel therapeutics are required. It has long been noted that patients with elevated levels of lactate dehydrogenase, extent of disease, central nervous system (CNS) disease at presentation, suboptimal response to a cytoreductive prophase, and advanced age represent a cohort with a worse prognosis [28, 29, 57]. Recent investigations regarding the biology of Burkitt lymphoma have identified other markers of poor prognosis. Deletions of 13q and gain of 7q [58], cellular FLICE (FADD-like IL-1beta-converting enzyme)-inhibitory protein (c-FLIP) levels [59] and minimal residual disease (MRD) detection by long-distance polymerase chain reaction assay detecting the (8;14)(q24;q32) translocation and [60] have all recently been identified as indicators of inferior outcome, possibly identifying subgroups of patients that may benefit from intensification of therapy [61].

Monoclonal antibodies and other biologic reagents continue to provide promise as novel addition therapy for patients with Burkitt lymphoma. The addition of the anti-CD20 monoclonal antibody rituximab to existing treatment regimens such as HyperCVAD has been found to be especially beneficial in older patients [62]. As discussed previously dose-adjusted EPOCH plus rituximab (DA-EPOCH-R) has produced durable remissions with minimal toxicity in a number of adult patients, and a confirmatory multicenter study is currently underway [39].

The anti-CD22 monoclonal antibody epratuzumab is also being studied as adjuvant therapy. Studies of its use in several Burkitt lymphoma cell cultures have revealed cytotoxicity [63]. Investigations into using epratuzumab concomitantly with rituximab in Burkitt lymphoma cell lines have revealed possible synergy, but clinical trials are still evolving [64].

Transcriptional regulation via epigenetic mechanism is yet another possible target of future therapeutics. Histone deacetylase inhibitors such as depsipeptide have recently been shown to have additive cytotoxicity when combined with standard therapy in Burkitt lymphoma cell lines [65].

Conclusion

The treatment of Burkitt lymphoma has evolved over the last 50 years as further understanding of the biological characteristics of the tumor has been obtained. High intensity, short duration chemotherapy with CNS prophylaxis is now the standard of care, with special consideration of treatment toxicities such as acute tumor lysis syndrome. Continued investigations regarding the biology of the tumor cells, and attempts to reduce the intensity of chemotherapy while maintaining excellent disease-free survival should continue the gains first obtained by Dr. Denis Burkitt in the 1950s.

Denis Parsons Burkitt (1911–1993)

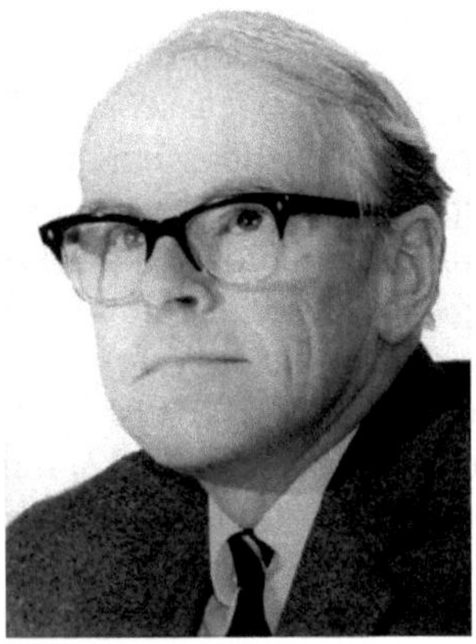

Born in Enniskillen, in what is now Northern Ireland, Burkitt entered university to study engineering. A tutor wrote a letter to his father in which he expressed grave doubts as to whether Burkitt would ever be able to obtain a degree [66]. His deep Christian faith drove him to serve his fellow man by becoming a physician. After completing his training in surgery, he volunteered for the Colonial Medical Service in West Africa early in 1941. He mentioned a sense of vocation in his application but this did not evoke the response he expected "this surprisingly seemed to scare them, using the pretext that I had lost an eye in an accident as a child they rejected my offer without even an interview. This was a profound disappointment, but when I eventually reached Africa, God, in his mercy enabled me with my one eye to see things which my predecessors had missed with two" [67].

> I put in for two research grants, which together amounted to $75.00. That was all we had for the first 18 months of our study—a study which formed the basis from which hundreds, if not thousands, of scientific papers have subsequently been published. We used most of the funds for postage stamps, and for leaflets that were sent all over Africa.
>
> After requesting grants from several of the large research facilities, we were able to amass about $1500 with which we bought an old Ford station wagon. With the remainder

> for pocket money, three of us set off to cover about 10,000 miles, visiting 57 hospitals in 10 countries of east, central and south Africa. I had two missionary doctors traveling with me, Ted Williams and Cliff Nelson, chosen for their good company as well as their professional/mechanical and other knowledge. This was, after all, my summer holiday [4].

The trip was done on a shoestring budget, which Denis made light of daily. Indeed, the research grant for the project was a mere £25. "Of course, we'll have the hotel room without the bath. For a quid or two it's a cinch to walk down the hall." Or, "Is a box of biscuits and a cup of tea in the car while we're travelling okay with you two again today instead of a fancy, expensive lunch?" His humour kept our spirits buoyed up as well. We'll never forget statements such as, "This must be the safest ever safari in Africa. Here we are three doctors, each with our private stock of medicines making a beeline from one hospital to the next". Ted, after looking over countless giant anthills, asked, "I wonder how many anthills there are in Africa?" "Easy," shot back Denis, "count the ants and divide by 50,000" [66].

References

1. Pagano L et al (2009) Clinical aspects and therapy of sporadic Burkitt lymphoma. Mediterr J Hematol Infect Dis 1(2):e2009030
2. Burkitt D (1958) A sarcoma involving the jaws in African children. Br J Surg 46(197):218–223
3. Bendiner E (1990) A missionary, heart and soul. Hosp Pract 25(7), 166–172, 175–176, 179–180 passim
4. Levine PH (1987) Epstein-Barr virus and human disease. In: Experimental biology and medicine. Humana Press, Clifton, xxxi, 530 p
5. O'Conor GT (1961) Malignant lymphoma in African children. II. A pathological entity. Cancer 14:270–283
6. Burkitt DP, Wright DH (1970) Burkitt's lymphoma. Livingstone, Edinburgh, xi, 251 p
7. Burkitt D, O'Conor GT (1961) Malignant lymphoma in African children. I. A clinical syndrome. Cancer 14:258–269
8. Burkitt DP, Kyalwazi SK (1967) Spontaneous remission of African lymphoma. Br J Cancer 21(1):14–16
9. Ziegler JL (1982) Burkitt's Lymphoma. CA Cancer J Clin 32(3):144–161
10. Oettgen HF, Burkitt D, Burchenal JH (1963) Malignant lymphoma involving the jaw in African children: treatment with Methotrexate. Cancer 16:616–623
11. Burkitt D, Hutt MS, Wright DH (1965) The African lymphoma: preliminary observations on response to therapy. Cancer 18:399–410
12. Burkitt D (1966) African lymphoma. Observations on response to vincristine sulphate therapy. Cancer 19(8):1131–1137
13. Pizzo PA, Poplack DG (2002) Principles and practice of pediatric oncology, 4th edn. Lippincott Williams & Wilkins, Philadelphia, xv, 1692 p
14. Morrow RH, Pike MC, Kisuule A (1967) Survival of Burkitt's lymphoma patients in Mulago Hospital, Uganda. Br Med J 4(5575):323–327
15. Magrath I (2009) Lessons from clinical trials in African Burkitt lymphoma. Curr Opin Oncol 21(5):462–468
16. Ziegler JL et al (1970) Treatment of Burkitt's tumor with cyclophosphamide. Cancer 26(2):474–484
17. Ziegler JL et al (1972) Intensive chemotherapy in patients with generalized Burkitt's lymphoma. Int J Cancer 10(2):254–261

18. Olweny CL et al (1980) Long-term experience with Burkitt's lymphoma in Uganda. Int J Cancer 26(3):261–266
19. Olweny CL et al (1976) Treatment of Burkitt's lymphoma: randomized clinical trial of single-agent versus combination chemotherapy. Int J Cancer 17(4):436–440
20. Olweny CL et al (1977) Cerebrospinal irradiation of Burkitt's lymphoma. Failure in preventing central nervous system relapse. Acta Radiol Ther Phys Biol 16(3):225–231
21. Ziegler JL, Bluming AZ (1971) Intrathecal chemotherapy in Burkitt's lymphoma. Br Med J 3(5773):508–512
22. Anderson JR et al (1983) Childhood non-Hodgkin's lymphoma. The results of a randomized therapeutic trial comparing a 4-drug regimen (COMP) with a 10-drug regimen (LSA2-L2). N Engl J Med 308(10):559–565
23. Anderson JR et al (1993) Long-term follow-up of patients treated with COMP or LSA2L2 therapy for childhood non-Hodgkin's lymphoma: a report of CCG-551 from the Childrens Cancer Group. J Clin Oncol 11(6):1024–1032
24. Patte C et al (1986) Improved survival rate in children with stage III and IV B cell non-Hodgkin's lymphoma and leukemia using multi-agent chemotherapy: results of a study of 114 children from the French Pediatric Oncology Society. J Clin Oncol 4(8):1219–1226
25. Patte C et al (2001) The Societe Francaise d'Oncologie Pediatrique LMB89 protocol: highly effective multiagent chemotherapy tailored to the tumor burden and initial response in 561 unselected children with B-cell lymphomas and L3 leukemia. Blood 97(11):3370–3379
26. Patte C et al (1991) High survival rate in advanced-stage B-cell lymphomas and leukemias without CNS involvement with a short intensive polychemotherapy: results from the French Pediatric Oncology Society of a randomized trial of 216 children. J Clin Oncol 9(1):123–132
27. Jaglowski SM et al (2009) Lymphoma in adolescents and young adults. Semin Oncol 36(5):381–418
28. Patte C et al (2007) Results of the randomized international FAB/LMB96 trial for intermediate risk B-cell non-Hodgkin lymphoma in children and adolescents: it is possible to reduce treatment for the early responding patients. Blood 109(7):2773–2780
29. Cairo MS et al (2007) Results of a randomized international study of high-risk central nervous system B non-Hodgkin lymphoma and B acute lymphoblastic leukemia in children and adolescents. Blood 109(7):2736–2743
30. Soussain C et al (1995) Small noncleaved cell lymphoma and leukemia in adults. A retrospective study of 65 adults treated with the LMB pediatric protocols. Blood 85(3):664–674
31. Divine M et al (2005) Burkitt lymphoma in adults: a prospective study of 72 patients treated with an adapted pediatric LMB protocol. Ann Oncol 16(12):1928–1935
32. Magrath I et al (1996) Adults and children with small non-cleaved-cell lymphoma have a similar excellent outcome when treated with the same chemotherapy regimen. J Clin Oncol 14(3):925–934
33. Adde M et al (1998) Additional chemotherapy agents improve treatment outcome for children and adults with advanced B-cell lymphomas. Semin Oncol 25(2 Suppl 4):33–39, discussion 45–8
34. Mead GM et al (2002) An international evaluation of CODOX-M and CODOX-M alternating with IVAC in adult Burkitt's lymphoma: results of United Kingdom Lymphoma Group LY06 study. Ann Oncol 13(8):1264–1274
35. Thomas DA et al (1999) Hyper-CVAD program in Burkitt's-type adult acute lymphoblastic leukemia. J Clin Oncol 17(8):2461–2470
36. Fayad L, Thomas D, Romaguera J (2007) Update of the MD Anderson Cancer Center experience with hyper-CVAD and rituximab for the treatment of mantle cell and Burkitt-type lymphomas. Clin Lymphoma Myeloma 8(Suppl 2):S57–S62
37. Kaplan LD et al (1997) Low-dose compared with standard-dose m-BACOD chemotherapy for non-Hodgkin's lymphoma associated with human immunodeficiency virus infection. National Institute of Allergy and Infectious Diseases AIDS Clinical Trials Group. N Engl J Med 336(23):1641–1648
38. Noy A (2010) Controversies in the treatment of Burkitt lymphoma in AIDS. Curr Opin Oncol 22(5):443–448

39. Dunleavy K et al (2007) Efficacy and toxicity of dose-adjusted EPOCH-rituximab in adults with newly diagnosed Burkitt lymphoma. J Clin Oncol 25(18S):8035
40. The NCCN Clinical Practice Guidelines in Oncology (NCCN Guidelines®) Non-Hodgkin's Lymphoma (Version 3.2012). © 2012 National Comprehensive Cancer Network, Inc. Available at: NCCN.org. Accessed [August 30, 2012]. To view the most recent and complete version of the NCCN Guidelines®, go on-line to NCCN.org
41. Cheson BD et al (2007) Revised response criteria for malignant lymphoma. J Clin Oncol 25(5):579–586
42. Seam P, Juweid ME, Cheson BD (2007) The role of FDG-PET scans in patients with lymphoma. Blood 110(10):3507–3516
43. Abeloff MD (2008) Abeloff's clinical oncology, 4th edn. Churchill Livingstone/Elsevier, Philadelphia, xxx, 2555 p
44. Brenner DJ, Hall EJ (2007) Computed tomography – an increasing source of radiation exposure. N Engl J Med 357(22):2277–2284
45. Sodickson A et al (2009) Recurrent CT, cumulative radiation exposure, and associated radiation-induced cancer risks from CT of adults. Radiology 251(1):175–184
46. Berrington de Gonzalez A et al (2009) Projected cancer risks from computed tomographic scans performed in the United States in 2007. Arch Intern Med 169(22):2071–2077
47. Ladenstein R et al (1997) High-dose chemotherapy with autologous bone marrow rescue in children with poor-risk Burkitt's lymphoma: a report from the European Lymphoma Bone Marrow Transplantation Registry. Blood 90(8):2921–2930
48. Sweetenham JW et al (1996) Adult Burkitt's and Burkitt-like non-Hodgkin's lymphoma – outcome for patients treated with high-dose therapy and autologous stem-cell transplantation in first remission or at relapse: results from the European Group for Blood and Marrow Transplantation. J Clin Oncol 14(9):2465–2472
49. Cohen LF et al (1980) Acute tumor lysis syndrome. A review of 37 patients with Burkitt's lymphoma. Am J Med 68(4):486–491
50. Ngu VA (1972) Chemotherapy of Burkitt's tumor at the University of Ibadan, Nigeria. JAMA 222(9):1166
51. Jeha S (2001) Tumor lysis syndrome. Semin Hematol 38(4 Suppl 10):4–8
52. Cairo MS, Bishop M (2004) Tumour lysis syndrome: new therapeutic strategies and classification. Br J Haematol 127(1):3–11
53. Howard SC, Jones DP, Pui CH (2011) The tumor lysis syndrome. N Engl J Med 364(19):1844–1854
54. Coccia P (2011) The more things change, the more they stay the same. Oncology 25(4):381–382
55. Blum KA, Lozanski G, Byrd JC (2004) Adult Burkitt leukemia and lymphoma. Blood 104(10):3009–3020
56. Yustein JT, Dang CV (2007) Biology and treatment of Burkitt's lymphoma. Curr Opin Hematol 14(4):375–381
57. Woessmann W et al (2005) The impact of the methotrexate administration schedule and dose in the treatment of children and adolescents with B-cell neoplasms: a report of the BFM Group Study NHL-BFM95. Blood 105(3):948–958
58. Poirel HA et al (2009) Specific cytogenetic abnormalities are associated with a significantly inferior outcome in children and adolescents with mature B-cell non-Hodgkin's lymphoma: results of the FAB/LMB 96 international study. Leukemia 23(2):323–331
59. Safa A, Pollok K (2011) Targeting the anti-apoptotic protein c-FLIP for cancer therapy. Cancers 3:1639–1671
60. Mussolin L et al (2003) Prospective analysis of minimal bone marrow infiltration in pediatric Burkitt's lymphomas by long-distance polymerase chain reaction for t(8;14)(q24;q32). Leukemia 17(3):585–589
61. Mussolin L et al (2011) Minimal disseminated disease in high-risk Burkitt's lymphoma identifies patients with different prognosis. J Clin Oncol 29(13):1779–1784
62. Thomas DA et al (2006) Chemoimmunotherapy with hyper-CVAD plus rituximab for the treatment of adult Burkitt and Burkitt-type lymphoma or acute lymphoblastic leukemia. Cancer 106(7):1569–1580

63. Tuscano JM et al (1999) CD22 cross-linking generates B-cell antigen receptor-independent signals that activate the JNK/SAPK signaling cascade. Blood 94(4):1382–1392
64. Carnahan J et al (2007) Epratuzumab, a CD22-targeting recombinant humanized antibody with a different mode of action from rituximab. Mol Immunol 44(6):1331–1341
65. Kano Y et al (2007) Cytotoxic effects of histone deacetylase inhibitor FK228 (depsipeptide, formally named FR901228) in combination with conventional anti-leukemia/lymphoma agents against human leukemia/lymphoma cell lines. Invest New Drugs 25(1):31–40
66. Nelson CL, Temple NJ (1994) Tribute to Denis Burkitt. J Med Biogr 2(3):180–183
67. Coakley D (2006) Denis Burkitt and his contribution to haematology/oncology. Br J Haematol 135(1):17–25
68. National Cancer Institute. Physician Data Query (PDQ). Childhood Non-Hodgkin Lymphoma Treatment. 8/14/2012. Accessed at http://www.cancer.gov/cancertopics/pdq/treatment/child-non-hodgkins/HealthProfessional on August 30, 2012
69. National Cancer Institute. Physician Data Query (PDQ). Adult Non-Hodgkin Lymphoma Treatment. 8/14/2012. Accessed at http://www.cancer.gov/cancertopics/pdq/treatment/adult-non-hodgkins/HealthProfessional on August 30, 2012

Chapter 15
Animal Models of Burkitt's Lymphoma

Alexandra Vrazo, Maria Chauchard, Osman Cen, and Richard Longnecker

Introduction

Burkitt's lymphoma (BL) is a high-grade B-cell malignancy occurring most frequently in children in areas with holoendemic and hyperendemic malaria (about 5–10 cases per 100,000 children), and with lesser frequency in all other parts of the world. BL is classified as an aggressive non-Hodgkin's lymphoma (NHL) derived from germinal center B-cells, based on cellular morphology, the expression of BCL-6 and CD10, and the hallmark MYC translocation. BL can be subdivided into three different clinical variants based on epidemiological observations: endemic BL (eBL), sporadic BL (sBL), and immunodeficiency-associated BL (iBL). Although there is considerable overlap, unique clinical features have been described in each of these variants. While eBL primarily affects children between the ages of 4 and 7 years, sBL is seen in both children and young adults with a median age of 30 years [1–3]. For all three types of BL, males are more commonly affected than females with an approximate ratio of 2 to 1. eBL is most commonly observed in Equatorial Africa and Papua New Guinea, with frequent involvement of the jaw, facial bones, and kidneys, although ileal, cecal, ovarian, and breast involvement has also been reported [1–4]. The particularly high incidence of BL in Equatorial Africa (50-fold higher than in the USA) and the geographic distribution of this tumor, corresponding to the distribution of endemic malaria, have led to its designation as eBL. In contrast, in other geographic areas, most patients present with abdominal and nodal involvement with no specific geographic distribution [1–8]. This clinical variant, designated sBL, accounts for 1–2% of all adult lymphomas, and 30–50% of pediatric lymphomas in Western Europe and the USA. Five-year mortality of sBL in the USA showed demonstrates a positive correlation with age, with pediatric cases having an

A. Vrazo • M. Chauchard • O. Cen • R. Longnecker (✉)
Department of Microbiology-Immunology, Northwestern University Feinberg School of Medicine, Chicago, IL 60611, USA
e-mail: r-longnecker@northwestern.edu

E.S. Robertson (ed.), *Burkitt's Lymphoma*, Current Cancer Research,
DOI 10.1007/978-1-4614-4313-1_15, © Springer Science+Business Media New York 2013

approximately 25% mortality rate, adult cases 50%, and geriatric cases 70% [6]. iBL typically involves the lymph nodes and bone marrow [9]. This subtype is frequently observed in the setting of HIV infection and, unlike other HIV-related lymphomas, it is frequently observed in patients with CD4 counts over 200 cells/μL.

The three forms of BL are characterized from other NHL by histological analysis. Features characteristic to BL include medium-sized cells with abundant, basophilic cytoplasm, often containing lipid vacuoles; round nuclei with clumped chromatin and multiple nucleoli, and a diffuse, monotonous pattern of infiltration. A "starry sky" appearance has been described in BL because of a high proliferation rate of tumor cells, frequent apoptosis, and numerous macrophages containing ingested apoptotic debris from tumor cells. BL cells express surface IgM, BCL-6, CD19, CD20, CD22, CD10, and CD79a and are negative for CD5, CD23, and TdT [10].

The molecular hallmark of BL is the ectopic expression of the *MYC* oncogene due to reciprocal chromosomal translocations [11–14]. Eighty percent of BL cases harbor t(8;14)(q24;q32) translocations, resulting in the juxtaposition of the *MYC* gene on chromosome 8 with immunoglobulin heavy chain (*IgH)* enhancer elements on chromosome 14, which drive c-Myc mRNA and protein production. In the remaining 20% of BL cases, translocations occurring between chromosomes 2 and 8, t(2;8)(p12;q24), or chromosomes 8 and 22, t(8;22)(q24;q11), place *MYC* adjacent to either κ or λ light chain (*IgL*) loci and enhancer elements, respectively. As heavy chain and light chain loci are specifically active in mature B cells, *MYC* transcription is favored in B cells harboring the translocation. *MYC* encodes the c-Myc transcription factor, which was first discovered nearly 30 years ago as a cellular homologue of the avian retroviral oncogene v-Myc [15]. Since then, c-Myc has been recognized as one of the most commonly activated oncoproteins in human cancers. Functions of genes in the c-Myc target gene network include the regulation of cell cycle progression, proliferation, differentiation, and apoptosis [16–18]. Under normal conditions, c-Myc is activated in response to mitogenic factors and is repressed upon exposure to anti-proliferative signals. Overexpression of c-Myc contributes to proliferation by inducing the activity of cyclins, while at the same time repressing the activity of the cyclin inhibitor p27 [19].

Even though translocation of *MYC* is generally considered a hallmark for BL, other genetic alterations contribute to lymphomagenesis. Overexpression of c-Myc not only drives cells into the cell cycle, but also leads to apoptosis by activation of the pro-death p53 pathway. Like other tumors, development of BL often occurs upon disruption of one of the tumor suppressor pathways that normally induce apoptosis in response to oncogenic stimuli. Indeed, mutation of the sequence encoding the master tumor suppressor, p53, is frequently found in BL biopsies and cell lines [20–22]. One study found that 41% of BL biopsies contained a P53 mutation [23]. In addition, pro-survival signals can also be provided by other aberrantly activated oncogenes, such as RAS or BCL-2.

It should be noted that some studies have identified a very small number of BL cases (<10% of sBL) that do not show any *MYC* translocation, yet still overexpress c-Myc. This phenomenon has been linked to downregulation of miRNAs that negatively regulate c-Myc mRNA translation [24, 25]. In contrast, cases of BL with *MYC* translocations also show higher expression levels of these miRNAs.

This gives two distinct mechanisms by which BL cells may come to overexpress c-Myc: (1) the translocation of *MYC* to an Ig locus, and (2) downregulation of miRNAs which regulate translation of c-Myc mRNA.

EBV and Burkitt's Lymphoma

EBV is a member of the gammaherpes family of double-stranded DNA viruses. Worldwide, more than 90% of individuals become infected with EBV at some point during their lifetime. Though most infected individuals remain healthy, infection with EBV may promote the development of a number of human pathologies and malignancies. EBV transforms normal primary human B lymphocytes into continuously growing immortalized cells, lymphoblastoid cell lines (LCLs) [26]. In addition, though all BL variants have similar phenotypes, it has been suggested that the three subtypes may have different pathogenetic mechanisms due to the degree of association with EBV. About 95% of eBL cases are associated with EBV [2]. In contrast, only 5–15% of sBL and 30–40% of HIV-associated BL are EBV positive [27]. The differential association patterns and the detection of clonal EBV genomes and latency proteins in BL suggest that EBV may have a mechanistic role in pathogenesis of some forms of BL [28]. A number of latency proteins with growth-promoting or survival functions are detected in EBV-associated BL, including Epstein–Barr nuclear antigen 1 (EBNA1), latent membrane protein 2A (LMP2A), or the EBV-encoded RNAs [29–32]. Thus, EBV may promote BL development by protecting pre-tumor B cells with an MYC translocation from apoptosis.

Animal Models

Animal models are powerful tools for studying the contribution of known or candidate oncogenes to human diseases, and for studying the effectiveness of potential therapeutics in a model system. Nonhuman primate models have been used to understand the biology of EBV infection and lymphomagenesis and, more specifically, to develop therapeutic strategies for use in humans. To model BL in the mouse, several lineages of Myc transgenic mice have been generated, where c-Myc expression can be restricted to the B-cell lineage using a B-cell-specific promoter and enhancer. Transgenic animals have also been critical for studying the role of EBV latent gene products in BL, as there is strong evidence for a causative or perhaps cooperative viral role in the development of BL. Since EBV is a strict human pathogen, its study is limited in vivo by the inability of mice to be infected with EBV, and the lack of homology between EBV latent proteins and those of a related herpes virus, *Murid herpesvirus 68* (MHV68). To overcome these restrictions, transgenic mice expressing EBV latent proteins have been crossed with Myc transgenic mice to generate models of EBV-associated BL, so that the relative contribution of viral proteins to development and progression of BL-like can be assessed.

Additionally, Myc and EBV-Myc mouse models have been used to test specific inhibitors of the pathways deregulated in murine BL with the hope of future use in humans. In addition, the recent generation of humanized mice, defined as immunodeficient mouse strains reconstituted with human hematopoietic cells, has provided a convenient model to recapitulate EBV infection in mice.

Nonhuman Primate Models of EBV-Associated Lymphoproliferation

The recognition of viral-induced spontaneous lymphomas in nonhuman Old World primates came in 1973 at the USSR Academy of Medical Sciences at Sukhumi, USSR, in a group of experimental baboons [33]. The etiologic agent was baboon lymphocryptovirus (LCV), a virus in the same *Lymphocryptovirus* genus as EBV. LCV infection is ubiquitous in adult Old World nonhuman primates where it is associated with spontaneous lymphomas in the host and can immortalize B cells in culture. To use LCV as a model for EBV, Moghaddam et al. [34] infected Old World rhesus macaques with rhesus LCV and demonstrated that many features of rhesus LCV infection were similar to EBV infection of humans; acute and persistent infections were initiated, lifelong antibody responses were maintained, LCV could be isolated from peripheral blood leukocytes of healthy animals, and LCV was shed from the oropharynx [35]. More recently, the first EBV-related LCV naturally infecting a New World primate, the common marmoset (*Callithrix jacchus*), has been described [36]. The inability of LCV to model a Burkitt's-like lymphoma led researchers to assess the outcome of infecting nonhuman primates with EBV. However, the development of lymphomas in EBV-infected nonhuman primates has been largely variable and is dependent on the EBV strain, the type of primate, and the route of infection. Many examples exist of certain primates refractive to EBV infection, or once infected, unable to develop tumors. In one study, no tumors were observed in 42 rhesus macaques, 4 chimpanzees, and one cynomolgus macaque infected with EBV and followed for 8 years, despite serological testing indicating that 14 of 47 animals had been successfully infected with EBV [37].

More success has been achieved with EBV infection of callitrichids, including cottontop tamarins (*Saguinus oedipus*) and common marmosets (*Callithrix jacchus*). Marmosets and tamarins are susceptible to persistent and acute infection with EBV, and replicate many of the characteristics of human EBV infection and develop EBV lymphoproliferative disorders [38–40]. The ability of marmosets to be infected with EBV has permitted testing of a vaccine against the EBV envelope glycoprotein gp350 in infected animals, which decreased viral load in saliva and blood [41, 42]. In terms of EBV-induced lymphomas, tamarins are currently the most tractable primate model available. Early studies indicated lymphoma development in some, but not all, cottontop tamarins infected with cell-free EBV, with tumors presenting in the lymph nodes near the site of inoculation by 46 days [43–45]. Later experiments infecting animals with higher EBV titers resulted in lymphoma generation in 100%

of infected tamarins [46]. Histological analysis found that these lymphomas were of B cell origin of immunoblastic and follicular center cell types, demonstrating mono- and oligoclonality. The EBV latency proteins LMP1, EBNA1, and EBNA2 were detected, reiterating the similarity between EBV-associated lymphoproliferations arising in humans and classifying these tumors as being more similar to post-transplant lymphoproliferative disorder (PTLD) than a Burkitt's-like lymphoma [47].

Based on the ability of EBV to induce lymphomas in cottontop tamarins, these animals have been used to test the effectiveness of the EBV envelope glycoprotein gp350/220 as a candidate vaccine to prevent EBV-associated lymphomas [47–51]. The candidate vaccine was sufficient to prevent lymphoma development, but not EBV infection, as EBV gene products were detected at low levels in healthy lymphoid tissue of immunized animals, and antibodies to gp350/220 were raised, but did not neutralize EBV.

The use of nonhuman primates to study EBV infection and associated lymphomas is feasible. However, there are a number of reasons why primates as models for lymphoma have fallen out of favor since the 1980s. As discussed previously, not all cottontop tamarins develop lymphoma unless inoculated with a high titer of virus, and the kinetics of lymphoma development are not consistent. In addition, handling and care of nonhuman primates can be cost prohibitive. Furthermore, cottontop tamarins are a highly endangered species with a narrow natural habitat in northwest Colombia [52]. These considerations and the evolution of molecular biology techniques in the late 1980s led many researchers to use transgenic mice to investigate the involvement of the *MYC* translocation and EBV gene products in the genesis of BL. Currently, primates are still occasionally used to model the humoral response to EBV infection and to EBV vaccine candidates [53].

MYC Transgenic Mouse Models

The discovery of the canonical *MYC* translocation to one of the immunoglobulin gene loci indicated the importance of c-Myc upregulation in the initiation or maintenance of BL [11, 14, 54]. Successive research aiming to study the role of c-Myc in lymphomagenesis led to the generation of a Myc transgenic mouse strain as a BL model [55]. Several Myc-expressing transgenic mouse lines have been developed, where transgene expression is driven by a B-cell-specific promoter to ensure expression of c-Myc is limited to the B-cell compartment. These models have helped define the role of c-Myc and the immunoglobulin enhancer region in the development of lymphomas, as well as in normal cellular function, and will be discussed here.

Eμ-*myc* Mice

The first Myc transgenic mouse models were reported in 1985 [55, 56]. To mimic the t(8:14) chromosomal translocation of *MYC* to the *IgH* locus detected in 80% of

BL cases, the murine form of *MYC* was expressed as a minigene construct under the control of the intronic enhancer region (Eμ) of the immunoglobulin heavy chain (*IgH*) gene (Eμ-*myc*), or under the control of the SV40 promoter and the κ light chain enhancer region (Eκ-SV-*myc*). The bone marrow of young (4–7 week) Eμ-*myc* mice was dominated by large pre-B cells, and most abnormally, pre-B cells composed almost 25% of splenic B cells, indicating a brief proliferative phase during which time B-cell expansion was controlled by apoptosis [57]. Eμ-*myc* mice developed spontaneous aggressive tumors, with a median onset at 9 weeks and an average morbidity or mortality by 12 weeks with an overall tumor incidence of 86% [58]. In the same study, the average morbidity or mortality of the Eκ-SV-*myc* lineage was 23 weeks, with tumor development in 35%. Massive lymph node enlargement and moderate enlargement of the spleen and thymus was observed, with variable invasion of other tissues, such as the liver and large intestine. Although heterogeneity in tumors was observed, most tumor cells were sIg^- with *IgL* in the germline conformation, although a small proportion (20%) were sIg^+ and had rearranged *IgL* genes [59]. Most tumor cells were monoclonal, suggesting a single cell of origin for each tumor. These features lead to the classification of tumors arising in Eμ-*myc* mice as lymphoblastic lymphoma with a leukemic component, based on the composition of pre-B lymphocytes or a mix of pre-B/B lymphocytes, unlike the more mature B-cell phenotype observed in human BL.

The short latent period for Eμ-*myc* tumors indicates that other mutations contribute to tumorigenesis in this murine model of BL, in a similar fashion to human BL where lesions in apoptotic pathways are critical for aiding Myc-induced lymphomagenesis. Disruption of the p53-ARF-MDM2 pathway occurs in approximately 80% of Eμ-*myc* tumors, similar to that observed in human BL [20, 60]. In addition, the BCL-2 pro-survival family of proteins have been implicated in Myc-driven lymphomagenesis; Eμ-*myc* mice crossed with *bcl-2* transgenic mice give rise to rapidly developing tumors [61].

Eμ-*myc* mice have been used extensively as a model of BL-like tumor development and therapeutics. The demonstration that Myc suppression can cause tumor regression [62] has supported the development of therapeutic strategies targeting Myc. However, the presence of leukemias and pre-/pro-B-cell origin indicates that these tumors could present a murine analogue of acute lymphoblastic leukemia rather than a BL analogue. Immature tumors may be a function of copy number, with higher levels of Myc expression favoring immature tumors, and single copies of Myc (such as those used in the Myc-YAC mice, discussed later) developing more mature IgM^+ tumors [63].

Igλ-MYC Mice

To reflect BL chromosomal breakpoints seen in 20% of BL which result in fusion to the *IgL* locus, Kovalchuk et al. [64] constructed a *MYC* transgene isolated from the human BL line IARC-BL60, under the control of a 12 kb genomic portion of *IgL* including the enhancer. All Igλ-MYC mice developed lymphoma with a variable

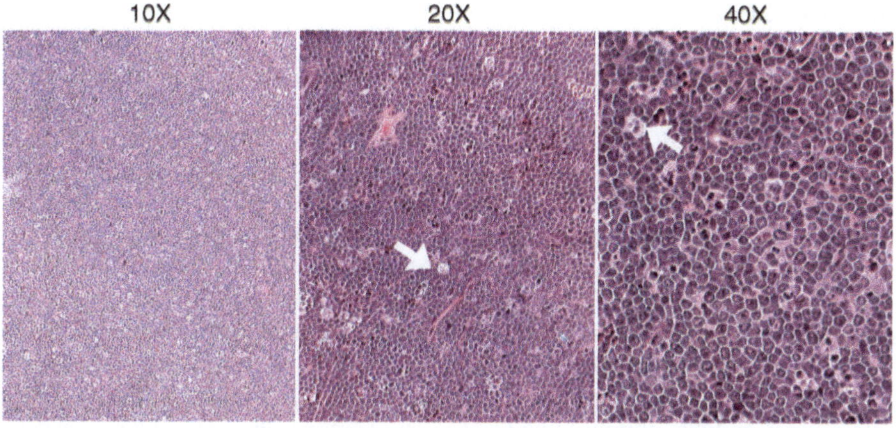

Fig. 15.1 Hematoxylin and eosin (H&E) stained section of tumoral lymph node of a λ-MYC transgenic mouse. A monotonous population of medium-sized tumoral lymphoid cells with high proliferative activity and apoptotic activity is observed. The tumor cells are monomorphic with round nuclei, multiple nucleoli, and basophilic cytoplasm. The "starry sky" appearance seen under low power is due to scattered tingible body-laden macrophages ingesting debris of apoptotic tumor cells (*white arrow*)

onset between 1 and 7 months, succumbing to mostly cervical lymph node tumors at 17 weeks of age, on average [64–66]. Histologic analysis of Igλ-MYC mice presenting with lymphadenopathy showed the loss of normal architecture with a dense infiltrate of monomorphic lymphocytes with many mitotic figures. Large numbers of metallophilic macrophages imparted a "starry sky" appearance to tumor tissues composed of nearly 100% B cells, similar to human BL. The tumor immunophenotype was also similar to human BL in that tumor cells expressed IgM, B220, CD19, and CD43, and were negative for CD5, CD23, CD38, and T cell markers. Tumor cells had rearranged *IgL* genes and were monoclonal, having developed from an initial polyclonal population of B cells. Tumor cells were immature and had not been selected by antigen, as identified by non-mutated V regions. Later studies indicated a variable expression of sIgM on tumor cells of Igλ-MYC mice, with ~60% $sIgM^+$ [67], indicating that lymphomagenesis in Igλ-MYC mice requires cooperation from other genetic lesions rather than altered BCR signaling (as discussed later in the MYC-BCR model). In a similar manner to E*μ-myc* tumors, 60% of Igλ-MYC tumors were found to contain p53 mutations [65].

The Igλ-MYC model was the first murine model to demonstrate "starry sky" tumor histology, similar to that seen in human BL (Fig. 15.1). One consideration with the Igλ-MYC model and the Eμ-Myc model is the multiplicity of transgene copies per cell, as it is well known that increasing the gene dosage of oncogenes can ameliorate and accelerate tumor development in a linear fashion. A second consideration is that these translocations reproduce only one element of BL; either the *IgH* Eμ translocation or the more rare *IgL* translocation.

Myc-YAC Mice

A concern arising with the use of transgenic mice relying on heterologous enhancer regions is that translocations of Myc into the region of a known Ig enhancer have seldom been reported, and the position of the breakpoint in the predominant t(8;14) translocation can vary. In addition, the types of BL generated in transgenic models can vary phenotypically, which may be a function of the mouse strain or the transgene construct. This variance of immature and mature B-cell tumors can, however, be relevant in BL, as sporadic BL demonstrates a more mature follicular B-cell phenotype, whereas endemic BL demonstrates an immature center cell phenotype. To identify possible oncogene activation signals driving Myc expression in BL, a 220 kb region of the human *IgH* locus containing V, D, J, and C (μ and δ) was cloned head to tail with a human *MYC* fragment isolated from the BL cell line Raji into a yeast artificial chromosome (YAC). To overcome the issues with transgene dosage, single copy clones were injected into BALB/c blastocysts to generate chimeric mice, termed Myc-YAC mice. Tumor incidence was 100% in Myc-YAC mice, with an onset at 6 weeks of age [63]. Splenomegaly was observed, although tumor masses were generally detected in non-lymphoid regions, such as the skull, the abdomen, and the chest. The location of tumors in the Myc-YAC model is reminiscent of BL detection at extranodal sites in humans, including the jaw, abdomen, or central nervous system [2]. Tumor cells were generally pre-B-cell lymphomas with a phenotype of $B220^+CD19^+IgM^+IgD^+CD43^{+/-}$ [68]. Tumor cells were clonal and had rearranged $V_H(D)J_H$, but had not hypermutated V_H, suggesting an early origin of the malignant cells. Tumors in this model therefore may represent BL in the leukemic phase of the disease. The Myc-YAC model was the first to give insight that the regulation of translocated oncogenes may occur through Ig-specific enhancers located in the core region of the *IgH* locus. Concerns with the Myc-YAC approach include the absence of the Eα enhancer, the unusual location of *MYC* in the *IgH* locus, and the head-to-tail orientation of *MYC* to *IgH*, which is not observed in human BL or mouse plasmacytomas.

iMyc$^{E\mu}$ Mice

In attempting to reproduce the t(8:14) translocation in human BL and the t(12;15) translocation in mouse plasmacytoma in vivo while using the minimum 3′ enhancer region, Park et al. [69] constructed an intronless murine *MYC* cDNA containing the orientation of *MYC* and *IgH* observed in these two malignancies, which was inserted downstream of J_H. An advantage in using the endogenous *MYC* gene is the ability to study promoter shift and cytogenetic alterations involved in tumorigenesis. iMyc$^{E\mu}$ mice developed IgM^+ BL-like lymphoblastic B-cell lymphomas, BCL-6$^+$ diffuse large B-cell lymphomas (DLBCLs), and CD138$^+$ plasmacytomas with onset at 6 months of age and an overall incidence of 68% by 21 months. The BL-like tumor demonstrated "starry sky" histology with a phenotype of $IgM^+IgD^+B220^+CD19^+CD5^-$. The tumor cells were clonal, but did not demonstrate significant levels of mutated V_H

sequences, suggesting an immature cell of origin. Interestingly, the Myc transcript exhibited the P2 to P1 promoter shift exhibited in human BL. The point mutations in the *MYC* transactivation domain that are observed in 60% of human BL [70] were not identified in this model. Similar to other Myc mouse models, alterations in the p53-ARF-MDM2 axis were observed in ~50% of the BL-like tumors arising in this model. Genomic instability was present in all BL-like tumors analyzed, with translocations, deletions, and tetraploidization seen. A consideration with the iMyc$^{E\mu}$ model is the long latency period observed in tumor development, which may be a result of the knocked-in allele inhibiting J_H rearrangements. As a result, a concern with this model is that the transgene may have been inserted into heterochromatin, possibly explaining the transgene expression at a lower level than other Myc models.

IgH-3′E-myc Mice

The recognition that the 3′ locus control region (LCR) downstream of the *IgH* locus is active in human BL cells provided a rationale for developing a mouse model expressing Myc under the control of the 3′ LCR. The 3′ LCR contains four B-cell-specific transcriptional enhancers that are active over a long range during class-switch recombination and terminal B-cell differentiation [71, 72]. To test whether the 3′ LCR played a role in BL, Wang and Boxer designed a truncated 3′ enhancer cassette by insertional targeting into the 5′ region of the murine c-*MYC* locus [73]. Healthy IgH-3′E-myc mice had a higher frequency of B220$^+$CD19$^+$ B cells in the spleen, and an increase in a B220$^+$IgM$^+$IgD^{low} population. However, the frequency of pro-B cells was not perturbed as in other Myc models. Premalignant B cells of IgH-3′E-myc demonstrated a growth advantage in vitro as shown by enhanced proliferation, cell cycle progression, and apoptosis. Lymphadenopathy and splenomegaly were observed in mice from 10 to 12 months of age, and mean age at death was 379 days for heterozygotes and 314 days for homozygotes. Tumor histology in IgH-3′E-myc demonstrated a "starry sky" appearance with medium-sized cells with basophilic cytoplasm and round nuclei, and infiltration in lung, kidney, and intestine was also observed. Most tumor cells displayed a mature B-cell phenotype of IgM$^+$CD19$^+$B220$^+$CD23$^-$CD34$^-$. Alterations in apoptotic pathways were also observed in tumors from IgH-3′E-myc mice, with an increase in BCL-X_L, BCL-2, and MDM2 protein, or stabilization of p53. In addition, the P2 to P1 Myc promoter shift was observed in tumor cells. The long latent period for lymphoma onset may be indicative of poor Myc expression due to the knock-in disrupting upstream or downstream regulatory elements of Myc [74, 75]. However, the IgH-3′E-myc model was instrumental in indicating the importance of the 3′ LCR of the *IgH* locus in the modulation of Myc expression in BL.

c-*myc*-3′ LCR Mice

The previous Myc models of BL discussed herein describe the use of different schemes to mimic BL in the mouse, which resulted in the identification of the minimal *IgH* locus elements necessary to elicit Myc overexpression. In fact, this region has been identified as being active in human BL and is always conserved on the c-*MYC*-translocated chromosome in all forms of BL, unlike other *IgH*-derived regions previously used as transgenes [72]. To avoid the long latencies observed with IgH-3′E-myc mice, Truffinet et al. [76] generated mice harboring a single copy of a c-*myc*-3′ IgH LCR transgene. In young transgenic mice, B-cell maturation was normal, although immunoglobulin production was impaired. Disease onset manifesting as lymphadenopathy occurred at 12 weeks, and overall tumor incidence was 80% at 34 weeks of age, with a mean mortality at 23 weeks of age. The majority of tumors developing in c-myc-3′ mice were aggressive Burkitt's-like lymphoblastic B-cell lymphomas, although diffuse anaplastic plasmacytomas ($B220^{-}IgM^{low}CD138^{-}$) were observed with longer latency periods. Histology of the Burkitt's-like tumor demonstrated a "starry sky" appearance, and tumor cells displayed a mature B-cell phenotype of $B220^{+}IgM^{+}IgD^{+}CD43^{-}CD138^{-}$. Tumor cells were clonal in origin, and V_H sequencing indicated that no hypermutation had occurred, but by contrast, AID was expressed and had promoted hypermutation of sequences upstream of c-Myc due to inclusion of the 3′ *IgH* region. These mutations may have had a deleterious effect on the ability of negative regulators of c-Myc to bind, resulting in the higher protein levels of c-Myc detectable in the tumor cells [77].

Currently, these c-myc-3′ "minilocus" mice are the closest reproduction to BL in the mouse, as they contain the key features of human BL; tumors displaying a mature phenotype driven by B-cell lineage-specific Myc deregulation promoted by the 3′ LCR of *IgH*. In addition, the generation of mature B-cell lymphomas in these mice compared to previous models may be explained by the recent finding that the 3′ *IgH* regulatory region is required for peripheral B-cell lymphomas, such as BL, with translocations associated with class-switch recombination, such as the *MYC* translocation [78]. The importance of the *IgH* regulatory region has been tested as a therapeutic strategy in Myc-overexpressing tumors in vivo, and is discussed later.

MYC-BCR^{HEL} Transgenic Mice

Many B-cell lymphomas (BCLs), including BL, express a BCR such as IgM on the cell surface. Forty years ago, it was proposed that antigen stimulation may contribute to the generation of B-cell lymphomas, and since then, several lines of evidence have supported this hypothesis [79–81]. In some BCLs, the BCR has been selected by antigen, or may bind a known pathogen, such as a viral antigen, or an autoantigen in the context of autoimmunity [82, 83]. To explore whether constitutive or antigen-activated BCR stimulation cooperated with *MYC* in the genesis of BL, Refaeli et al. [84] used E*μ*-*myc* mice and MMTV-rtTA/TRE-*MYC* mice. In the latter, the *MYC* transgene is expressed in the B-cell lineage and is controlled by a tetracycline responsive element, such that expression can be repressed by administration of tetracycline or doxycycline [62]. These Myc transgenic mice were crossed to mice expressing a transgenic mature BCR specific for the model antigen hen egg lysozyme (HEL), and crossed to mice that expressed soluble HEL (sHEL) to provide an antigenic stimulus.

Tumors composed of mature, naïve B cells generated from a limited number of clones arose in Eμ-*MYC*/BCR^{HEL} and MMTV-rtTA/TRE-*MYC*/BCR^{HEL} mice around 18 weeks of age. The acceleration in latency from E*μ-myc* tumors in the absence of soluble HEL, with onset at 22 weeks, was attributed to the transgenic mature BCR being expressed from an early age, as has been observed in other ligand-independent BCR models [85]. E*μ-myc*/BCR^{HEL} tumors were similar to human B-cell chronic lymphocytic leukemia (B-CLL) in that tumor histology showed an absence of "starry sky" morphology with a surface phenotype of B220$^+$CD19$^+$IgM$^+$CD21$^+$PNA$^-$CD5$^-$.

The greatest acceleration of tumorigenesis was observed when the BCR was constitutively stimulated by antigen in the context of overexpressed MYC. All E*μ-myc*/BCR^{HEL}/sHEL and MMTV-rtTA/TRE-*myc*/BCR^{HEL}/sHEL mice developed aggressive tumors with a "starry sky" appearance, with large, activated B220$^+$CD19$^+$IgM$^+$CD21$^+$PNA$^+$CD5$^-$ lymphocytes with clumped chromatin. However, tumors in E*μ-myc*/BCR^{HEL}/sHEL and MMTV-rtTA/TRE-*myc*/BCR^{HEL}/sHEL differed in the rate of appearance and anatomical presentation, with the former arising in the lymph nodes and spleen at 7 weeks of age on average, and the latter arising as unilateral jaw tumors at 10 weeks of age, with later spread to most organs. Multiclonality was observed, suggesting that several clones were selected in which additional tumorigenic events had occurred.

The studies with MYC-BCR transgenic models have provided a role for both antigen stimulation and *MYC* overexpression in the establishment and maintenance of B-cell lymphomas. These animals have also shown potential in studies for potential treatment options targeting Myc-overexpressing tumors. Firstly, the inhibition of *MYC* expression by doxycycline administration decreased the tumor burden in MMTV-rtTA/TRE-*myc*/BCR^{HEL}/sHEL mice, and secondly, the administration of shRNA to components of the BCR in E*μ-myc*/BCR^{HEL} and E*μ-myc*/BCR^{HEL}/sHEL tumor cell lines resulted in an acute competitive disadvantage when tumor cells were transferred in to Rag1$^{-/-}$ mice.

Other MYC Transgenic Models

N-Myc, a cellular homolog of c-Myc, can substitute for c-Myc in certain cellular functions as shown by targeted gene replacement experiments. N-Myc is required during neurogenesis and is amplified in neuroblastoma. Despite the lack of N-myc deregulation in BL, the finding that N-myc may regulate c-Myc provided a rationale to assess the formation of lymphomas in N-myc transgenic mice. B-cell lymphomas developed in mice transgenic for N-Myc under the control of the *IgH* enhancer Eμ and either the N-Myc, SV40, or Ig V_H promoter (Eμ-N-Myc mice) [86]. Here, onset occurred as early as 10 weeks of age and tumors developed by 13–18 weeks on average in the lineage with the highest expression of the Eμ-N-Myc transgene. Most tumors were clonal and had rearranged *IgM* genes, with a minority also rearranging *Igκ* giving the tumors a pre-B and immature B-cell phenotype. Interestingly, c-Myc was never upregulated in tumors and was nearly undetectable, suggesting that N-Myc may negatively regulate c-Myc.

The function of *MYC* point mutations described in human BL has also been studied in mice. Retroviral vectors carrying the wild-type *MYC* gene, or the P57S and T58A point mutations, were used to infect hematopoietic stem cells, which were then reconstituted into immunodeficient host mice [87]. P57S and T58A were shown to accelerate lymphomagenesis compared to wild-type *MYC* and were able to uncouple apoptosis from proliferation by failing to induce the pro-apoptotic protein Bim. Studies with these mice may be particularly important for the understanding of Burkitt's lymphoma development, in the context of mutated Myc.

Models of EBV-Associated BL

The association of EBV latency with BL has provided a rationale for exploration of the role of the virus in lymphomagenesis. As EBV does not infect mice, and MHV68 encodes non-homologous latency proteins, crossing mice transgenic for an EBV protein with a Myc model to study the involvement of EBV proteins in Myc tumorigenesis has proved valuable in both understanding the mechanisms of EBV-induced lymphomagenesis and the similarities and differences between latent protein function in humans and in mice.

EμEBNA1 Mice

EBV latent infection involves host cell immortalization, and a number of EBV proteins have been hypothesized to be critical to this function. The viral protein EBNA1, which tethers the viral genome to chromatin, is consistently expressed in BL. EBNA1 may contribute to pathogenesis by inducing chromosomal instability through induction of reactive oxygen species, leading to activated telomerase and chromosomal translocations such as that of MYC [88–90]. In addition, EBNA1 can induce Rag1 and Rag2 expression, which may further help facilitate the *Ig-MYC* translocation [91, 92].

EBNA1 may also play a role in inducing aberrant proliferation in BL. The first example of EBNA1 directly affecting cell proliferation came with the generation of C57BL/6 mice transgenic for expression of EBNA1 under the control of the polyomavirus promoter and the *IgH* enhancer region Eμ (EμEBNA-1 mice) [93]. The expression of EBNA1 in two EμEBNA-1 lineages with varying EBNA1 expression causes B-cell lymphomas with associated leukemias, with onset at 2 months of age and mortality between 4 and 12 months. The lymphoma phenotype bears resemblance to the E*μ-myc* tumors and was also representative of B cells at different stages of development [55]. Bone marrow lymphocytes from the EμEBNA-1 mice were shown to have a higher rate of proliferation and survival ex vivo as a result of upregulating BCL-X_L and MDM2 [94]. Interestingly, trisomy of chromosome 15 leading to Myc overexpression was observed in EμEBNA-1 tumors, suggesting a cooperative role for Myc and EBNA1 in lymphomagenesis [95].

When crossed with E*μ-myc* mice, EBNA1 did not significantly increase Myc-driven lymphomagenesis from 63 days on average [95]. However, when crossed with Eμ-N-Myc mice which have a longer latency of ~310 days, Eμ-N-Myc/EBNA1 mice developed tumors significantly faster, at ~94 days [86, 95]. In these models, the levels of EBNA1 were stable in the absence or presence of c-Myc or N-Myc, indicating that EBNA1 did not act as an oncogene by upregulation, but instead cooperated with Myc to accelerate lymphomagenesis. Based on the findings that Eμ-EBNA1 transgenic tumors express increased BCL-X_L and MDM2 protein levels, the upregulation of these anti-apoptotic proteins by EBNA1 is a likely mechanism contributing to tumorigenesis in this model [94].

However, later studies indicated that the contribution of EBNA1 to lymphomagenesis in animal models may be strain-specific, as Kang et al. [96] developed three lineages where EBNA1 was expressed in B cells of Friend leukemia virus B (FVB) mice, and observed no acceleration in tumor development over non-transgenic mice. The variation in EBNA1-induced tumor development suggests that EBNA1 may induce as-yet unrecognized strain-specific target genes to cooperate in tumorigenesis. As previously discussed, EBNA1 also induces chromosomal instability by inducing reactive oxygen species [88–90]. Since EBV has been detected at a high frequency along with the 1q chromosomal translocation in BL [97], EBNA1 transgenic mice on the C57BL/6 background may be useful for studies of EBV-induced chromosomal aberrations contributing to lymphoma development.

LMP2A/λ-MYC Mice

The EBV-encoded gene product LMP2A is expressed in B cells during latent infection and is one of the few EBV gene products consistently detected in primary BL biopsies [29, 98–100]. The presence of LMP2A in all forms of latency, as well as in disease, emphasizes the importance of LMP2A expression in both latency and latency-associated malignancies. LMP2A functions as a B-cell receptor (BCR) mimic by constitutively associating with Lyn and Syk kinases through an immunoreceptor tyrosine-based activation motif (ITAM) [101–104]. LMP2A protects human and murine B cells from apoptosis by activating the Ras/Akt pathway and upregulating anti-apoptotic molecules, including BCL-2 and BCL-X_L through NF-κB [105–108].

Although LMP2A transgenic mice do not develop lymphoma, they display altered B-cell signaling and development, such that in the absence of a functional BCR, LMP2A signaling allows B cells to survive. These features taken together with findings with a Myc model where the BCR was constitutively active indicate a contributing role for BCR engagement in the development of BL [84]. The presence of LMP2A in EBV-positive BL along with the Myc translocation may therefore constitute a molecular mechanism underlying BL development, and has provided rationale for the development of a murine model of LMP2A-positive BL to study the role of LMP2A in lymphomagenesis.

LMP2A mice were crossed with Igλ-MYC mice to generate LMP2A/λ-MYC double transgenic mice, which demonstrated splenomegaly from an early age, with absence of normal lymphoid architecture [65, 66]. LMP2A/λ-MYC pretumor spleens contain a fivefold increase in B220⁺ B cells, which are mostly in the cell cycle and more resistant to apoptosis compared to Myc B cells. LMP2A/λ-MYC mice present with accelerated lymphadenopathy and splenomegaly and develop detectable lymphoma around 6–8 weeks of age, whereas the Igλ-MYC mice typically take 15–20 weeks to develop lymphoma. LMP2A/λ-MYC tumors show a "starry sky" morphology and tumor B cells are $IgM^{-}CD43^{+}$, indicating a pro-B/pre-B-cell origin.

Tumor development in LMP2A/λ-MYC mice is dissimilar from known mechanisms of Myc tumorigenesis, as p53 pathway alterations are not observed, and the pro-apoptotic protein BIM is induced in LMP2A/λ-MYC tumor cells. One explanation for the acceleration in LMP2A-expressing tumors is the high expression of the survival protein BCL-X_L as compared to Igλ-MYC tumors alone, which is consistent with the detection of elevated BCL-X_L expression in LMP2A-expressing B cells [106]. The LMP2A/λ-MYC BL model is the first example of an EBV protein not known to be oncogenic cooperating with Myc. This model can be used to study the role of LMP2A in Myc-induced Burkitt's-like lymphoma development and has been used to design therapeutic regimens targeting LMP2A-altered cellular pathways [109, 110].

LMP1/λ-MYC Mice

LMP1 is detected in a number of B-cell malignancies and is essential for B-cell immortalization in vitro [111–114]. LMP1 is a transmembrane protein with C-terminal signal domains that mimics signaling of the TNF receptor family member CD40 to constitutively activate JNK, p38 and IRF7 as well as the canonical and non-canonical NF-κB pathways, leading to the activation and proliferation of the B cell [115–122]. While LMP1 has been shown to upregulate Myc expression in cultured B cells, the requirement for cell proliferation on LMP1 expression can be overcome by expressing Myc [123, 124]. This observation may explain the absence of LMP1 detection in endemic BL, with a potential model being that the immune system may target LMP1-expressing cells for destruction, and only those cells that have undergone the *MYC* translocation are able to survive the loss of LMP1 [29, 99, 123, 125, 126]. However, LMP1 has been detected in a handful of AIDS-associated EBV-positive BL biopsies, suggesting that the immunosuppression associated with HIV infection may allow LMP1-expressing cells to survive [127]. In addition, one study showed that a small handful of sporadic BL biopsies were LMP1 positive [128], and another that a number of endemic BL biopsies were LMP1 positive [100]. LMP1 may therefore play a role in early proliferative stages of BL development.

The contribution of LMP1 to B-cell tumorigenesis in vivo has been studied in mice. Kulwichit et al. [118] generated several lineages of LMP1 BALB/c transgenic mice, with the coding region of LMP1 under the control of the mouse IgH enhancer Eμ and a V_H promoter. LMP1 transgenic mice developed B-cell lymphoma, with varying incidence among lineages, with up to 42% of mice presenting with tumors between 12 and 18 months, to 52% of mice over 18 months presenting with tumors. Histology of LMP1-expressing tumors revealed B-cell follicular lymphomas (FL) ($B220^{+}IgG^{+}CD3^{-}$) in enlarged spleen with dissemination to liver, lungs, or cervical lymph nodes. LMP1 lymphomas displayed evidence of clonal J_H rearrangements, which correlated with the expression of LMP1. Antiapoptotic and growth pathways were also activated in LMP1 tumors, with overexpression of BCL-2, A20, and c-Myc, as is common with most human FL. Later work indicated that pre-tumor LMP1-expressing B cells from transgenic mice are phenotypically normal, but are hyperproliferative in response to stimuli, suggesting a role for antigen stimulation contributing to LMP1-driven tumors [129].

Mating LMP1 mice with Igλ-MYC mice generated a greatly accelerated tumor phenotype, resulting in tumor onset between 4 and 9 weeks of age. Tumors initially presented as an enlarged spleen two- to fivefold larger than LMP1 or Myc transgenic spleen, with dissemination to cervical and mesenteric lymph nodes. Tumor cells were of B-cell origin with an immature surface phenotype of $B220^{+}CD19^{+}IgM^{-}IgD^{-}GL7^{+}CD23^{-}CD43^{+}$ (A. Vrazo, unpublished observations). LMP1/Igλ-MYC mice may be useful in evaluating the cooperation of these pathways in the early stages of BL development, and in non-BL-like lymphomas, such as AIDS-associated non-Hodgkin's lymphomas, which frequently express both c-Myc and LMP1.

Eμ-EBER1/E*μ-myc* Mice

EBV expresses two small non-coding RNAs, the EBV-encoded RNAs (EBERs), which are highly conserved among primate homologues of EBV. EBER1 and EBER2 are 166- and 172-nucleotide single-stranded RNAs, respectively, and are the most abundant RNA species in most EBV-infected cells and disease conditions. While their function and mechanism of action is unclear, there is evidence for EBERs in inducing the expression of cytokines such as IL-10, which can enhance B-cell growth [130]. EBER1 is detected in primary BL biopsies as well as BL and lymphoblastoid cell lines, which provides rationale for assessment of the contribution of EBER1 to lymphomagenesis [131, 132]. A murine model expressing EBER1 under the immunoglobulin heavy chain intronic enhancer Eμ (Eμ-EBER1) was recently developed which indicated that EBER1 is tumorigenic in vivo albeit with a long latency period [133]. The Eμ-EBER1 model is the first demonstration that a non-coding viral gene has oncogenic potential. Young Eμ-EBER1 mice have normal $B220^{+}$ B-cell numbers, but EBER1 eventually promotes lymphoid hyperplasia and lymphomagenesis, which presents as initial splenomegaly with mesenteric lymph node involvement. Tumor incidence was 58% in the highest EBER1-expressing line of mice by 2 years of age, and tumors were $B220^{+}$ B-cell lymphomas with clonal *IgH* rearrangements, or histiocytic sarcomas. Intriguingly, c-Myc was upregulated in several Eμ-EBER1 tumors, and activation of Myc target DNA sequences was also observed, suggesting that EBER1 may function in BL tumorigenesis by cooperating with c-Myc.

Based on the findings that the EBER1 promoter contains a Myc binding site that may indicate the upregulation of EBER by c-Myc [134], Eμ-EBER1 mice were crossed with E*μ-myc* mice [133]. No acceleration of onset was observed, and tumors that arose in Eμ-EBER1/E*μ-myc* mice were phenotypically similar to E*μ-myc* tumors, with extensive lymph node involvement. In sum, the Eμ-EBER1 model will be useful for studying the biology of EBER1 and the potential cross-regulation between EBER1 and Myc.

Therapeutic Models

Modeling cancers such as Burkitt's lymphoma in the mouse has been an effective system to examine the etiology of cancer in vivo. As such, mouse models of cancer represent valuable tools to examine the effectiveness of new therapeutics. To evaluate the effectiveness of therapeutics targeted to gene products altered in BL or their pathways, such as Myc or EBV LMP2A, immunocompetent transgenic models have been used. For assessment of therapeutics against xenografts derived from human BL cell lines, immunodeficient mice are primarily used, as they are unable to reject the xenograft. Recently, advances in humanized immunodeficient mice have resulted in mice engrafted with human hematopoietic systems, which can be infected with EBV, permitting extensive analysis of lymphoma development and progression. Given that mice have been historically refractive to EBV infection, the advent of humanized mice is a large step in understanding the biology of EBV and the mechanisms associated with BL tumorigenesis in an animal model.

Immunocompetent Mouse Models

Many immunocompetent mouse models of BL, including the transgenic mice discussed above, have been used to study the effectiveness of preclinical therapies, including conditional oncogene inactivation, small drug molecules, and immunotherapeutic agents. Based on the observation that Myc-driven tumors often become resistant to chemotherapeutics because of acquisition of mutations that impair BCL-2-regulated apoptosis, small molecule antagonists of BCL-2 have been tested in Myc models. The small molecule ABT-737 mimics BH3-only proteins, which are antagonists of the pro-survival BCL-2 family. ABT-737 was extremely effective with low-dose cyclophosphamide against lymphomas transplanted into C57BL/6 recipients derived from E*μ-myc* or E*μ-myc*/*bcl-2* mice [135]. Tumor regression in this model demonstrated that ABT-737 could be useful in human BL that overexpresses BCL-2 family proteins.

The inhibition of pathways constitutively activated by EBV gene products that cooperate with Myc in lymphomagenesis has also been demonstrated using small molecule inhibitors. A small molecule inhibitor of the mammalian target of rapamycin (mTOR), aberrantly activated by LMP2A, increased tumor regression in LMP2A/Myc tumors compared to Myc tumors, identifying a potential therapeutic for LMP2A-expressing BL [110]. Similarly, LMP2A-induced Lyn activation was effectively inhibited by dasatinib in the LMP2A/Myc model. These findings suggest that small molecule inhibitors could be effectively used in EBV-associated BL to specifically target pathways activated by LMP2A [136].

The ability to conditionally induce or repress expression of a single oncoprotein such as Myc could be a specific and effective therapy for human BL. The tetracycline regulatory system has been used to generate mice conditionally expressing human Myc in hematopoietic cells, which developed T-cell lymphomas and acute myeloid leukemias [62]. Targeted inactivation of the *MYC* transgene by administration of doxycycline to repress the *Tet* element resulted in extensive differentiation, proliferative arrest, and regression of tumors. Whether the induced regression of Myc could lead to epigenetic changes that may revoke the ability of Myc to maintain tumorigenesis is unclear. The ability to repress a single oncogene to bring about tumor regression suggests that with some modification to the transgene construct, similar results could be observed in a B-cell-specific murine model of BL.

Immunodeficient and Humanized Mouse Models

The advent of immunodeficient murine models lacking components of the humoral and cellular immune systems has been critical in permitting the study of allogeneic and xenogeneic tumor transplants. Studies of effectiveness of candidate therapeutic agents have been extensively carried out, and a prospective benefit of these mice may be in the development of a rapid treatment protocol for individual patients. More recently, an increasing need for in vivo studies of human cells, tissues, and organs without putting patients at risk has led to the development of humanized mice on existing immunodeficient backgrounds. Humanized mice, defined as mice engrafted with human tissues, hematopoietic stem cells (HSCs), or peripheral blood mononuclear cells (PBMCs), allow researchers to examine in vivo biological processes, including the safety and effectiveness of candidate therapeutic agents and vaccines. The development of humanized mice engrafted with human B cells has greatly aided with models of EBV infection, as murine B cells are not susceptible to EBV infection. In the context of BL, both immunodeficient and humanized models have been used to study BL-specific therapeutics.

Severe combined immunodeficiency (SCID) mice and their derivative strains result from a loss of function mutation in the protein kinase, DNA activated, catalytic polypeptide (*Prkdc*) gene [137]. Prkdc functions in double strand break repair during V(D)J recombination, thus loss of Prkdc function ablates B- and T-cell maturation. By subcutaneously transplanting human tumor cells into SCID mice as xenografts, researchers can characterize the biology, aggressiveness, and metastatic nature of a tumor in vivo. In one report, newly identified BL cell lines were engrafted in SCID mice in this manner, and demonstrated a high level of metastasis to spleen, bone marrow, and ovaries [138].

Tumor regression following administration of therapeutics has been extensively studied with SCID mice. To selectively target Myc under the control of the Eμ enhancer, a peptide nucleic acid to Eμ (PNAEμWT) was administered to SCID mice engrafted with the BRG and Ramos BL cell lines [139]. PNAEμWT was able to block expression of c-Myc in tumors arising from the BRG cell line, which expresses Myc under the control of the Eμ enhancer. By also demonstrating that this PNA construct was nontoxic with an extended half-life in vivo, this therapeutic model provided evidence that PNA administration may be tractable in human patients.

Recombinant monoclonal antibodies have also been effective in SCID models of BL to specifically target cells expressing BL markers, such as CD74 and CD52. Lapalombella et al. [140] used alemtuzumab, a monoclonal antibody against CD52, to enhance complement-mediated cytotoxicity against $CD52^{+}$ Raji xenografts in SCID mice and to delineate the mechanism of alemtuzumab action. Chang et al. [141] used an immunotoxin, an anti-CD74 antibody coupled to a cytotoxic ribonuclease from frog oocytes, such that initial anti-CD74 binding and internalization by BL cells would result in targeted cell death. The modified antibody was nontoxic, had good bioavailability, and led to survival in SCID mice engrafted with the human $CD74^{+}$ BL cell lines Raji and Daudi.

SCID mice have been used in EBV-specific BL therapies. For example, the proteasome inhibitor bortezomib activates lytic EBV gene expression and induces apoptosis of EBV-expressing cells [142]. Bortezomib treatment prolonged the survival of SCID mice inoculated with LCLs [143], and when used as a pretreatment, enhanced the sensitivity of the EBV-positive Rael BL cell line to radiation therapy in SCID mice [144]. Humanized SCID mice, engrafted with human peripheral blood lymphocytes (hu-PBL-SCID), have provided a valuable model to study EBV-associated neoplasia. Humanized mice also allow EBV researchers to examine the role of different forms of viral infection in the context of pressure exerted by a functioning human immune system. This is advantageous as many viral and host factors likely control whether EBV-infected cells proliferate into lymphomas, and the comparative contributions of each factor are, for the most part, unknown. The initial description of hu-PBL-SCID mice came in 1990, when EBV-seronegative or seropositive PBLs were transferred into SCID mice, which were later infected with EBV [145, 146]. The mice developed oligo- or polyclonal $CD19^{+}CD23^{low}CD10^{-}CD20^{+}$ B-cell lymphomas, expressing LMP1, EBNA1, and EBNA2 [147, 148]. However, low levels of human cell engraftment in SCID mice due to enhanced NK cell activity and generation of B- and T-cells during aging (known as "leakiness") drove researchers to develop improved immunodeficient models.

SCID mice were crossed with non-obese diabetic (NOD) mice to generate NOD-SCID mice, which had lower levels of NK cell activity, and as such could support higher levels of engraftment with human tissues. Islas-Ohlmayer et al. [149] used NOD-SCID mice to engraft human $CD34^{+}$ hematopoietic stem cells in order to provide a complete humanized microenvironment in which to study the outcome of EBV infection. Engrafted mice were successfully infected with EBV strain B95-8, and developed $CD19^{+}CD20^{+}CD30^{+}$ large cell immunoblastic lymphomas in the spleen at 5 weeks postinfection. Tumor cells in this model expressed EBV proteins in a type II latency program (EBNA1, LMP1, and LMP2A).

A breakthrough came in 2005 with the development of a highly immunodeficient, non-leaky strain based on the combination of the *Prkdc*^{scid} mutation, the NOD/ShiLtJ background, and the knockout of the IL2 receptor gamma chain locus (*Il2rg*) [150]. The NOD/SCID/gamma (NSG) strain lack mature B, T, and NK cells as the *Il2rg* gene encodes the common cytokine receptor chain used during B, T, and NK development and function. As such, the NSG strain can be injected with primary BL isolates or BL cell lines to assess the effectiveness of targeting dysregulated pathways with therapeutics.

NSG mice are improved over previously described strains used for humanized models, with high levels of engraftment of human HSCs and PBMCs. NSG mice have been recently used to improve the engraftment of human tissues to study EBV-induced lymphoproliferative diseases. Yajima et al. [151] infected NSG mice reconstituted with CD34$^+$ hematopoietic cells with two different titers of EBV, and observed lymphoproliferative disease in the high-titer group with a latency III profile (EBNA1, 2, LMP1, 2A, 2B, and EBER were expressed), and asymptomatic persistent infection in the low-titer group. Antiviral antibodies and antiviral CD8$^+$ T-cell responses were also generated in this model, despite lower levels of T-cell action common to NSG mice.

A shortcoming of the NSG model in the context of EBV infection is that human T cells mature on mouse thymus, which may result in nonoptimal T-cell selection and dampening of T-cell responses to infection. To address this, NSG mice can be sublethally irradiated, and human fetal liver and thymus can be implanted under the renal capsule of NSG mice, followed by an intravenous injection of CD34$^+$ hematopoietic cells from the same fetal liver source. These mice mount HLA class-II-restricted T-cell responses to EBV infection [152]. Contrary to results seen in previous humanized mice lacking thymic material, EBV latency types IIa and IIb was established, instead of latency III. This observation is consistent with T-cell elimination of latency III-expressing cells. Interestingly, 55% of EBV-infected NSG mice developed CD20$^+$ DLBCL, which expressed type II EBV latent genes. Although a Burkitt's lymphoma-like tumor has yet to be observed in humanized mice, the ability to model EBV-induced neoplasia and target EBV-specific therapies without putting patients at risk will be of great use in the future.

Future Directions

The phenotype of Burkitt's lymphoma as a germinal center-derived neoplasma where chromosome translocations active during class-switch recombination permit the *MYC* translocation have prompted questions regarding the stage at which germinal center B cells become BL cells. In order to more accurately model BL in mice, Myc activation could be postponed to the germinal center by placing Myc under the control of a tetracycline-responsive element and a germinal center-specific promoter, for example. To model EBV-associated BL, inducible *MYC* transgenes could be combined with EBNA1 or LMP2A transgenes targeted to B cells.

With the aim of understanding the pathways involved in lymphoma development and the role of EBV infection, whole genome sequencing including transcriptome or exome could be used to study the genome expression profile of tumor cells. In a similar manner to recent advances with gene expression profiling identifying subtypes of tumors that respond differently to therapeutic strategies, the use of whole genome sequencing could identify novel biomarkers as drug targets in murine BL models. These gene expression profiles could then be validated in human BL [153–156].

The ability to alter the species tropism of EBV to infect murine B cells would be valuable, as it would bypass the need for immunodeficient mice. The human CD21 (hCD21) molecule, which is expressed preferentially on human B lymphocytes, is the receptor for EBV adsorption before viral fusion and entry [157]. Introduction of the hCD21 gene has made canine and rat cells susceptible to EBV infection and stably EBV-infected cell clones could be isolated from these non-primate cells [158]. Those results prompted the authors to generate a transgenic rat expressing the hCD21 gene, which could become an animal model for EBV infection [159]. Unfortunately, splenic B cells expressing hCD21 were susceptible to EBV infection, but unlike human B lymphocytes, EBV infection was abortive and was not followed by blastogenesis, cellular DNA synthesis, or proliferation. The efficiency of EBV infection was very low compared to human infection because of the absence of HLA Class II expression, known to be necessary for EBV entry into the cell after adsorption [160, 161]. Murine cell lines are also typically resistant to infection by EBV. Expression of the two human B-cell receptors for EBV (hCD21 and HLA-DR) on the surface of murine B cells allowed efficient viral entry that led to the establishment of latent EBV infection and long-term persistence of the viral genome [162]. Latent gene expression in these cells resembled the latency II program in that EBNA1 and LMP1 were detected whereas EBNA2 and the EBNA3s were not expressed. Transgenic mice bearing hCD21 and HLA-DR could therefore offer a novel system to study aspects of EBV infection and disease that have previously been difficult to investigate due to the species tropism of EBV.

Currently, EBV-positive lymphomas arising in humanized mice do not resemble BL, but one potential strategy to drive BL-like tumor development could utilize humanized strains engrafted with $CD34^+$ stem cells. These mice could be infected with a tetracycline-regulated *MYC* transgene that could be switched on later during B-cell development. Infection with EBV before or after tetracycline administration could help answer the long-standing question of whether EBV produces a cellular environment that enables the *MYC* translocation, or whether EBV maintains the survival of cells that have undergone an otherwise deleterious Myc translocation in the genesis of BL.

Conclusion

The study of Burkitt's lymphoma in humans has been traditionally hindered by the availability of tumor tissues, the inhibitory effects of therapeutics on tumor growth, and ethical concerns with human studies. Animal models have been crucial in

Table 15.1 Mouse models of Burkitt's lymphoma

Transgenic models

Strain	Enhancer	Tumor phenotype and histology	References
Eμ-*myc*; Eκ-*myc*	Eμ (IgH); Eκ (Igκ)	Pre-/pro-B lymphoma, leukemia	[55]
λ-MYC	λ (Igλ)	Pre-/pro-B lymphoma; "starry sky"; $IgM^{+/-}B220^{+}CD43^{+}CD23^{-}$	[64]
Myc-YAC	Eμ (IgH)	Pre-B-cell lymphomas; $IgM^{+}IgD^{+}B220^{+}CD43^{+/-}$	[63]
$iMyc^{E\mu}$	Eμ (IgH)	Immature B-cell lymphomas; "starry sky"; $B220^{+}IgM^{+}IgD^{+}CD5^{-}$	[69]
IgH-3′E-myc	3′ LCR (IgH)	Mature B-cell lymphomas; "starry sky"; $B220^{+}IgM^{+}CD23^{-}CD34^{-}$	[73]
c-Myc-3′ IgH	3′ LCR (IgH)	Mature B cell lymphomas; "starry sky"; $B220^{+}IgM^{+}IgD^{+}CD43^{-}$	[76]
MYC/BCR^{HEL}	Tet-o-Myc/ Eμ SRα	Mature B-cell lymphomas; "starry sky"; $B220^{+}$ $IgM^{+}CD21^{+}CD5^{-}$	[84]
Eμ–EBER1	Eμ	Lymphoid hyperplasia and B lymphoma	[133]
Eμ–Myc/ EBER1	Eμ/Eμ	Pre-/pro-B-cell lymphoma	[133]
Eμ–EBNA1	Eμ	Pre-/pro-B lymphoma with leukemia	[93]
Eμ–Myc/ EBNA1	Eμ/Eμ	Pre-/pro-B lymphoma with leukemia	[93, 95]
LMP1	Eμ	Follicular B lymphomas; $B220^{+}IgG^{+}CD3^{-}$	[118]
LMP1/Myc	Eμ/ Eμ	Accelerated pre-/pro-B lymphomas; $B220^{+}IgM^{-}CD43^{+}$	(Vrazo, unpublished observations)
LMP2A	Eμ	No lymphoma; altered BCR signaling	[163]
LMP2A/Myc	Eμ/Igλ	Accelerated pro-B lymphomas; "starry sky"; $IgM^{-}CD43^{+}$	[65, 66]

Immunodeficient and humanized models

Strain	Description	Experimental protocol	References
SCID; NOD/ SCID	*Prkdc*^{scid} mutation ablates B- and T-cell development	Allogeneic/xenogeneic tumor transplant; therapeutics; humanization; EBV infection	[164, 149]
NSG	*Prkdc*^{scid} mutation, NOD, *Il2rg* knockout ablates B, T, NK cells	Allogeneic/xenogeneic tumor transplant; therapeutics; humanization; EBV infection	[165]

overcoming these constraints to better understand the biology, growth, and treatment of BL (see Table 15.1 for a summary). Transgenic mice overexpressing Myc in B cells to model the canonical t(8;14) translocation in human BL have greatly improved our understanding of the mechanisms involved in lymphomagenesis, as well the mechanism of *MYC* regulation by elements within the 3′ locus control region of the immunoglobulin enhancer. Transgenic Myc models have also allowed the identification of additional genetic lesions occurring in BL, such as the alteration of the p53–ARF–MDM2 axis, and the overexpression of BCL-2 family proteins, which have been further validated in human BL. Double transgenic mice expressing Myc with an EBV latent protein detected in human BL have been vital in investigating the role of single EBV gene products in the modulation of cellular pathways contributing to BL development and progression in vivo. Immunocompetent transgenic mice have allowed for the study of small molecule agonists and antagonists to pathways involved in lymphomagenesis, including BCL-2 and mTOR, and the outcome of conditional ablation of Myc on tumor growth. These analyses may provide valuable cellular targets for tailored therapeutic intervention in LMP2A- or BCL-2-expressing lymphomas. When evaluating transgenic models, one should keep in mind that human BL is highly heterogeneous, so the presence of only one or two major alterations may not be the most accurate model of the disease.

Of the primate models discussed herein, the cottontop tamarin is the most tractable as a model of EBV-induced lymphoma despite the absence of a true BL phenotype. Primates that are susceptible to EBV infection may be of use for studies characterizing the EBV-specific immune response and the biology of infection. Lastly, primates infected with EBV may be useful in preclinical vaccine trials, similar to proof-of-principal studies with simian immunodeficiency virus (SIV) vaccines in rhesus macaques. Caveats precluding large-scale studies with cottontop tamarins or other primates include the extent to which these animals are endangered, and the large amounts of space and resources needed for their care.

For xenograft tumor studies, immunodeficient SCID mice and derivative strains are the model of choice as the lack of adaptive and cellular immune responses abrogates xenograft rejection. SCID-derivative mice have been used in such diverse assays as the characterization of novel BL cell lines, tumor-targeted recombinant monoclonal antibodies, Myc-specific peptides, and EBV-specific radiotherapies. The SCID model system may provide faster translational value to identify altered cellular pathways and effective therapeutic agents, and therefore may be more useful for development of a rapid treatment protocol for individual patients.

Humanized mice based on the *Prkdc*^{scid} strain have largely replaced concerns associated with primate models in that biology of EBV infection and lymphomagenesis can be modeled in the context of a functioning human immune system. Initial studies where human PBLs were injected into SCID mice followed by EBV infection have been largely superseded by studies with NOD/SCID and NSG mice, which demonstrate improved engraftment of a human hematopoietic system. In these mice, CD34$^+$ human hematopoietic stem cells can engraft, differentiate, and be infected with EBV to drive lymphoma development. The patterns of EBV latent gene product expression observed in tumors of these mice are more similar to those observed in human tumor biopsies. In summary, despite the challenges and limitations of attempting to model Burkitt's lymphoma in animal models, the potential power of these models will continue to be realized with the development of new genetic techniques that allow researchers to more accurately represent pathways deregulated in BL.

Acknowledgements The authors gratefully acknowledge the assistance of their colleagues and funding sources (National Cancer Institute and National Institute of Allergy and Infectious Diseases) and apologize to those investigators whose contributions were not included in this chapter due to space limitations.

References

1. Burkhardt B, Zimmermann M, Oschlies I, Niggli F, Mann G, Parwaresch R, Riehm H, Schrappe M, Reiter A (2005) The impact of age and gender on biology, clinical features and treatment outcome of non-Hodgkin lymphoma in childhood and adolescence. Br J Haematol 131:39–49
2. Magrath I (1990) The pathogenesis of Burkitt's lymphoma. Adv Cancer Res 55:133–270
3. Rochford R, Cannon MJ, Moormann AM (2005) Endemic Burkitt's lymphoma: a polymicrobial disease? Nat Rev Microbiol 3:182–187
4. Sandlund JT, Downing JR, Crist WM (1996) Non-Hodgkin's lymphoma in childhood. N Engl J Med 334:1238–1248
5. Levine PH, Connelly RR, McKay FW (1985) Burkitt's lymphoma in the USA: cases reported to the American Burkitt Lymphoma Registry compared with population-based incidence and mortality data. IARC Sci Publ 60:217–224
6. Mbulaiteye SM, Anderson WF, Bhatia K, Rosenberg PS, Linet MS, Devesa SS (2010) Trimodal age-specific incidence patterns for Burkitt lymphoma in the United States, 1973–2005. Int J Cancer 126:1732–1739
7. Mbulaiteye SM, Biggar RJ, Bhatia K, Linet MS, Devesa SS (2009) Sporadic childhood Burkitt lymphoma incidence in the United States during 1992–2005. Pediatr Blood Cancer 53:366–370
8. Ogwang MD, Bhatia K, Biggar RJ, Mbulaiteye SM (2008) Incidence and geographic distribution of endemic Burkitt lymphoma in northern Uganda revisited. Int J Cancer 123:2658–2663
9. Roithmann S, Tourani JM, Andrieu JM (1991) AIDS-associated non-Hodgkin lymphoma. Lancet 338:884–885
10. WHO (2008) WHO Classification of Tumours of Haematopoietic and Lymphoid Tissues. Lyon, IARC
11. Dalla-Favera R, Bregni M, Erikson J, Patterson D, Gallo RC, Croce CM (1982) Human c-myc onc gene is located on the region of chromosome 8 that is translocated in Burkitt lymphoma cells. Proc Natl Acad Sci U S A 79:7824–7827
12. Hecht JL, Aster JC (2000) Molecular biology of Burkitt's lymphoma. J Clin Oncol 18:3707–3721
13. Klein G (1983) Specific chromosomal translocations and the genesis of B-cell-derived tumors in mice and men. Cell 32:311–315
14. Taub R, Kirsch I, Morton C, Lenoir G, Swan D, Tronick S, Aaronson S, Leder P (1982) Translocation of the c-myc gene into the immunoglobulin heavy chain locus in human Burkitt lymphoma and murine plasmacytoma cells. Proc Natl Acad Sci U S A 79:7837–7841
15. Watson DK, Reddy EP, Duesberg PH, Papas TS (1983) Nucleotide sequence analysis of the chicken c-myc gene reveals homologous and unique coding regions by comparison with the transforming gene of avian myelocytomatosis virus MC29, delta gag-myc. Proc Natl Acad Sci U S A 80:2146–2150
16. Dang CV, O'Donnell KA, Zeller KI, Nguyen T, Osthus RC, Li F (2006) The c-Myc target gene network. Semin Cancer Biol 16:253–264
17. Pelengaris S, Khan M, Evan G (2002) c-MYC: more than just a matter of life and death. Nat Rev Cancer 2:764–776

18. Zeller KI, Zhao X, Lee CW, Chiu KP, Yao F, Yustein JT, Ooi HS, Orlov YL, Shahab A, Yong HC et al (2006) Global mapping of c-Myc binding sites and target gene networks in human B cells. Proc Natl Acad Sci U S A 103:17834–17839
19. Alarcon RM, Rupnow BA, Graeber TG, Knox SJ, Giaccia AJ (1996) Modulation of c_myc activity and apoptosis in vivo. Cancer Res 56(19):4315–4319
20. Bhatia KG, Gutierrez MI, Huppi K, Siwarski D, Magrath IT (1992) The pattern of p53 mutations in Burkitt's lymphoma differs from that of solid tumors. Cancer Res 52:4273–4276
21. Farrell PJ, Allan GJ, Shanahan F, Vousden KH, Crook T (1991) p53 is frequently mutated in Burkitt's lymphoma cell lines. EMBO J 10:2879–2887
22. Gaidano G, Ballerini P, Gong JZ, Inghirami G, Neri A, Newcomb EW, Magrath IT, Knowles DM, Dalla-Favera R (1991) p53 mutations in human lymphoid malignancies: association with Burkitt lymphoma and chronic lymphocytic leukemia. Proc Natl Acad Sci U S A 88:5413–5417
23. Newcomb EW (1995) P53 gene mutations in lymphoid diseases and their possible relevance to drug resistance. Leuk Lymphoma 17:211–221
24. Chang TC, Yu D, Lee YS, Wentzel EA, Arking DE, West KM, Dang CV, Thomas-Tikhonenko A, Mendell JT (2008) Widespread microRNA repression by Myc contributes to tumorigenesis. Nat Genet 40:43–50
25. O'Donnell KA, Wentzel EA, Zeller KI, Dang CV, Mendell JT (2005) c-Myc-regulated microRNAs modulate E2F1 expression. Nature 435:839–843
26. Henle W, Diehl V, Kohn G, Zur Hausen H, Henle G (1967) Herpes-type virus and chromosome marker in normal leukocytes after growth with irradiated Burkitt cells. Science 157:1064–1065
27. Kelly GL, Rickinson AB (2007) Burkitt lymphoma: revisiting the pathogenesis of a virus-associated malignancy. Hematology Am Soc Hematol Educ Program 277–284
28. Lindahl T, Adams A, Bjursell G, Bornkamm GW, Kaschka-Dierich C, Jehn U (1976) Covalently closed circular duplex DNA of Epstein-Barr virus in a human lymphoid cell line. J Mol Biol 102:511–530
29. Bell AI, Groves K, Kelly GL, Croom-Carter D, Hui E, Chan AT, Rickinson AB (2006) Analysis of Epstein-Barr virus latent gene expression in endemic Burkitt's lymphoma and nasopharyngeal carcinoma tumour cells by using quantitative real-time PCR assays. J Gen Virol 87:2885–2890
30. Kennedy G, Komano J, Sugden B (2003) Epstein-Barr virus provides a survival factor to Burkitt's lymphomas. Proc Natl Acad Sci U S A 100:14269–14274
31. Komano J, Maruo S, Kurozumi K, Oda T, Takada K (1999) Oncogenic role of Epstein-Barr virus-encoded RNAs in Burkitt's lymphoma cell line Akata. J Virol 73:9827–9831
32. Ruf IK, Rhyne PW, Yang H, Borza CM, Hutt-Fletcher LM, Cleveland JL, Sample JT (1999) Epstein-Barr virus regulates c-MYC, apoptosis, and tumorigenicity in Burkitt lymphoma. Mol Cell Biol 19:1651–1660
33. Lapin BA (1973) The epidemiologic and genetic aspects of an outbreak of leukemia among Hamadryas baboons of the Sukhumi monkey colony. Bibl Haematol 39:263–268
34. Moghaddam A, Rosenzweig M, Lee-Parritz D, Annis B, Johnson RP, Wang F (1997) An animal model for acute and persistent Epstein-Barr virus infection. Science 276: 2030–2033
35. Moghaddam A, Koch J, Annis B, Wang F (1998) Infection of human B lymphocytes with lymphocryptoviruses related to Epstein-Barr virus. J Virol 72:3205–3212
36. Cho Y-G, Ramer J, Rivailler P, Quink C, Garber RL, Beier DR, Wang F (2001) An Epstein-Barr-related herpesvirus from marmoset lymphomas. Proc Natl Acad Sci 98:1224–1229
37. Levine PH, Leiseca SA, Hewetson JF, Traul KA, Andrese AP, Granlund DJ, Fabrizio P, Stevens DA (1980) Infection of rhesus monkeys and chimpanzees with Epstein-Barr virus. Arch Virol 66:341–351
38. Cox C, Chang S, Karran L, Griffin B, Wedderburn N (1996) Persistent Epstein-Barr virus infection in the common marmoset (Callithrix jacchus). J Gen Virol 77(Pt 6):1173–1180

39. Falk L, Deinhardt F, Wolfe L, Johnson D, Hilgers J, de-The G (1976) Epstein-Barr virus: experimental infection of Callithrix jacchus marmosets. Int J Cancer 17:785–788
40. Wedderburn N, Edwards JM, Desgranges C, Fontaine C, Cohen B, de The G (1984) Infectious mononucleosis-like response in common marmosets infected with Epstein-Barr virus. J Infect Dis 150:878–882
41. Cox C, Naylor BA, Mackett M, Arrand JR, Griffin BE, Wedderburn N (1998) Immunization of common marmosets with Epstein-Barr virus (EBV) envelope glycoprotein gp340: effect on viral shedding following EBV challenge. J Med Virol 55:255–261
42. Mackett M, Cox C, Pepper SD, Lees JF, Naylor BA, Wedderburn N, Arrand JR (1996) Immunisation of common marmosets with vaccinia virus expressing Epstein-Barr virus (EBV) gp340 and challenge with EBV. J Med Virol 50:263–271
43. Deinhardt F, Falk LA, Wolfe LG (1974) Transformation of nonhuman primate lymphocytes by Epstein-Barr virus. Cancer Res 34:1241–1244
44. Miller G, Shope T, Coope D, Waters L, Pagano J, Bornkamn G, Henle W (1977) Lymphoma in cotton-top marmosets after inoculation with Epstein-Barr virus: tumor incidence, histologic spectrum antibody responses, demonstration of viral DNA, and characterization of viruses. J Exp Med 145:948–967
45. Shope T, Dechairo D, Miller G (1973) Malignant lymphoma in cottontop marmosets after inoculation with Epstein-Barr virus. Proc Natl Acad Sci U S A 70:2487–2491
46. Cleary ML, Epstein MA, Finerty S, Dorfman RF, Bornkamm GW, Kirkwood JK, Morgan AJ, Sklar J (1985) Individual tumors of multifocal EB virus-induced malignant lymphomas in tamarins arise from different B-cell clones. Science 228:722–724
47. Young LS, Finerty S, Brooks L, Scullion F, Rickinson AB, Morgan AJ (1989) Epstein-Barr virus gene expression in malignant lymphomas induced by experimental virus infection of cottontop tamarins. J Virol 63:1967–1974
48. Morgan AJ, Finerty S, Lovgren K, Scullion FT, Morein B (1988) Prevention of Epstein-Barr (EB) virus-induced lymphoma in cottontop tamarins by vaccination with the EB virus envelope glycoprotein gp340 incorporated into immune-stimulating complexes. J Gen Virol 69(Pt 8):2093–2096
49. Morgan AJ, Mackett M, Finerty S, Arrand JR, Scullion FT, Epstein MA (1988) Recombinant vaccinia virus expressing Epstein-Barr virus glycoprotein gp340 protects cottontop tamarins against EB virus-induced malignant lymphomas. J Med Virol 25:189–195
50. Niedobitek G, Agathanggelou A, Finerty S, Tierney R, Watkins P, Jones EL, Morgan A, Young LS, Rooney N (1994) Latent Epstein-Barr virus infection in cottontop tamarins. A possible model for Epstein-Barr virus infection in humans. Am J Pathol 145:969–978
51. Ragot T, Finerty S, Watkins PE, Perricaudet M, Morgan AJ (1993) Replication-defective recombinant adenovirus expressing the Epstein,ÄîBarr virus (EBV) envelope glycoprotein gp340/220 induces protective immunity against EBV-induced lymphomas in the cottontop tamarin. J Gen Virol 74:501–507
52. Mittermeier RA, Wallis J, Rylands AB, Ganzhorn JU, Oates JF, Williamson EA, Palacios E, Heymann EW, Kierulff CM, Yongcheng L et al (2009) Primates in peril: the world's 25 most endangered primates 2008–2010. Primate Conservation 24:1–57
53. Orlova N, Fogg MH, Carville A, Wang F (2011) Antibodies to lytic infection proteins in lymphocryptovirus-infected rhesus macaques: a model for humoral immune responses to Epstein-Barr virus infection. Clin Vaccine Immunol 2011 Sep;18(9):1427–1434
54. Gelmann EP, Psallidopoulos MC, Papas TS, Dalla-Favera R (1983) Identification of reciprocal translocation sites within the c-myc oncogene and immunoglobulin mu locus in a Burkitt lymphoma. Nature 306:799–803
55. Adams JM, Harris AW, Pinkert CA, Corcoran LM, Alexander WS, Cory S, Palmiter RD, Brinster RL (1985) The c-myc oncogene driven by immunoglobulin enhancers induces lymphoid malignancy in transgenic mice. Nature 318:533–538
56. Adams JM, Cory S (1985) Myc oncogene activation in B and T lymphoid tumours. Proc R Soc Lond B Biol Sci 226:59–72

57. Adams JM, Harris AW, Strasser A, Ogilvy S, Cory S (1999) Transgenic models of lymphoid neoplasia and development of a pan-hematopoietic vector. Oncogene 18:5268–5277
58. Harris AW, Pinkert CA, Crawford M, Langdon WY, Brinster RL, Adams JM (1988) The E mu-myc transgenic mouse. A model for high-incidence spontaneous lymphoma and leukemia of early B cells. J Exp Med 167:353–371
59. Prasad VS, Temple MJ, Davisson MT, Akeson EC, Sidman CL (1996) Heterogeneity of B-lymphoid tumors in E mu-myc transgenic mice. Cytometry 23:131–139
60. Eischen CM, Weber JD, Roussel MF, Sherr CJ, Cleveland JL (1999) Disruption of the ARF-Mdm2-p53 tumor suppressor pathway in Myc-induced lymphomagenesis. Genes Dev 13:2658–2669
61. Strasser A, Harris AW, Bath ML, Cory S (1990) Novel primitive lymphoid tumours induced in transgenic mice by cooperation between myc and bcl-2. Nature 348:331–333
62. Felsher DW, Bishop JM (1999) Reversible tumorigenesis by MYC in hematopoietic lineages. Mol Cell 4:199–207
63. Butzler C, Zou X, Popov AV, Bruggemann M (1997) Rapid induction of B-cell lymphomas in mice carrying a human IgH/c-mycYAC. Oncogene 14:1383–1388
64. Kovalchuk AL, Qi CF, Torrey TA, Taddesse-Heath L, Feigenbaum L, Park SS, Gerbitz A, Klobeck G, Hoertnagel K, Polack A et al (2000) Burkitt lymphoma in the mouse. J Exp Med 192:1183–1190
65. Bieging KT, Amick AC, Longnecker R (2009) Epstein-Barr virus LMP2A bypasses p53 inactivation in a MYC model of lymphomagenesis. Proc Natl Acad Sci U S A 106:17945–17950
66. Bultema R, Longnecker R, Swanson-Mungerson M (2009) Epstein-Barr virus LMP2A accelerates MYC-induced lymphomagenesis. Oncogene 28:1471–1476
67. Bieging KT, Fish K, Bondada S, Longnecker R (2011) A shared gene expression signature in mouse models of EBV-associated and non-EBV-associated Burkitt lymphoma. Blood 118(26):6849–6859
68. Palomo C, Zou X, Nicholson IC, Butzler C, Bruggemann M (1999) B-cell tumorigenesis in mice carrying a yeast artificial chromosome-based immunoglobulin heavy/c-myc translocus is independent of the heavy chain intron enhancer (Emu). Cancer Res 59:5625–5628
69. Park SS, Kim JS, Tessarollo L, Owens JD, Peng L, Han SS, Tae Chung S, Torrey TA, Cheung WC, Polakiewicz RD et al (2005) Insertion of c-Myc into Igh induces B-cell and plasma-cell neoplasms in mice. Cancer Res 65:1306–1315
70. Chang DW, Claassen GF, Hann SR, Cole MD (2000) The c-Myc transactivation domain is a direct modulator of apoptotic versus proliferative signals. Mol Cell Biol 20:4309–4319
71. Laurencikiene J, Tamosiunas V, Severinson E (2007) Regulation of epsilon germline transcription and switch region mutations by IgH locus 3′ enhancers in transgenic mice. Blood 109:159–167
72. Madisen L, Groudine M (1994) Identification of a locus control region in the immunoglobulin heavy-chain locus that deregulates c-myc expression in plasmacytoma and Burkitt's lymphoma cells. Genes Dev 8:2212–2226
73. Wang J, Boxer LM (2005) Regulatory elements in the immunoglobulin heavy chain gene 3′-enhancers induce c-myc deregulation and lymphomagenesis in murine B cells. J Biol Chem 280:12766–12773
74. Mautner J, Joos S, Werner T, Eick D, Bornkamm GW, Polack A (1995) Identification of two enhancer elements downstream of the human c-myc gene. Nucleic Acids Res 23:72–80
75. Remmers EF, Yang JQ, Marcu KB (1986) A negative transcriptional control element located upstream of the murine c-myc gene. EMBO J 5:899–904
76. Truffinet V, Pinaud E, Cogne N, Petit B, Guglielmi L, Cogne M, Denizot Y (2007) The 3′ IgH locus control region is sufficient to deregulate a c-myc transgene and promote mature B cell malignancies with a predominant Burkitt-like phenotype. J Immunol 179:6033–6042
77. Vincent C, Truffinet V, Fiancette R, Petit B, CognÈ N, CognÈ M, Denizot Y (2009) Uncoupling between Ig somatic hypermutation and oncogene mutation in mouse lymphoma. Biochimica et Biophysica Acta 1793:418–426

78. Gostissa M, Yan CT, Bianco JM, Cogné M, Pinaud E, Alt FW (2009) Long-range oncogenic activation of Igh, Äìc-myc translocations by the Igh 3[prime] regulatory region. Nature 462:803–807
79. Chapman CJ, Mockridge CI, Rowe M, Rickinson AB, Stevenson FK (1995) Analysis of VH genes used by neoplastic B cells in endemic Burkitt's lymphoma shows somatic hypermutation and intraclonal heterogeneity. Blood 85:2176–2181
80. Chapman CJ, Wright D, Stevenson FK (1998) Insight into Burkitt's lymphoma from immunoglobulin variable region gene analysis. Leuk Lymphoma 30:257–267
81. Dameshek W, Schwartz RS (1959) Leukemia and auto-immunization – some possible relationships. Blood 14:1151–1158
82. De Re V, De Vita S, Marzotto A, Rupolo M, Gloghini A, Pivetta B, Gasparotto D, Carbone A, Boiocchi M (2000) Sequence analysis of the immunoglobulin antigen receptor of hepatitis C virus-associated non-Hodgkin lymphomas suggests that the malignant cells are derived from the rheumatoid factor-producing cells that occur mainly in type II cryoglobulinemia. Blood 96:3578–3584
83. Quinn ER, Chan CH, Hadlock KG, Foung SK, Flint M, Levy S (2001) The B-cell receptor of a hepatitis C virus (HCV)-associated non-Hodgkin lymphoma binds the viral E2 envelope protein, implicating HCV in lymphomagenesis. Blood 98:3745–3749
84. Refaeli Y, Young RM, Turner BC, Duda J, Field KA, Bishop JM (2008) The B cell antigen receptor and overexpression of MYC can cooperate in the genesis of B cell lymphomas. PLoS Biol 6:e152
85. Bannish G, Fuentes-Panana EM, Cambier JC, Pear WS, Monroe JG (2001) Ligand-independent signaling functions for the B lymphocyte antigen receptor and their role in positive selection during B lymphopoiesis. J Exp Med 194:1583–1596
86. Dildrop R, Ma A, Zimmerman K, Hsu E, Tesfaye A, DePinho R, Alt FW (1989) IgH enhancer-mediated deregulation of N-myc gene expression in transgenic mice: generation of lymphoid neoplasias that lack c-myc expression. EMBO J 8:1121–1128
87. Hemann MT, Bric A, Teruya-Feldstein J, Herbst A, Nilsson JA, Cordon-Cardo C, Cleveland JL, Tansey WP, Lowe SW (2005) Evasion of the p53 tumour surveillance network by tumour-derived MYC mutants. Nature 436:807–811
88. Gruhne B, Sompallae R, Marescotti D, Kamranvar SA, Gastaldello S, Masucci MG (2009) The Epstein-Barr virus nuclear antigen-1 promotes genomic instability via induction of reactive oxygen species. Proc Natl Acad Sci U S A 106:2313–2318
89. Gruhne B, Sompallae R, Masucci MG (2009) Three Epstein-Barr virus latency proteins independently promote genomic instability by inducing DNA damage, inhibiting DNA repair and inactivating cell cycle checkpoints. Oncogene 28:3997–4008
90. Schulz TF, Cordes S (2009) Is the Epstein-Barr virus EBNA-1 protein an oncogen? Proc Natl Acad Sci U S A 106:2091–2092
91. Kuhn-Hallek I, Sage DR, Stein L, Groelle H, Fingeroth JD (1995) Expression of recombination activating genes (RAG-1 and RAG-2) in Epstein-Barr virus-bearing B cells. Blood 85:1289–1299
92. Srinivas SK, Sixbey JW (1995) Epstein-Barr virus induction of recombinase-activating genes RAG1 and RAG2. J Virol 69:8155–8158
93. Wilson JB, Bell JL, Levine AJ (1996) Expression of Epstein-Barr virus nuclear antigen-1 induces B cell neoplasia in transgenic mice. EMBO J 15:3117–3126
94. Tsimbouri P, Drotar ME, Coy JL, Wilson JB (2002) bcl-xL and RAG genes are induced and the response to IL-2 enhanced in EmuEBNA-1 transgenic mouse lymphocytes. Oncogene 21:5182–5187
95. Drotar ME, Silva S, Barone E, Campbell D, Tsimbouri P, Jurvansu J, Bhatia P, Klein G, Wilson JB (2003) Epstein-Barr virus nuclear antigen-1 and Myc cooperate in lymphomagenesis. Int J Cancer 106:388–395
96. Kang MS, Lu H, Yasui T, Sharpe A, Warren H, Cahir-McFarland E, Bronson R, Hung SC, Kieff E (2005) Epstein-Barr virus nuclear antigen 1 does not induce lymphoma in transgenic FVB mice. Proc Natl Acad Sci U S A 102:820–825

97. Polito P, Cilia AM, Gloghini A, Cozzi M, Perin T, De Paoli P, Gaidano G, Carbone A (1995) High frequency of EBV association with non-random abnormalities of the chromosome region 1q21-25 in aids-related Burkitt's lymphoma-derived cell lines. Int J Cancer 61(3):370–374
98. Ong KW, Teo M, Lee V, Ong D, Lee A, Tan CS, Vathsala A, Toh HC (2009) Expression of EBV latent antigens, mammalian target of rapamycin, and tumor suppression genes in EBV-positive smooth muscle tumors: clinical and therapeutic implications. Clin Cancer Res 15:5350–5358
99. Tao Q, Robertson KD, Manns A, Hildesheim A, Ambinder RF (1998) Epstein-Barr virus (EBV) in endemic Burkitt's lymphoma: molecular analysis of primary tumor tissue. Blood 91:1373–1381
100. Xue SA, Labrecque LG, Lu QL, Ong SK, Lampert IA, Kazembe P, Molyneux E, Broadhead RL, Borgstein E, Griffin BE (2002) Promiscuous expression of Epstein-Barr virus genes in Burkitt's lymphoma from the central African country Malawi. Int J Cancer 99:635–643
101. Fruehling S, Longnecker R (1997) The immunoreceptor tyrosine-based activation motif of Epstein-Barr virus LMP2A is essential for blocking BCR-mediated signal transduction. Virology 235:241–251
102. Fruehling S, Swart R, Dolwick KM, Kremmer E, Longnecker R (1998) Tyrosine 112 of latent membrane protein 2A is essential for protein tyrosine kinase loading and regulation of Epstein-Barr virus latency. J Virol 72:7796–7806
103. Longnecker R, Druker B, Roberts TM, Kieff E (1991) An Epstein-Barr virus protein associated with cell growth transformation interacts with a tyrosine kinase. J Virol 65:3681–3692
104. Rovedo M, Longnecker R (2008) Epstein-Barr virus latent membrane protein 2A preferentially signals through the Src family kinase Lyn. J Virol 82:8520–8528
105. Mancao C, Hammerschmidt W (2007) Epstein-Barr virus latent membrane protein 2A is a B-cell receptor mimic and essential for B-cell survival. Blood 110:3715–3721
106. Portis T, Longnecker R (2004) Epstein-Barr virus (EBV) LMP2A mediates B-lymphocyte survival through constitutive activation of the Ras/PI3K/Akt pathway. Oncogene 23:8619–8628
107. Swanson-Mungerson M, Bultema R, Longnecker R (2010) Epstein-Barr virus LMP2A imposes sensitivity to apoptosis. J Gen Virol 91:2197–2202
108. Swanson-Mungerson MA, Caldwell RG, Bultema R, Longnecker R (2005) Epstein-Barr virus LMP2A alters in vivo and in vitro models of B-cell anergy, but not deletion, in response to autoantigen. J Virol 79:7355–7362
109. Bieging KT, Swanson-Mungerson M, Amick AC, Longnecker R (2010) Epstein-Barr virus in Burkitt's lymphoma: a role for latent membrane protein 2A. Cell Cycle 9:901–908
110. Cen O, Longnecker R (2011) Rapamycin reverses splenomegaly and inhibits tumor development in a transgenic model of Epstein-Barr virus-related Burkitt's lymphoma. Mol Cancer Ther 10:679–686
111. Izumi KM, Kaye KM, Kieff ED (1994) Epstein-Barr virus recombinant molecular genetic analysis of the LMP1 amino-terminal cytoplasmic domain reveals a probable structural role, with no component essential for primary B-lymphocyte growth transformation. J Virol 68:4369–4376
112. Izumi KM, Kaye KM, Kieff ED (1997) The Epstein-Barr virus LMP1 amino acid sequence that engages tumor necrosis factor receptor associated factors is critical for primary B lymphocyte growth transformation. Proc Natl Acad Sci U S A 94:1447–1452
113. Kaye KM, Izumi KM, Kieff E (1993) Epstein-Barr virus latent membrane protein 1 is essential for B-lymphocyte growth transformation. Proc Natl Acad Sci U S A 90:9150–9154
114. Kaye KM, Izumi KM, Mosialos G, Kieff E (1995) The Epstein-Barr virus LMP1 cytoplasmic carboxy terminus is essential for B-lymphocyte transformation; fibroblast cocultivation complements a critical function within the terminal 155 residues. J Virol 69:675–683
115. Cahir-McFarland ED, Carter K, Rosenwald A, Giltnane JM, Henrickson SE, Staudt LM, Kieff E (2004) Role of NF-kappa B in cell survival and transcription of latent membrane protein 1-expressing or Epstein-Barr virus latency III-infected cells. J Virol 78:4108–4119

116. Devergne O, Cahir McFarland ED, Mosialos G, Izumi KM, Ware CF, Kieff E (1998) Role of the TRAF binding site and NF-kappaB activation in Epstein-Barr virus latent membrane protein 1-induced cell gene expression. J Virol 72:7900–7908
117. Izumi KM, Cahir McFarland ED, Ting AT, Riley EA, Seed B, Kieff ED (1999) The Epstein-Barr virus oncoprotein latent membrane protein 1 engages the tumor necrosis factor receptor-associated proteins TRADD and receptor-interacting protein (RIP) but does not induce apoptosis or require RIP for NF-kappaB activation. Mol Cell Biol 19:5759–5767
118. Kulwichit W, Edwards RH, Davenport EM, Baskar JF, Godfrey V, Raab-Traub N (1998) Expression of the Epstein-Barr virus latent membrane protein 1 induces B cell lymphoma in transgenic mice. Proc Natl Acad Sci U S A 95:11963–11968
119. Luftig M, Prinarakis E, Yasui T, Tsichritzis T, Cahir-McFarland E, Inoue J, Nakano H, Mak TW, Yeh WC, Li X et al (2003) Epstein-Barr virus latent membrane protein 1 activation of NF-kappaB through IRAK1 and TRAF6. Proc Natl Acad Sci U S A 100:15595–15600
120. Luftig M, Yasui T, Soni V, Kang MS, Jacobson N, Cahir-McFarland E, Seed B, Kieff E (2004) Epstein-Barr virus latent infection membrane protein 1 TRAF-binding site induces NIK/IKK alpha-dependent noncanonical NF-kappaB activation. Proc Natl Acad Sci U S A 101:141–146
121. Mosialos G, Birkenbach M, Yalamanchili R, VanArsdale T, Ware C, Kieff E (1995) The Epstein-Barr virus transforming protein LMP1 engages signaling proteins for the tumor necrosis factor receptor family. Cell 80:389–399
122. Wang D, Liebowitz D, Kieff E (1985) An EBV membrane protein expressed in immortalized lymphocytes transforms established rodent cells. Cell 43:831–840
123. Dirmeier U, Hoffmann R, Kilger E, Schultheiss U, Briseno C, Gires O, Kieser A, Eick D, Sugden B, Hammerschmidt W (2005) Latent membrane protein 1 of Epstein-Barr virus coordinately regulates proliferation with control of apoptosis. Oncogene 24:1711–1717
124. Polack A, Hortnagel K, Pajic A, Christoph B, Baier B, Falk M, Mautner J, Geltinger C, Bornkamm GW, Kempkes B (1996) c-myc activation renders proliferation of Epstein-Barr Virus (EBV)-transformed cells independent of EBV nuclear antigen 2 and latent membrane protein 1. Proc Natl Acad Sci U S A 93:10411–10416
125. Chen F, Zou JZ, di Renzo L, Winberg G, Hu LF, Klein E, Klein G, Ernberg I (1995) A subpopulation of normal B cells latently infected with Epstein-Barr virus resembles Burkitt lymphoma cells in expressing EBNA-1 but not EBNA-2 or LMP1. J Virol 69:3752–3758
126. Kelly GL, Milner AE, Baldwin GS, Bell AI, Rickinson AB (2006) Three restricted forms of Epstein-Barr virus latency counteracting apoptosis in c-myc-expressing Burkitt lymphoma cells. Proc Natl Acad Sci U S A 103:14935–14940
127. Schlaifer D, Brousset P, Attal M, Massip P, Payen C, Marchou B, Huguet F, Muller C, Laurent G, Pris J et al (1994) bcl-2 proto-oncogene and Epstein-Barr virus latent membrane protein-1 expression in AIDS-related lymphoma. Histopathology 25:77–82
128. Mansoor A, Stetler Stevenson M, Li RZ, Frekko K, Weiss W, Ahmad M, Khan AH, Mushtaq S, Saleem M, Raffeld M et al (1997) Prevalence of Epstein-Barr viral sequences and EBV LMP1 oncogene deletions in Burkitt's lymphoma from Pakistan: epidemiological correlations. Hum Pathol 28:283–288
129. Uchida J, Yasui T, Takaoka-Shichijo Y, Muraoka M, Kulwichit W, Raab-Traub N, Kikutani H (1999) Mimicry of CD40 signals by Epstein-Barr virus LMP1 in B lymphocyte responses. Science 286:300–303
130. Samanta M, Iwakiri D, Takada K (2008) Epstein-Barr virus-encoded small RNA induces IL-10 through RIG-I-mediated IRF-3 signaling. Oncogene 27:4150–4160
131. Jat P, Arrand JR (1982) In vitro transcription of two Epstein-Barr virus specified small RNA molecules. Nucleic Acids Res 10:3407–3425
132. Minarovits J, Hu LF, Marcsek Z, Minarovits-Kormuta S, Klein G, Ernberg I (1992) RNA polymerase III-transcribed EBER 1 and 2 transcription units are expressed and hypomethylated in the major Epstein-Barr virus-carrying cell types. J Gen Virol 73(Pt 7):1687–1692
133. Repellin CE, Tsimbouri PM, Philbey AW, Wilson JB (2010) Lymphoid hyperplasia and lymphoma in transgenic mice expressing the small non-coding RNA, EBER1 of Epstein-Barr virus. PLoS One 5:e9092

134. Niller HH, Salamon D, Ilg K, Koroknai A, Banati F, Bauml G, Rucker O, Schwarzmann F, Wolf H, Minarovits J (2003) The in vivo binding site for oncoprotein c-Myc in the promoter for Epstein-Barr virus (EBV) encoding RNA (EBER) 1 suggests a specific role for EBV in lymphomagenesis. Med Sci Monit 9:HY1–HY9
135. Mason KD, Vandenberg CJ, Scott CL, Wei AH, Cory S, Huang DC, Roberts AW (2008) In vivo efficacy of the Bcl-2 antagonist ABT-737 against aggressive Myc-driven lymphomas. Proc Natl Acad Sci U S A 105:17961–17966
136. Dargart JL, Fish K, Gordon LI, Longnecker R, Cen O (2012) Dasatinib therapy results in decreased B cell proliferation, splenomegaly, and tumor growth in a murine model of lymphoma expressing Myc and Epstein-Barr virus LMP2A. Antiviral Res 95(1):49–56
137. Bosma GC, Custer RP, Bosma MJ (1983) A severe combined immunodeficiency mutation in the mouse. Nature 301:527–530
138. Abe M, Suzuki O, Tasaki K, Abe R, Wakasa H (1996) Establishment and characterization of new human Burkitt's lymphoma cell lines (HBL-7 and HBL-8) that are highly metastatic in SCID mice: a metastatic SCID mouse model of human lymphoma lines. Pathol Int 46:630–638
139. Boffa LC, Cutrona G, Cilli M, Matis S, Damonte G, Mariani MR, Millo E, Moroni M, Roncella S, Fedeli F et al (2007) Inhibition of Burkitt's lymphoma cells growth in SCID mice by a PNA specific for a regulatory sequence of the translocated c-myc. Cancer Gene Ther 14:220–226
140. Lapalombella R, Zhao X, Triantafillou G, Yu B, Jin Y, Lozanski G, Cheney C, Heerema N, Jarjoura D, Lehman A et al (2008) A novel Raji-Burkitt's lymphoma model for preclinical and mechanistic evaluation of CD52-targeted immunotherapeutic agents. Clin Cancer Res 14:569–578
141. Chang CH, Sapra P, Vanama SS, Hansen HJ, Horak ID, Goldenberg DM (2005) Effective therapy of human lymphoma xenografts with a novel recombinant ribonuclease/anti-CD74 humanized IgG4 antibody immunotoxin. Blood 106:4308–4314
142. Shirley CM, Chen J, Shamay M, Li H, Zahnow CA, Hayward SD, Ambinder RF (2011) Bortezomib induction of C/EBPbeta mediates Epstein-Barr virus lytic activation in Burkitt lymphoma. Blood 117:6297–6303
143. Zou P, Kawada J, Pesnicak L, Cohen JI (2007) Bortezomib induces apoptosis of Epstein-Barr virus (EBV)-transformed B cells and prolongs survival of mice inoculated with EBV-transformed B cells. J Virol 81:10029–10036
144. Fu DX, Tanhehco Y, Chen J, Foss CA, Fox JJ, Chong JM, Hobbs RF, Fukayama M, Sgouros G, Kowalski J et al (2008) Bortezomib-induced enzyme-targeted radiation therapy in herpesvirus-associated tumors. Nat Med 14:1118–1122
145. Cannon MJ, Pisa P, Fox RI, Cooper NR (1990) Epstein-Barr virus induces aggressive lymphoproliferative disorders of human B cell origin in SCID/hu chimeric mice. J Clin Invest 85:1333–1337
146. Okano M, Taguchi Y, Nakamine H, Pirruccello SJ, Davis JR, Beisel KW, Kleveland KL, Sanger WG, Fordyce RR, Purtilo DT (1990) Characterization of Epstein-Barr virus-induced lymphoproliferation derived from human peripheral blood mononuclear cells transferred to severe combined immunodeficient mice. Am J Pathol 137:517–522
147. Mosier DE, Picchio GR, Baird SM, Kobayashi R, Kipps TJ (1992) Epstein-Barr virus-induced human B-cell lymphomas in SCID mice reconstituted with human peripheral blood leukocytes. Cancer Res 52:5552s–5553s
148. Mosier DE, Picchio GR, Kirven MB, Garnier JL, Torbett BE, Baird SM, Kobayashi R, Kipps TJ (1992) EBV-induced human B cell lymphomas in hu-PBL-SCID mice. AIDS Res Hum Retroviruses 8:735–740
149. Islas-Ohlmayer M, Padgett-Thomas A, Domiati-Saad R, Melkus MW, Cravens PD, Martin Mdel P, Netto G, Garcia JV (2004) Experimental infection of NOD/SCID mice reconstituted with human CD34+ cells with Epstein-Barr virus. J Virol 78:13891–13900
150. Shultz LD, Lyons BL, Burzenski LM, Gott B, Chen X, Chaleff S, Kotb M, Gillies SD, King M, Mangada J et al (2005) Human lymphoid and myeloid cell development in NOD/LtSz-

scid IL2R gamma null mice engrafted with mobilized human hemopoietic stem cells. J Immunol 174:6477–6489
151. Yajima M, Imadome K, Nakagawa A, Watanabe S, Terashima K, Nakamura H, Ito M, Shimizu N, Honda M, Yamamoto N et al (2008) A new humanized mouse model of Epstein-Barr virus infection that reproduces persistent infection, lymphoproliferative disorder, and cell-mediated and humoral immune responses. J Infect Dis 198:673–682
152. Ma SD, Hegde S, Young KH, Sullivan R, Rajesh D, Zhou Y, Jankowska-Gan E, Burlingham WJ, Sun X, Gulley ML et al (2011) A new model of Epstein-Barr virus infection reveals an important role for early lytic viral protein expression in the development of lymphomas. J Virol 85:165–177
153. Dave SS, Fu K, Wright GW, Lam LT, Kluin P, Boerma EJ, Greiner TC, Weisenburger DD, Rosenwald A, Ott G et al (2006) Molecular diagnosis of Burkitt's lymphoma. N Engl J Med 354:2431–2442
154. Hummel M, Bentink S, Berger H, Klapper W, Wessendorf S, Barth TF, Bernd HW, Cogliatti SB, Dierlamm J, Feller AC et al (2006) A biologic definition of Burkitt's lymphoma from transcriptional and genomic profiling. N Engl J Med 354:2419–2430
155. Piccaluga PP, De Falco G, Kustagi M, Gazzola A, Agostinelli C, Tripodo C, Leucci E, Onnis A, Astolfi A, Sapienza MR et al (2011) Gene expression analysis uncovers similarity and differences among Burkitt lymphoma subtypes. Blood 117:3596–3608
156. Staudt LM, Dave S (2005) The biology of human lymphoid malignancies revealed by gene expression profiling. Adv Immunol 87:163–208
157. Fingeroth JD, Weis JJ, Tedder TF, Strominger JL, Biro PA, Fearon DT (1984) Epstein-Barr virus receptor of human B lymphocytes is the C3d receptor CR2. Proc Natl Acad Sci U S A 81:4510–4514
158. Yang L, Maruo S, Takada K (2000) CD21-mediated entry and stable infection by Epstein-Barr virus in canine and rat cells. J Virol 74:10745–10751
159. Yang L, Ikeda H, Lai Y, Yoshiki T, Takada K (2003) Epstein-Barr virus infection of rat lymphocytes expressing human CD21 results in restricted latent viral gene expression and not in immunoblastic transformation. J Med Virol 70:126–130
160. Haan KM, Kwok WW, Longnecker R, Speck P (2000) Epstein-Barr virus entry utilizing HLA-DP or HLA-DQ as a coreceptor. J Virol 74:2451–2454
161. Li Q, Spriggs MK, Kovats S, Turk SM, Comeau MR, Nepom B, Hutt-Fletcher LM (1997) Epstein-Barr virus uses HLA class II as a cofactor for infection of B lymphocytes. J Virol 71:4657–4662
162. Haan KM, Aiyar A, Longnecker R (2001) Establishment of latent Epstein-Barr virus infection and stable episomal maintenance in murine B-cell lines. J Virol 75:3016–3020
163. Caldwell RG, Wilson JB, Anderson SJ, Longnecker R (1998) Epstein-Barr virus LMP2A drives B cell development and survival in the absence of normal B cell receptor signals. Immunity 9:405–411
164. Agliano A, Martin-Padura I, Mancuso P, Marighetti P, Rabascio C, Pruneri G, Shultz LD, Bertolini F (2008) Human acute leukemia cells injected in NOD/LtSz-scid/IL-2Rgamma null mice generate a faster and more efficient disease compared to other NOD/scid-related strains. Int J Cancer 123(9):2222–2227
165. Cocco M, Bellan C, Tussiwand R, Corti D, Traggiai E, Lazzi S, Mannucci S, Bronz L, Palummo N, Ginanneschi C, Tosi P, Lanzavecchia A, Manz MG, Leoncini L (2008) CD34+ cord blood cell-transplanted Rag2-/- gamma(c)-/- mice as a model for Epstein-Barr virus infection. Am J Pathol 173(5):1369–1378

Chapter 16
Summary and Conclusion: Thinking About Latent BL

Beverly E. Griffin

Denis Parsons Burkitt 1911–1993

Denis Burkitt first published his research in "The British Journal of Surgery" in 1958. This went unnoticed. It was his article, co-written with Greg O'Conor, "Malignant tumours in African children: A clinical syndrome" published in Cancer in 1961, that made a mark in the medical world.

Irish by birth, Trinity by the Grace of God—A Life Celebrated. A Symposium, Published by Trinity College, Dublin, 2011.

1. Burkitt D, A sarcoma involving the jaws in African children. Br J Surg, 218–223, 1958.
2. Burkitt D, O' Conor. Malignant tumours in African children: A clinical syndrome. Cancer 14, 258–269, 1961.
3. Cancer in Africa. Clifford P, Linsell DA, Timms GL. 1968. E. Africa Med. J. Nairobi:

   (a) Cancer in Africa. Patterns of cancer distribution in Tanzania, Burkitt D, Slavin G. 3, 13–17. Also, in the same volume.
   (b) Epidemiological, anatomical, virological and serological observation of the lymphomas of African Children, Dalldorf G, Bergamini F, Frost P, Couaux T. 17, 125–131.
   (c) Notes on the hypothesis that mosquitoes may be concerned in transmission of a causative agent in Burkitt's tumour, McCrae AWR. 18, 133–141.
   (d) Further membrane immunofluorescent studies on Burkitt's lymphoma biopsy cells and established tissue culture lines, Klein G, Clifford P. 20, 155–165.

B.E. Griffin (✉)
Department of Medicine at St. Mary's, Imperial College, Norfolk St, London W2 1RT, UK
e-mail: b.griffin@imperial.ac.uk; tomas.lindahl@cancer.org.uk;
bgriffin12z@hotmail.com; Pascale.Kropf@lshtm.ac.uk

E.S. Robertson (ed.), *Burkitt's Lymphoma*, Current Cancer Research,
DOI 10.1007/978-1-4614-4313-1_16, © Springer Science+Business Media New York 2013

(e) Burkitt's tumour in the United States, Ziegler JL, Carbone PP, Berard CW, Thomas LB. 28, 239–250.
(f) Cell Proliferation in Burkitt's tumours, Cooper EH, Frank GL, Wright DH. 30, 259–263.
(g) Abstract: Survival of patients with Burkitt's tumour in east and west Mengo districts of Uganda, Morrow RH, Pike MC, 453–455.

4. (a) De-The G, Geser A, Day NE, Tukei PM, Williams EH et al. Epidemiological evidence for causal relationship between Epstein–Barr virus and Burkitt's lymphoma from Ugandan prospective study. Nature 274, 756–761, 1978.
   (b) Geser A, de The G, Lenoir G, Day NE, Williams EH. Final case reporting from the Ugandan prospective study of the relationship between EBV and Burkitt's lymphoma. Int J Cancer 15, 397–400, 1982.

5. Wright D H. What is Burkitt's Lymphoma and when is it Endemic? Blood, 93, 758, 1999.
6. Epstein–Barr Virus. Ed. E.S. Robertson, Caister Academic Press. Chapters 1 and 33, Norfolk. England.

   (a) Epstein MA. The origins of EBV Research: Discovery and Characterization of the virus. 1–14, 2005.
   (b) Rickinson A. Epstein-Barr virus: Summary, Conclusions and a Forward Look. 711–753, 2005.

Background

Burkitt's lymphoma is a medical topic that requires a special interest. This disease—largely of children—is not easily dealt with since it grows so rapidly, the fastest proliferating human tumour. What is required is a combined effort in this field, as a disease that should not be ignored but to be given increased focus and attention. Although EBV has about 100 separate genes in order for it to replicate and survive, these are not the genes that mainly support the tumour. Here, only a handful of genes are required that, so far as we know, are mainly composed of the EBV Ebna1 (or EBNA1), and in some cases also of a lytically associated membrane gene (EBV LMP1), two small RNAs not expressed for generating proteins, and recently just being sorted out, is a group of small, virally coded RNAs, known as microRNAs (miRNAs) which as yet are not well understood. The rest of the viral genes or other factors not yet known to us act within the host cell to create "a malignancy". What is required for the growth of this virus in the host depends also on other EBV genes that help maintain the virus and are expressed from a supercoiled circular viral DNA, within the malignancy. This deals with how the virus replicates, and continues to function, but is retained apart from the tumour per se, as far as we know. This may be part of the problem in understanding this tumour.

Lytic replication of EBV may lyse the infected cells and so destroy the tumour, but the growth cycle of this virus may also contribute to its destruction on its own.

Information existing in the supercoiled virus within a single cell implies that we need more data from the virus, not merely the major genes required for replication of the virus, but also about the latent virus causal for the entity, BL. It may be necessary to separate out the malignancy from the alternative growth function of the virus, and try to understand how we can distinguish the tumour functions from the lytic component of the viral DNA. Table 16.1 shows the viral gene expression patterns detected from frozen samples of BL biopsies from Africa.

This section of the summary takes in data from Kornberg and Baker, "DNA Replication", 1992 (Freeman and Co.), where EBV is briefly considered. First, EBV has "distinct replication origins". One, oriP, is responsible for maintaining the genome in a latent extrachromosomal state (i.e. that seen in the infected tumour cells) and the other, oriLyt, is responsible for amplification of the genome and progeny production (i.e. replication) during the lytic growth phase. The two origins are located quite separately, and apart, on the large double-stranded DNA genome. They require distinct viral products for their activities, and do efficiently promote different modes of replication. DNA synthesis from oriP is circle-to-circle, through several intermediates, and during lytic replication long concatemers are generated, indicative of a separate mechanism. These are then processed resulting in propagation of the latent circular, viral genome into new daughter cells, and linear dsDNA packaged into progeny virions. EBV is unique in the efficiency with which it can immortalize human B lymphocytes, and from 10% to 100% of infected peripheral B cells yield progeny that proliferate indefinitely with EBV maintained in a latent plasmid state.

Section 1

Turning to the heart of this subject, the major section of this chapter (approximately 95%) deals with references from 2005 and onward, and mainly with the tumour, BL. An early version (see [1]) was used, in a web site shown for an American's tumour provided by the family, on his death from Burkitt's. In [2], Vonka, used early suggestions and includes both early and later tumours, as well as Burkitt's arguments that "soulless piling up of corroborative observations is of far less value for a scientific program than is active effort to overthrow hypotheses and replaced them by others". This included Zur Hausen's thoughts on Burkitt's lymphoma which he studied then in the 1980s. In [3], Kazembe et al. examined a population of 92 patients with BL in rural Malawi some 5 years after being treated and apparently surviving the disease—73 patients were traced. Of these, 40% were alive, and 63.5% of surviving children identified had tumours only involving the head clinically, and 21% with the abdomen involved. Obtaining long-term tumour information of this sort seems rare, with most follow-up studies done mainly short term. Patients on the whole are followed for 1 year after recovery, rather than for 5-year survival. Turning to more recent information, Andrew Willy [4], a Glaxo/Smith/Kline Chief executive states that "pharmaceutical companies have a moral obligation

Table 16.1 Viral gene expression in African BL biopsies . From Xue and Griffin [74]

	EBNAI						*BARFI*						
Sample	Qp	Cp/Wp	*CSTs*	*IR4*	*IR2*	*BARFI*	Lytic	Latent	*BZLFI*	*LMPI*	*LMP2A*	*LMP2B*	*vIL-10*
SD	+	+	+	+	+	+	–	–	+	–	+	+	–
IB	+	–	+	+	+	+	+	–	+	–	+	–	+
LC	+	+	+	+	+	+	+	–	–	–	+	–	–
TJ	+	–	+	+	+	+	+	–	+	–	+(W)[a]	–	–
GE	+	–	+	+	+	+	+	–	–	–	+	–	–
BL-1[b]	+	–	+	+	+	+	+	+	+	+	+(W)[a]	–	+
BL-2[c]	+	–	+	+	–	–	–	–	–	–	–	–	–
BL-3	+	–	+	+	+	+	+	–	+	+	–	–	+
BL-4	+	–	+	+	+(W)[a]	+	–	–	–	+	–	–	–
BL-5	+	–	+	+	+	+	+	–	+	+	+	+	–
BL-6	+	–	+	+	+	+	+	+	+	+	+	–	–
BL-7	+	–	+	+	+	+	+	–	+	+	+	–	–
CC(control)	–	–	–	–	–	–	–	–	–	–	–	–	–

Summary of EBV transcriptional expression in tumour samples (taken from freshly frozen material)
[a]Weak
[b]HIV
[c]Probably not a BL

to conduct research and development into therapies for low-income countries", noting that the "financial returns are often limited". BL does not appear on his list of tumours, however. I did ask, and got a reply that "maybe yet they will change". He notes more promising results coming forth for the future of malaria prevention, so maybe that will be a link for the future also, with regard to BL, to which malaria is linked. Lastly in the 4th edition, of the WHO Classification of Tumors of Haematopoietic and Lymphoid Tissues, reviewed by Elaine Jaffe [5] in 2009. She noted that there is a greater appreciation now of the borderlands between BL and diffuse large B-cell lymphoma (DLBCL) and began to examine evidence of this positive approach, distinguishing between these two cell types, as discussed later here.

For more detailed reviews, two are specifically cited on BL (see [6, 7]). In the more recent review, Bornkamm [6] uses BL as a "paradigm in cancer research". He also treats, briefly, the question of "other viral genes, and animal models". Here, as often discovered also by others, mouse models are not finding answers that apply to this cancer in man. On the other hand, whereas BL affects most frequently young children (aged 2–14), the disease of adults appear to follow a comparable course. Thorley-Lawson and Allday raise many questions [7]. They are sceptical in feeling that the development of BL becomes more enigmatic than involving only c-Myc, EBV, and (even) malaria, but did not, I think, consider the role of HIV here (see below). They have not decided, one thinks, whether the BL cell is more a germinal centre, or a memory cell, or one or both. Boema et al. [8] include BL and DLBCL, and gave attention to c-Myc at (8q24), but translocations with the secondary genes coding for kappa light chain (IgK at 2p:12) or lambda light chain (IgL at 14:32), are not really mentioned. Indeed, through the literature, only c-Myc at 8q24 receives attention. This appears as a simple neglect, I think, but would we find other transpositions with changes in BL at the sites on chromosomes 2 and 22, like that on 14? The study by Lenses et al. [9] used a "middleman database" and defined a cytogenetic profile of "true BL". No differences were observed between children and adults in this work, nor in a "grey-zone" between the two Burkitt's (BL and DLBCL). Even with "gazing ahead" by reviewers, one is left with queries that may still be resolved, and may even vary among geographical sites. In another study, Orem et al. [10] turn to Africa, and report that both high incidence and mortality rates of BL are seen in East Africa, largely within Uganda. Here, the evidence for a causal relationship between EBV and BL in the endemic form is strong, but even malaria has not had a conclusive population study, and other possible risk factors, such as low socio-economic status, plant derivatives, pesticides, other infections, etc. are not yet convincingly proven. The emergence of a distinct subtype of BL in HIV-infected cells has, however, brought a new dimension where both HIV and BL are endemic. This previously "unknown" combination in children may be relevant for BL. However, they have been careful in making these general statements, until better proven. In the final two papers here, one argues in favour of EBERs in the pathogenesis of Burkitt's lymphoma—with different roles for the two separate RNAs [10]—and a separate study on sporadic paediatric and adult tumours sharing similar phenotypic and genotype features [11]. Two separate studies are interesting, and may be relevant.

Does geographical association of BL really differ in anatomical sites from various populations? In [12], a Chinese BL study specially notes that childhood and adult diseases appear similar in their behaviours. Does keeping these as "two diseases", then make sense, or have we, on the other hand, lost differences that are real, in different populations? Clearly, there is much yet to learn from the distributions of BL.

In the next studies, I turn again to the childhood disease in BL. First, there was an interesting essay from *The Lancet* [13] by John Phillips, who viewed this disease in December 2006 in Malawi. This won a small prize, as he wrote about a disease he has worked on over many years. He also worked with scientists at the Hammersmith Hospital (London UK) and Malawi, in a 2-year study, where a link between cyclophosphamide responsiveness or resistance in tumours was suggested to be due to EBV lysis-associated gene expression, see Labrecque et al. [14], and Fig. 16.1. Clinical data and EBV gene expression results supported the postulated association in these tumours. In another pilot study in "late" BL, a small group of patients with recurrent cyclophosphamide-resistant tumours was treated in Malawi. These did not respond to classical treatment when retreated, and instead were treated with a separate regimen of cyclophosphamide coupled to an HDAC inhibitor, sodium phenylbutyrate, as briefly described [15]. Of these retreated children, 2/4 did not respond, but the other two showed limited response to the combined drugs. After a lengthy, but interrupted treatment, one died of an alternative disease, but the second was still alive with only a small, second tumour. He did not, however, return to hospital for further treatment. In finishing this saga [16], there is now a new development in investigation of BL that allows tumour samples to be held at ambient room temperature (apparently for long times) and later examined, when needed. This is very useful for subsequent work being done in under conditions of limited resources, or sent elsewhere for examination. The effect of cyclophosphamide treatment of BL in children is still highly valuable and should be continued as is evidenced by its clear successes in children (Fig. 16.2).

In this section, two interesting papers on BL are noted: one deals with the cancer as a two-step disease (two pathogens, BL and malaria, interacting, Rochford et al. [17]), and the second [18], as an African disease first treated in 1960–7, and now updated to today [18]. These were selected, as dealing with general questions in BL. The first [17] looks at whether the risk is of suppression of EBV-specific T-cell immunity by the malaria parasite, *Plasmodium falciparum* that has been invoked for a long time, or is it the expansion of the B-cell pool in latently infected patients. One of the early BL patients in Uganda, seen in Albert Cook's material, in 1910 (taken from the Medical Library in Kampala), was clearly suffering from malaria. When de-The et al. were hunting for alternative causative factors for Burkitt's in the late 1970s, they pointed to malaria as an adjunct as a secondary interest (looking for differences between the USA and Africa). The Toll-like receptor, TLR-9, may be relevant in this regard (as discussed below), with expression of the receptor in normal and transformed cells. There, according to the review here [17], most research will require the development of EBV-specific immunity in BL. *The Lancet* article [18] urges collaboration between the HIV-1 and malaria programmes. Interestingly, this review brings together material from the USA, England and Uganda, and relates

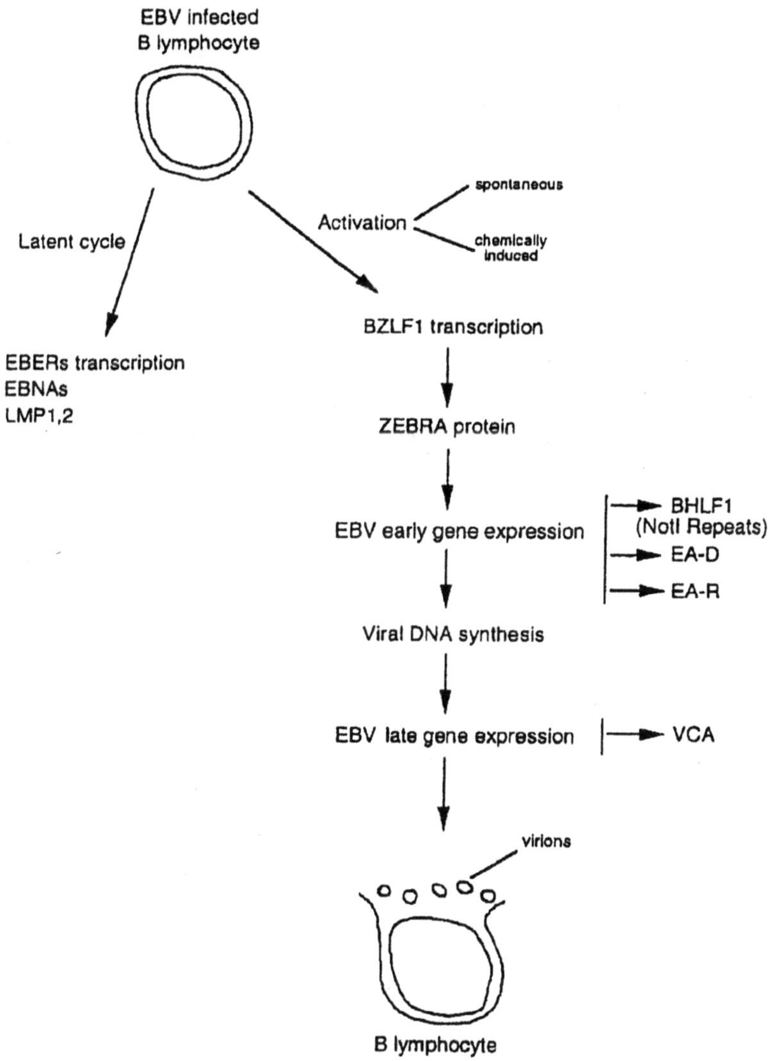

Fig. 16.1 Schematic diagram of the life cycle of EBV in B cells. In the latent cycle in B lymphocytes, viral gene expression is restricted to EBNAs and two small viral RNAs, EBER 1 and 2, and in addition, as far as we know, copies of EBV latent proteins, LMP1 and 2 [14], at the *left side* here. In some species, viral genes, as noted on the *right side*, are activated and expressed either spontaneous or chemically induce together with viral genes, and also micro-RNAs, as virion expression and ultimately as lysis

their work as "closely linked to Burkitt's lymphoma". It argues several issues, mostly that HIV is highly involved (90% of references) in this disease found in developed countries, but less than 60–70% in Africa and other geographic regions. They maintain "Africa is a long overdue moral imperative, and could be another milestone for a nascent paediatric oncology programme…saving the lives of

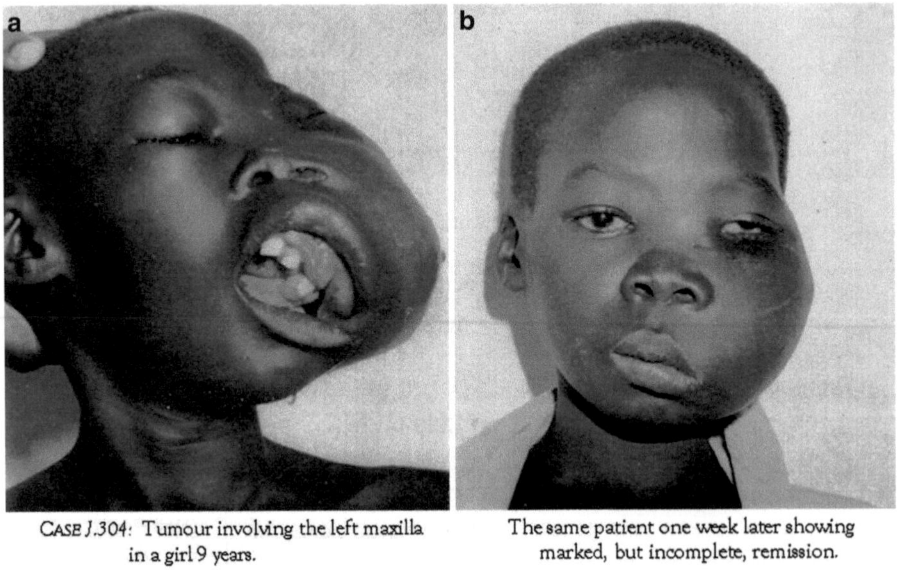

Fig. 16.2 Two cases of J.304, with a BL involving the left maxilla, in a girl aged 9 years (at the *left*) and then the same patient 1 week later, at *right*, having been treated with cyclophosphamide for 1 week, showing marked but incomplete remission. From Denis P. Burkitt, Possible Relationships between the African Lymphoma and Acute Leukaemia. Research Fund, Third Guest Lecture, London. Leukemia Research Fund, 1–28, 1967

thousands of African children dying from disease" which is indeed valid, and needed. It should also be more highly publicized for greater recognition as a major problem in oncology especially seen in children of the African continent.

Section 2

This section is tentatively divided into individual components that try to separate the disease, BL, into individual components, e.g. c-Myc, Epstein–Barr virus, Malaria, HIV, and other topics such as Bcl6 and Bcl2, ending with some comments such as needs for better therapy and more attention. We apologize that many articles have been deleted here but most are focused on developments since the last reviews in 2005. Reviews that precede this publication will have been covered in earlier ones.

The c-Myc Connection

Myc translocations are covered by pathways that include cell suicide or cancer, and are found in many tumours [19]. The c-Myc variant (as opposed to its families n-Myc or l-Myc) is found in BL at one of three chromosomal sites, at chromosome 8 (t8:14), at (t2:8) or (t8:22) alternative sites with the latter two (minor) sites involving IgH class switches. Oddly enough, even in the review by Allday [20] these two minor sites are rarely discussed in BL research, or even studied. However in a long-term study on lymphoblastoid cells lines in Korea, these have been found to be a resource for human study in genetic, immunological and pharmacogenomic studies—for long-term studies in cellular immortalization [21]. In an earlier paper on Myc, a paradox in the field of cancer biology, it was revealed by translocations that oncogenes, once thought to simply provide advantages to a cancer cell, actually put it at dire risk of cell suicide [22]. The precise mechanisms by which Myc target pathways are largely unresolved, but they are proposed to involve interactions to selectively repress the expression of Bcl2 that is specifically required for the survival of this type of death threat. This and its direct initiation also show that Bcl2 can be translated by c-Myc. On the other hand, germinal centres (GC) can be characterized by a unique transcription programme, distinct from other B-cell subsets. With a high expression of key transcription factors, such as GC in latent lymphomas, one comes to realize that BL and DLBCLs are suddenly recognized as different associations, or sub-sets, in alternative parts of the world [23].

Next a series of c-Myc-related lymphomas are dealt with more or less together as a topic, but differing in their findings [24–28]. Myc, as a transcription factor that regulates cell size, proliferation and apoptosis, is notably induced when normal cells are recruited into a cell cycle. Myc then also behaves as a basic helix–loop–helix zipper (that dimerises with Max) to bind with the DNA sequence, 5′-CACCTC, that acts as a C-Box, and activates transcription [24, 26]. In this mode, it also contributes to neoplastic transformation. Myc deregulation leads to a prime example for BL deregulation. Here also, they provide a symposium of the topics in a review that, in part, also helps with an unresolved summary, how to understand Myc-induced lymphomagenesis [27]. We also return to an older topic, molecular diagnosis of BL, where two works come together [28, 29] to review a "biological definition" of BL, from two difference points of view, and a further review itself [30], where the two arrays are discussed: the articles were complementary after differing in important ways, but reaching roughly the same conclusion: BL is not cured by the standard treatment for DLBCLs, nor is the aggressive treatment advocated for children in the west essentially safe. Children with BL in Africa may not tolerate the side effects of many intensive treatments. Diagnostic accuracy is essential to prevent their under- or over-treatment. The main diagnostic challenge is to distinguish one type of cell from another. Fairly clearly defined characteristics of BL are medium-sized cells that are CD10 and Bcl6 positive, and Bcl2 negative, while for DLBCL they are large cells with CD10 and Bcl6 negative, and Bcl2 positive. Two studies from the USA [28, 29] show that these characteristics may be used with FISH, real-time PCR, or immunologic methods, and allow the development of targeted therapies.

A paper from Brazil has pulled together a picture of Burkitt's lymphoma as a highly aggressive non-Hodgkin lymphoma, with a consistent Myc translocation [31]. It changes from area to area in Brazil, but is generally consistent. There is a higher than expected association with EBV in sporadic cases, with BL affecting males in 74%, and 26% female. This review is thorough, but records only expression of EBER1 and 2, and EBNA1, and at least BART microRNA, in part (see below), with no evidence about LMP-1 proteins, except in a few cases. They found a higher association with HIV-1. Also, Bcl6 is expressed as a major component, and is frequently discussed here as regards to the germinal center (GC) in BL, particularly in latent cells. The frequency is higher in paediatric cases, and lower in the South of Brazil.

In Malawi, East Africa, the cell type for children's BL seems controversial. From the recent paper on BL by Molyneux et al. [32], the cellular origin of the malignancy is unclear, with some workers arguing that it arises from a germinal central B-cell, while others are of the opinion that the tumour originates from a memory cell. EBV persists for the lifetime of the healthy individual and is found among young children, essentially 2–14 years of age. It is thought that this latent infection expresses only EBNA-1 similar to eBL, or a few other antigens of the EBV virus. In Africa, the tumour is noted essentially among the mainly rural population, and in Malawi, as elsewhere in Africa, the lake regions are prone to this disease. In the review in *The Lancet* [32], the observations on EBV-positive, compared to EBV-negative BL, have raised the alternative that whereas BL arises from the memory cells, maybe as a tumour BL originates from an earlier GC counterpart. This has not really been resolved, nor has the explanation of the higher frequency among young male children compared to females (approximately 2:1) been resolved. In most studies of BL, the children involved can be divided into two age groups (ages 1 or 2–9, as the larger part, and 10 and above, a minor part). Again, these tumours are almost always combined in studies. The two age groups have not really been clearly distinguished, although cells in the two BL groups sometimes appear different in terms of size and behaviour. In joint efforts, Italian/Ugandan studies have provided new interest in BLs [33]. They effectively divided their study into the three groups (endemic, sporadic and immunodeficiency-associated BLs), along with marker studies, and divided genes and substrates as being related to cell cycle control, B-cell receptor signalling, and tumour necrosis factor/nuclear factor kB pathways. In their work, they found that all BLs were related to GC cells, but differed in other findings, for example between eBLs, sBLs or IBLs, each type affecting different populations and presenting with different features. Bcl6 is expressed as a major component, and is frequently discussed here as regards germinal centre (GC) in BL, particularly in latent cells. The authors found a consistent set of genes differentially expressed in BL and normal B-cells, as a consequence of malignant transformation, and programs were altered, including those related to immune response, cell cycle regulations and BC-receptor signalling. They also offer novel evidence possibly relevant for its classification and future treatment, with subtypes of cells significantly different, suggesting different pathogenetic mechanisms and the role(s) of infectious agents. They also were involved in micro-RNAs that will promise interest for the future. It is an interesting study, and clearly needs follow-up. In the studies of Tumwine et al. [34, 35], also involving some of the same collaborators, they initially classify B-cell non-Hodgkin lymphomas using immunohistochemical markers to correlate BL types and patient outcomes. In these papers, they have compared different tumours, and again, show BL essentially to behave differently from other lymphomas (compared, e.g. with DLBMC), and they found the BLs to be Bcl-6 and Bcl-2 negative (see below), with Mum1/IRF4 essentially negative, as opposed to the Brazil study [31]. In a short study from China, on children's BL in 65 of 74 lymphomas described as BL [36], they found results, as far as I can tell, like those from [34, 35]. The children's tumours are often associated with an aggressive clinical behaviour and morphologic and immunohistochemistry behaviour differing little from the Uganda studies. Interesting, however, is the finding for MUM1, reportedly 23% positive among the Chinese BLs, as opposed to the Uganda data. Takada in earlier data on BL [37], and working on the Akata cells from Japanese materials, found expression of EBNA1, EBER, BARF0 and LMP 2A, with absence of EBNA2 and LMP1. These cells have an activated c-Myc chromosome. As he points out, the data show Akata to upregulate expression of Bcl-2 protein to protect cells from c-Myc-induced apoptosis and allow c-Myc to exert its oncogenic functions. (It is interesting to note that in this study Takada, in 2011, also notes a rare and extremely "unfavourable type of lymphoma", with translocations of both Bcl-2 and Myc. The patient, a 67-year-old diagnosed with Burkitt-like lymphoma which was first responsive to chemotherapy, then had a second relapse with a chemo-resistance and after 1 month, died. He had chromosomal t(14:18) and t(8:22) translocations, which has not previously been detected.)

Two further studies, from the USA and Brazil [38, 39], are put forward as studies of BL, but with slightly different findings from those of Ugandan BL (see also [31]). The BLs were highly aggressive lymphomas with endemic, sporadic and immunodeficiency-associated clinical variants. Classically, the immuno-phenotype of BL has been considered to be essentially a GC type. Here, they studied 222 cases of well-characterized BLs, with classic phenotype and c-Myc translocation, and found 90 cases (40.5%) of MUM1/IRF4 (multiple myeloma 1/interferon regulation factor 4 protein) positive. In their findings, MUM1 was found in the final histogenetic marker of the late-GC and post-GC cell, and the morphologic spectrum of positive cell ranged from that of a centrocyte to that of a plasmablast/plasma cell [38]. Mum1 is considered to be a key regulator of several steps in lymphoid/lymphoid and dendritic cell differentiation and maturation. It may be a promising target for the treatment of some of these neoplasms [39].

I turn now to a report by Hesseling et al. [40] of a 15-day chemotherapy schedule for resistant or relapsed endemic BL, where a 15-day chemotherapy schedule saved 36% of patients. In the same report predictors for mortality have recently also included anti-retroviral therapy (ART), started from 2007. This review was published in 2009, and perhaps it may continue with time [41]. Two studies that have looked further into factors to contribute to BL pathogenesis that may suggest the importance of this topic [42, 43], and another study on BL may indicate the importance of induction by HDAC (histone deacetylase inhibitors [44]). HDAC induction has exhibited effects interacting with drug exposure, as evidenced by increased site-specific histone acetylation. In the latter, where BL and lytically related diseases in replication may co-exist in a tumour, it may provide sites for latently infected cells to act, on their own, at the expense of the HDACs. In a small document, this review deals with a derivative from a B-cell, post-BC stage of differentiation, possible a memory B-cell precursor [45]. It is more related to the latter cells than other kinds of lymphoid cells and is thought to be, on the other hand, cells related to BL between memory or GC cells dealing with BLs in arguments given in Molyneux et al. [32] in *The Lancet*. It might be studied as such for its possible relationship to BL [45] in the absence of replicating cells.

The Malaria Connection

For more than 50 years scientists have been asking how *P. falciparum* malaria might be associated with EBV and BL, and we turn to two reviews on this topic here [17, 18]. A more recent review of malaria by Sumba et al. [46] correlated malnutrition, malaria and EBV. The identification of different levels of BL in nearby regions in western Kenya led the authors to ask whether the incidence of the disease was associated with factors such as malnutrition and malaria. They found that children with the lowest antioxidant GP (glutathione peroxidase), an indicator of malnutrition, had highest EBV viral loads and the highest incidence of malaria, consistent with other studies that suggested correlation between malaria transmission intensities. Further studies are needed to determine whether these GP levels or other malaria biomarkers, as proposed [47] will have a role in the aetiology of BL. On the other hand, 2,602 patient cases in Uganda, Ghana and Tanzania [48] were explored with malaria biomarkers from these countries. Malaria was found to peak at 2 years of age, and decreased sharply between 2 and 3, and were related with novel findings correlated with BL, with age-specific pattern of locally prevalent malarial genotypes of *P. falciparum*. The authors concluded that "malaria could be related with onset of BL". Elsewhere in W. Africa, the role of protective immunity to *P. falciparum*, in Ghana,1965–1994, was "unknown" [48], but confirmed for malaria antibodies in 92% of the cases. In this study, the absorbent immunoassays showed lower malaria antibodies than observed in children (aged up to 14) with BL. In a different type of study, Yuan and colleagues [49] assayed 61 parasite lines against drug compounds. Thirty-two reactive compounds were explored for growth inhibition of malarial parasites against 33 strains of malaria. The compounds generated differential chemical phenotypes linked to wild-type or mutant alleles that could be protonated at physiologic, or lower, pH. Their overall work focused on three limited responses and were cited with loci and genes associated with drug responses, providing an "unknown but with a genetic basis" to better delineate the nature of drug resistance in malaria. The compounds generated differential chemical phenotypes linked to wild-type or mutant alleles that could be protonated at physiologic, or lower, pH. Their overall work focused on three limited responses and were linked with loci and genes associated with drug responses, providing an "unknown but with a genetic basis" to better delineate the nature of drug resistance in malaria. This interesting route has not yet been tried on BL, although with other tumours and could be used now in cases of BL-resistant malignancies [50]. Finally, also in brief, a report on malaria in Zanzibar [51] examines how facilities and donors could be made available to cope with the few thousand malaria cases they normally encounter, focused overall on control of the disease. In Zanzibar, a British-American initiative has provided bed netting to wipe out malaria on this island. Further, a group of scientists in India, where BL is not common, has looked at peptide-based therapies as offering the potential for non-genotoxic, genotypic-specific alternatives, or adjuvants, centred on a range of traditional cancer treatments. Their list includes drugs that can be generally useful. They have treated their studies as an "application in tumour therapy". Their concluding remarks are worth considering here also, in the African situation of BL. Here, Bhutia and Maiti note [52] that the potential of peptides to serve as anticancer drugs has re-energized the scientific community in the search for better ways to combat tumours, allowing an appropriate drug to be delivered to a desired location in sufficient quantities in a timely fashion, as noted previously for cyclophosphamide in BL. In one further study in Malawi, 185 out of 258 HIV-infected children were alive, but recommended for anti-viral treatment in BL, identified here as WHO stages III and IV [53]. This offers the possibility that some other novel tumour therapy treatments might now ultimately be assessed in Africa for BL.

Further, a group of scientists in India, where BL is less common, has looked at peptide-based therapies as offering the potential for non-genotoxic, genotypic-specific alternatives, or adjuvants, and turned to a range of cancer traditional treatments. BL is not common in India, but this list includes drugs that can be generally useful. They have treated their studies as an "application in tumour therapy". Their concluding remarks are worth considering here also, in the African situation of BL.

Another question arises, on the role of the TLR9 gene in the relationship of malaria to BL. First, BL patients with EBV are mainly seen in areas that are endemic for malaria, bringing together the three related topics here on BL, where repeated immune activation by malaria may be an important pathogenic factor for this malignancy [18]. Toll-like receptors (TLRs) are key players in innate immunity, and B-cells express one of the marked Toll genes, TLR9 has special interests for BL. The expression of TLR9 increases transformation rates of ex vivo EBV-infected B-cells, and its effect on the EBV genome is now being actively studied. We cite here three TLR9 papers [54–56], and related ones. The paper by Fathallah et al. [54] shows that EBV suppresses by deregulating the transcript through LMP-1-mediated NF-kB activation. In their work, they reveal a mechanism used by BL to highlight the importance of the immune deregulation, as mediated by the tumour-inducing virus of EBV. Their data show that in addition to its key role in cells, malaria transforms EBV to synergize its gene, LMP1, in children living in malaria-endemic areas. Chene and colleagues, working with BL from Uganda, in a series of papers, show that EBV reactivation can be induced during malaria infections, and in itself act as a causative factor for BL [55]. They argue that acute and chronic malaria infections produce induction of polyclonal activation in the B-cell and a dramatic increase in levels of EBV in circulation. Considering a series of papers, working mainly on BL from Akara and other cells, Zauner and Nadal [56] argue for manipulation of host immune response towards favouring long-term survival of the virus, in its latent form. Considering this fact, they also argue that the load of the virus is elevated, but that TLR9 might suppress the lytic virus and lead to B-cell transformation, as an enforced latent gene expression. They further argue that TLR9 might allow EBV to gain access to a memory B-cell pool. All three of these studies [54–56] make ways of studying EBV with new ideas about therapy. In the last paper, Arama et al. look at TLR responses, not just TLR9, in West African children in Mali [57]. They focus on two different ethnic groups, one (the Fulani group) being better protected against *P. falciparum* malaria, as compared with a second, the Dogon (less protected). They focus on dendritic cells (DCs) and conclude that DC and TLR signalling may be important for the protective immunity against malaria, as observed in the Fulani tribe. This seems "early days" for BL and malaria, but it may be a new way forward in BL research.

The HIV Connection

"The globally coordinated efforts to strengthen health systems in Africa have been impressive, especially for treatment of *P. falciparum* malaria" and "HIV-1 infections". HIV-1 infection is associated with a 60-fold-increase of BL in adults in the west (sBL), and the effect of HIV-1 on eBL is controversial, with most being HIV negative [18]. Orem and colleagues [58], working in Uganda, stated that characteristics of children with BL and HIV have not been described there before (in 2009). Of 1,462 records of children at the Uganda Cancer Institute, 236 charts met the eligibility criteria for BL, of whom 158 children were HIV-negative and 78 were positive (61% male and 39% female, with mean age of 6.9 years). This finding is similar to children in general in HIV rates in Uganda. Although their treatment also suggested chemotherapy, most HIV+ children did not generally receive chemotherapy or, if treated, this was mainly for facial BL. There is a clear need for better characterization of children with BL to understand whether there is an HIV-related BL alongside endemic BL. In Malawi, there are two studies on this topic, one in 2008, the other in 2010 [59, 60]. The earlier study noted that HIV plus malaria may decrease the risk of BL, and the latter study [60] was unclear. They finally concluded that the "impact of HIV on the risk of cancer…remains uncertain". In South Africa [61], the numbers were larger (1897) and there were differences in age and tumour types. In all, DLBCL was the most frequent lymphoma and patients varied accord to tumour type. For BL, patients between the ages of 20 and 49 were very numerous, and there were more in the 0- to 9-year than the 10- to 19-year group, as is typical for BL. Instead of reviewing young BL children, the assumption was that these smaller children in SA generally reflected migration from east, central and West Africa, where this disease may account for 70% of all child cancers [61]. In trying to find good samples outside Africa, they also looked among small American samples [62], and these BLs (whether AIDS related, or not) comparing BL and DLBCL. In the USA, they were able to differentiate between BL and DLBCL using protein expression multiple markers [63], and could distinguish between the groups by immunohistochemistry. Then, they asked would anything of interest be found by analysing the entire HIV genome [64]? As used with RNA structure models, how does HIV-1 function in BL, and what could be reasonably useful for analysis? They asked whether AIDS-related BL, under the Surveillance, Epidemiology and End Results Programme (1973–2005), was useful [65]. They observed peaks near ages 10, 40 and 70 years for males (for females, 10 and 70 only). They noted that BL was a first indicator of AIDS onset, at least in the West. The notion that BL may be multimodal is controversial in that BL is unlike other malignancies, but is considered as isomorphic. However, paediatric and adult/geriatric types may (indeed) have different risk factors. The risk of BL during 1980–1989 was higher than later, when HIV infection with relatively higher CD4 lymphocyte counts was observed in men. The risk may have exceeded those of women, or non-Hispanic black men, in the USA. This study is the largest to assess age-specific incidence among persons with AIDS. They argue that diagnosis or separation between HIV relationships to age or CD4 lymphocyte counts may likely be random, and that low CD4 lymphocyte counts may suggest functional CD4 to be required for BL to develop. There were 456,635 males and the number of BL cases was 273, whereas for females there were 33 of 111,230 subjects. The incidence for 1980–89 was 29.4%, dropping down to 14.6% and 10.3% in 1990–95, and 18.8% in 1996–2005. It was interesting to observe the bimodal peaks for BL at different ages and suggests effects of non-cumulative risk factors at different ages.

In Africa, specific comprehensive cancer studies are only beginning to highlight the cancer prevention and treatment programmes, particularly also associated with AIDS-defining cancers (noted here as cervical cancer, Kaposi sarcoma and lymphoma). In reporting on the other "AIDS-defining" cancers, lymphoma and including particularly cases from Nigeria and Uganda, Brower [65] comments that BL, in particular, may even go undiagnosed and untreated. She suggested that this type of lymphoma might particularly be combined in programmes dealing with preponderance of 60% among BL patients. Others [66] propose current plans for a number of treatment trials of lymphoma in Uganda, Tanzania and Kenya, and one of these has now been reported [67], carried out in Uganda and Kenya. These were well documented. In terms of the subject patients and the fact that HIV is a real problem in East Africa, patients were carefully chosen. From 149 patients with confirmed lymphoma and positive HIV serology, 52 were enrolled and 49 ultimately received oral BL and HIV treatment. The overall response rate was 78%, and 33% of patients survived 5 years. They concluded that the dose-modified oral chemotherapy had comparable outcome (with others elsewhere) and is "pragmatic in sub-Saharan Africa". The collaboration has been successful and may now focus on optimizing combination of anti-retroviral therapy and chemotherapy. No doubt it has been worth continuing this study. In time, one can decide how effective this is, and how to progress.

The Contributions by Mi(micro)-RNAs

This component is essentially "work in progress", since miRNA is going into a second 5th year on BL [68–74] and has much yet to reveal. In the viral latent component, EBV appears in BL together with lytic EBV, and in the latter there are 11 components of lytic, expressed DNA. Most of the genome expressed during the latent cycle is involved with inhibition of the lytic cycle. In a surprising finding [68], miRNAs are not needed to control the viral genome in exit from latency. Rather, they indicate that miRNAs are associated with cellular transformation, and rather than regulating viral genes of the lytic phase are involved with inhibition or expression of the lytic cycle. EBV miRNA does not lead to increased activation as, for example, with KSHV, HCV and CMV. All the EBV tumour types of miRNAs, including Latency II-III, are largely associated with lytic infections, whereas Latency I, for BL, may be primarily associated with EBNA1 (see Fig. 16.1). We called attention to LMP1 and 2 for BL lymphoma in [14], in some cells. In the review [69], it was notable that more and more clearly, several reports suggest an interplay between virus and cellular mi-RNA involving several gene products. That virus-mediated mi-RNA dysregulation may be involved in several malignancies [70]. It has also come to attention that mi-RNA-9 is potentially relevant for malignant transformation in BL cases with no detectable Myc translocation. Thus deregulations of mi-RNA may be thus useful as a diagnostic tool, suggesting it as a novel candidate for tumour cell markers [71]. Mi-RNA is predicted to target as many as 300 different human transcripts, just as a single-RNA may be targeted by multiple mi-RNAs. Since mi-RNA expression is deregulated in several lymphomas, and unique mi-RNA signatures have been identified for prognosis and response to therapy, they become appealing as therapeutic targets. From previous and ongoing work in lymphomas, it is evident that deregulation of mi-RNA expression is one of the critical steps in pathogenesis of several lymphomas. Just as mouse variants as models for man have been shown as "not relevant to Burkitt's lymphoma in the past", in mi-RNA of man, profiling can successfully classify various lymphomas into therapeutic outcomes or survival categories. These aspects of BL, at least in Africa, are starting to look at new ways of assessing this disease, which may prove productive for the future. We must now wait.

Interestingly, other malignancies show homogenous mi-RNA profiles entirely distinct from BL and DLBCL. Differentially expressed mi-RNAs from these two tumour classes, including mi-155, segregates 17 mi-RNAs from being down-regulated in BL as compared with DLBCL, and 21 mi-RNAs showed a higher expression in BL as compared with DLBCL involved with inhibition of the lytic cycle. In this data set, the mi-RNAs can be separated using differences among the mi-RNAs. Mi-155 and four further mi-RNAs were down-regulated in DLBCL by RT-PCR. In different types of Burkitt's, eBL, sBL and HIV-BL within these variants, the "cut times" of the different mi-RNAs detected variance among their expressions [72]. Overall, molecular profiling of neoplasms is gaining increasing significance for the definition and characterizations of established tumour entities, and for the identification of new biological disease groups or subgroups. In summary, our analysis reveals that BL differs from DLBCL by a strong and characteristic mi-RNA signature that is enriched in mi-RNAs targeted on the NF-kB signalled pathway-associated mi-RNAs. Similar studies overall were also described by Piccaluga [33]. In an early study [73], Akao and colleagues found down-regulation of mi-143 and -145 RNAs in

B-cell malignancies. Although their model was mainly colon cancer, 8/9 B-cell lymphomas tested exhibited extremely low expression in human BLs. These could be expected to reach tumours efficiently and be used as a drug delivery system. They may differentiate B-cell malignant cells from normal cells, and contribute to carcinogenesis in B-cell malignancies, by a novel mechanism.

In our own studies, Xue and Griffin [74] (and earlier work), complexities associated with expression of EBV lytic origins of DNA replication, were studied. We had examined this region in two (145 and 102 bp) repetitive sequences in BL DNA, both encoding basic proteins, to understand why lytic replication—necessary for viral replication—and its controlling elements is so efficient. Studies uncovered a diverse family of promoters for both EBV BHLF1 and LF3, only one of these, the first, proving sensitive to chemical inducting agents. The other, abutting the replication core origin sequence of EBV, may play roles in the maintenance of viral latency. In this publication, the sequences of EBV exposed long regions of various small open reading frames (very long non-coding sequences) for subsequent work, possibly marking the two regions for future studies, as well as the mi-RNAs from these two regions.

Section 3

There are suggestions for a number of cellular components that might fall into chapters on BL. We select only a few of these at this time, briefly, for consideration.

BLIMP1 (or PRDMI)

This gene has been widely studied—but not necessarily with regard to BL. Blimp1 (or related to Blimp1a) is a transcription factor that is required for plasma cell differentiation, and associated with the germinal centre. It is also known otherwise as PRDMI gene [75, 76], whose loss contributes to lymphomagenesis by blocking plasma cell differentiation. The intimate association between terminal differentiation and EBV replication suggests that a switch from latency to lytic cycle is controlled by factors that normally regulate plasma cell differentiation. In [75], a striking overlap between the EBV LMP-1 gene and Blimp1a is shown between the two genes in germinal centre B cells. This is more associated with DLBCL than with childhood BL, but in tissue culture it is also identified in the latter as well. This multifunctional and complicated gene, altered in numerous cells, is highlighted here for the future, together also with the children's disease. It is also associated with deregulation of BCL6 [76], as below. One will need to know more about Blimp-1 in childhood BL, in future. We have tried to look at this tumour in BL in African children, in Malawi, but not yet found the materials that would help us in this study (see [16]). We thus raise it for others to comment on.

Bcl6

This protein is easily assessed both in childhood BL and other tumours related to BL (see [16]). In GC cells, most BL tumours appear to express this marker. There are two recent studies here that target cells controlling multiple pathways in normal germinal centre B cells. This transcription repressor has emerged as a critical regulator, and the B cells are selected based on the production of antibodies with high affinity for the antigen [77, 78]. Bcl6 can repress various functions in cell biology, including protection from DNA-induced apoptosis and inhibition of differentiation into plasma cells. It is a valid marker for BL. A recent study [78] results in a set of strictly defined biochemical and functional Bcl6 targets that have implication for the understanding of its activity as a transcription factor and of its role as an oncogene in lymphomagenesis. Bcl6 is expressed in all GC-derived malignancies, included BL, DLBCL, follicular lymphoma and a subset of Hodgkin lymphoma. Its finding suggests a potential synergic therapeutic activity between molecules aimed at inactivation of BCL6 and biologic agents leading to B-cell activation and differentiation. Stat3 mediated regulation of Blimp1, coordinated with Bcl6 down-regulation, acts to control human plasma cell differentiation [79]. In the single mouse cells cited here [80], T-cells that rapidly terminated proliferation and up-regulation of 1L-7 receptors, modulated Bcl6 response. The results suggest that because Bcl6 antibodies become low, after weeks of immunization, it is unclear how long Bcl6 remains in BL, over time. This is a topic; it seems, even now, for future work.

Bcl2

With Bcl2, a total of 1,260 cases of non-Hodgkin lymphoma were identified, between 1991 and 2007; of these, 54 cases (4%) were identified as having concurrent translocations involved Myc and Bcl2 [81]. These samples were acquired from patients having different diagnoses and treatment regimens. From their analysis, the authors concluded that Bcl2 and Myc-positive lymphomas have a very poor overall survival, unlike classical BL. From their analysis, both morphological and genetic information is important because diagnosis might be missed if genetic testing by karyotype and/or FISH analysis were not performed. They ultimately suggest that Bcl2-together with Myc translocations may be more common than previously appreciated, and it needs further study [81]. In Akata, EBV recognizes its own version of Bcl2 for an unknown pathway, enhancing the oncogenic potential of these cells [82]. The third lymphoma, also known as a "double-hit" lymphoma (DHL), is a rare neoplasm characterized by aggressive clinical behaviour, complex karyotypes and a spectrum of pathologic features overlapping with BL diffuse lymphoma, and B-lymphoblastic lymphoma/laeukemia [83]. The aggressive clinical behaviour and combination of genetic abnormalities seen in these tumours may warrant categorization as a separate entity. In total, except for Akata cells, most sBL did not agree with the characterization of these tumours, except their being mainly from adults, rather than for children. Indeed, in review [19], Bcl2 is noted occurring in memory cells, but rarely is Bcl6 found there. On the other hand, Bcl6 is expressed as a major component and is frequently discussed here as regards germinal centre (GC) in BL, particularly in latent cells.

EBV Vaccine

In November this year (2011), four authors propose a vaccine target for cancer prevention [84]. Infectious mononucleosis (IM) is marked as a key target for this, although cancers that range in different parts of the world are noted for the role(s) of tumours also associated with EBV. EBV-positive BL is the most common childhood tumour in equatorial African and, to some extent, also New Guinea. Of BL, the number of cases attributable to EBV per year is given as 6,600 in less-developed countries, as opposed to 100 cases in developed countries. They also note that the immune systems of models is limited by EBV not generally being pathogenic for animals, except for certain models like cotton-top monkeys or rhesus lymphocytovirus, that can be used for modelling candidate vaccines. On the basis of these observations, and the phase 2 EBV gp350 vaccine trial for the prevention of IM, the choice for EBV is limited. They thus propose a number of priorities (numbers 1–5) that can be envisaged for future research plans. These programs are ways for looking forward as regards BL, and the program for another EBV disease, found mostly in adults, nasopharyngeal carcinoma. It is worth much consideration, and they present the first positive plans for tumours associated with EBV.

In another recent development in 2011, Harold Varmus became head of the National Cancer Institute in the USA. This means perhaps more resources will be given to BL research and it will likely get better funding. One question asked him recently [85] was "should NCI not be doing something about the cost of cancer drugs?" and his reply was that "several of the drugs that are currently expensive, are to come off patent and that will result in price reductions", and "reducing the costs of some things that could put…to use in poorer countries" where the opportunities are still needed. For him, "some of them are truly low-hanging fruit and we ought to be doing something about this". Let us hope that the question is raised now with alternative drugs needed. And some of them, such as HDAC, may be useful for those children whose tumours need treatment, but this simple drug is still much too expensive. We shall wait to see.

Acknowledgments The author thanks Drs. John Phillips, Pascale Kropf and Ms. S. van Noorden for reading and considering this manuscript, and giving her relevant suggestions along the way. She also thanks her colleagues for the (DVD) manuscript, "Surviving Burkitts" and to many people in Malawi looking forward to the end of this malignancy which takes now away the lives of many young children there. For the film (DVD) we thank especially Stephanie and Wade who shared their son's life to this film, Dr. E. Molyneux who also oversaw this film and looked after the children, and finally a wonderful film producer, Alex Tweddle and his crew who produced this film, and my relations in the south of the USA and all friends who helped raise money for the film. Last but not least, a long-time college friend from India, but in this film the children to whom he has (and will continue) to support, with his efforts and his knowledge.

References

1. The Leroy Martin Family (1999) Burkitt's lymphoma resources. Web site. Nat Cancer Ins
2. Vonka V (2000) Causality in medicine: the case of tumours and viruses. Philos Trans R Soc Lond B Biol Sci 355:1831–1841
3. Kazembe P, Hesseling PB, Griffin BE, Lambert I, Wessels G, (2002) Long term survival of children with Burkitt lymphoma in Malawi after cyclophosphamide monotherapy. Med Pediatr Oncol 40:22–25
4. Witty A (2011) New strategies for innovation in global health: a pharmaceutical industry perspective. Health Aff 2011:118–126
5. Jaffe ES (2009) The 2008 WHO classification of lymphomas: implications for clinical practice and translational research. Hematology Am Soc Hematol Educ Program 523–531
6. Bornkamm GW (2009) Epstein-Barr and its role in the pathogenesis of Burkitt's: an unresolved issue. Semin Cancer Biol 19:351–365
7. Thorley-Lawson DA, Allday MJ (2008) The curious case of the tumour virus: 50 years of Burkitt's lymphoma. Nat Rev Microbiol 6:913–924
8. Boerma EG, Siebert R, Kluin PN, Baudis M (2009) Translocations involving 8q24 Burkitt lymphoma and other malignant lymphomas: a historical review of cytogenetics in the light of todays knowledge. Leukemia 23:225–234
9. Lenses D, Leoncini L, Hummel M, Volinia S, Liu C (2011) The different epidemiologic subtypes of Burkitt Lymphoma share a homogenous micro RNA profile distinct from diffuse large B-cell lymphoma. Leukemia 25(12):1869–1876
10. Orem J, Mbidda EK, Lambert B, de Sanjos S, Weiderpass E (2007) Burkitt's lymphoma in Africa, a review of the epidemiology and etiology. Afr Health Sci 7:166–175
11. Iwakiri D, Takada K (2010) Role of EBERs in the pathogenesis of EBV infection. Adv Cancer Res 107:119–136
12. Chuang S-S, Huang W-T, Hsieh P-P, Jung Y-C, He H et al (2008) Sporadic paediatric and adult Burkitt lymphomas share similar phenotypic and genotypic features. Histopathology 52: 427–435
13. Phillips JA (2008) Is Burkitt's lymphoma sexy enough? Lancet 368:2251–2252
14. Labrecque LG, Lampert I, Xue S-A, Kazembe G, Phillips J et al (1999) Expression of Epstein-Barr virus lytically related genes in African Burkitt's lymphoma: correlations with patient response to therapy. Int J Cancer 81:6–11
15. Xue S-A, Griffin BE (2009) Update on the Epstein-Barr Virus-associated malignancy, endemic Burkitt's lymphoma. In: Yoshida K (ed) Molecular biology of tumor virus gene products. Research Signpost, Kerala
16. Van Noorden S, Lampert IA, Xue S-A, Lykidin D, Phillips JA et al (2011) Burkitt's lymphoma: maximizing the use of fine needle aspirates by long-term preservation for diagnosis and research. Trans R Soc Trop Med Hyg 105(2):86–94
17. Rochford R, Cannon MJ, Moormann AD (2005) Endemic Burkitt's lymphoma: a polymicrobial disease? Nat Rev Microbiol 3:182–187
18. Mbulaiteye SM, Talisuna AO, Ogwang MD, McKenzie FE, Ziegler JL et al (2010) African Burkitt's lymphoma: could collaboration with HIV-1 and malaria programmes reduce the high mortality rate. Lancet 375:2010–2014
19. Nilsson JA, Cleveland JL (2003) Myc pathways promoting cell suicide and cancer. Oncogene 22:9007–9021

20. Allday MJ (2009) How does Epstein-Barr virus (EBV) complement the activation of Myc in the pathogenesis of Burkitt's lymphoma. Semin Cancer Biol 19:366–376
21. Reardon S (2011) A world of chronic disease. Science 333:558–559
22. Jeon AP, Nam HY, Shim SM, Han BG (2009) Sustained viral activity of Epstein-Barr virus contributes to cellular immortalization of lymphoblastoid cell lines. Mol Cell 27:143–148
23. Scheller H, Tobollik S, Kutzera A, Eder M, Unterlehberg J et al (2010) c-Myc overexpression promotes a germinal center-like program in Burkitt's lymphoma. Oncogene 29:888–897
24. Zeller KI, Zhao S, Lee CW, Chiu KP, Yao F et al (2006) Global mapping of c-Myc binding sites and target gene networks in human cells. Proc Natl Acad Sci U S A 103:17834–17839
25. Anastasiadou E, Vaeth S, Cuomo L, Boccellato F, Vincenti S et al (2009) Epstein-Barr virus infection leads to partial phenotypic reversion of terminally differentiated malignant B cells. Cancer Lett 284:165–174
26. Kim J, Lee J-H, Lyer VR (2008) Global identification of MYC target genes reveals its direct role in mitochondrial biogenesis and its e-box usage in vivo. PLoS One 3:e1798
27. Klapperoth K, Wirth T (2010) Advancers in the understanding of Myc-induced lymphomagenesis. Br J Haematol 149:484–497
28. Hummel M, Bentink S, Berger H, Klapper W, Wessendorf S et al (2006) A biologic definition of Burkitt's lymphoma from transcriptional and genomic profiling. N Engl J Med 354: 2419–2430
29. Dave SS, Fu K, Wright GW, Lam LT, Kluin P et al (2006) Molecular diagnosis of Burkitt's lymphoma. N Engl J Med 354:2431–2442
30. Harris NL, Homing SJ (2006) Burkitt's lymphoma, the message from microarrays. N Engl J Med 354:2495–2498
31. Queiroga EM, Gualco G, Weiss LM, Dittmer DP, Araujo I et al (2008) Burkitt lymphoma in Brazil is characterized by geographically distinct clinicopathologic features. Am J Clin Pathol 130:946–956
32. Molyneux EM, Rochford R, Griffin BE, Newton R, Jackson G et al (2012) Burkitt's lymphoma. Lancet 379(9822):1234–1244
33. Piccaluga PP, Di Falco G, Kustagi M, Gazzola A, Agostinelli C et al (2011) Gene expression analysis uncovers similarity and differences among Burkett lymphoma subtypes. Blood 117: 3596–3608
34. Tumwine LK, Campidelli C, Righi S, Neda S, Byarugaba W et al (2008) B-cell non-Hodgkin lymphomas in Uganda: an immunohistochemical appraisal on tissue microarray. Hum Pathol 39:817–823
35. Tumwine LK, Agostinelli C, Campidelli C, Othieno E, Wabaiga H et al (2009) Immunohistochemical and other prognostic factors in B cell non Hodgkin lymphoma patients, Kampala, Uganda. BMC Clin Pathol 9:11
36. Yang WP, Zhu CD, Gong LP, Lu BB, Zou Y et al (2009) Clinicopathologic and immunohistochemical study of intra-abdominal non-Hodgkin B-cell lymphoma occurring in children. Zhonghua Bing Li Xue Za Zhi 38:759–764 (abstract in English)
37. Takada K (2001) Role of Epstein-Barr virus in Burkitt's Lymphoma. Curr Top Microbiol Immunol 258:141–151
38. Gualco G, Queiroga EM, Weiss LM, Klumb CE, Harrington WJ et al (2009) Frequent expression of multiple myeloma 1/interferon regulatory factor 4 in Burkitt lymphoma. Hum Pathol 40:565–571
39. Gualco G, Weiss LM, Bacchi CE (2010) MumI/IRF4: a review. Appl Immunohistochem Mol Morphol 18:301–310
40. Hesseling PB, Molyneux E, Kamiza S, Broadhead R (2008) Rescue chemotherapy for patients with resistant or relapsed endemic Burkitt's lymphoma. Trans R Soc Trop Med Hyg 102:602–607
41. Fatzer BC, Hosseinipour MC, Kamthuzi P, Hyde L, Bramson B et al (2009) Predictors for mortality and loss to follow-up among children receiving anti-retroviral therapy in Lilongwe, Malawi. Trop Med Int Health 14:862–869

42. Xue S-A, Labrecque LG, Lu QL, Ong SK, Lampert IA et al (2002) Promiscuous expression of Epstein-Barr virus genes in Burkitt's lymphoma from the central African country Malawi. Int J Cancer 99:635–643
43. Kelly GT, Long HM, Stylianou J, Thomas WAE, Leese A et al (2009) An Epstein-Barr virus anti-apoptotic protein constitutively expressed in transformed cells and implicated in Burkitt lymphomagenesis: the Wp/BHR1 link. PLoS Pathog 5:e1000341
44. Daigle D, Megyola C, El-Guidy A, Gradoville Y, Tuck D et al (2010) Upregulation of STAT 3 marks Burkitt lymphoma cells refectory to Epstein-Barr virus lytic cycle induction by HDAC inhibitors. J Virol 84:993–1004
45. Novak U, Basso K, Pasqualucci L, Dalla-Favara R, Bhagat G (2011) Genomic analysis of non-splenic marginal zone lymphomas (MZL) indicates similarities between nodal and extranodal MZL and supports their derivation from memory B-cells. Br J Haematol 155(3):362–365
46. Sumba PO, Kabiru EW, Namuyenga E, Fiore N, Otieno RO et al (2010) Microgeographic variations in Burkitt's lymphoma incidence correlate with differences in malnurition, malaria and Epstein-Barr virus. Br J Cancer 103(11):1736–1741
47. Emmanuel B, Kawira E, Ogwang MD, Wabinga H, Magatti J et al (2010) African Burkitt lymphoma: age-specific risk and correlations with malaria biomarkers. Am J Trop Med Hyg 84:397–401
48. Guech-Ongey M, Yagi M, Palacpag NM, Emmanuel B, Talisuna AO et al (2012) Antibodies reactive to Plasmodium falciparum serine repeat antigen in children with Burkitt lymphoma from Ghana. Int J Cancer 130(8):1908–1914
49. Yuan J, Cheng KC, Johnson RL, Huang R, Pattaradilokrat S et al (2011) Chemical genomic profiling for antimalarial therapies, response signatures, and molecular targets. Science 333:724–729
50. Ogwang MD, Zhao W, Ayers LM, Mbulaiteye SM (2011) Accuracy of Burkitt lymphoma diagnosis in constrained pathology settings: importance to epidemiology. Arch Pathol Lab Med 135:445–450
51. Smith DS, Cohen JM, Moonen B, Tatem AJ, Sabot OJ et al (2011) Solving the Sisyphean problem of Malaria in Zanzibar. Science 332:1384–1385
52. Bhutia SK, Maiti TK (2008) Targeting tumors with peptides from natural sources. Trends Biotechnol 26:210–217
53. Fetzer BC, Hosseinipour MC, Kamthuzi P, Hyde L, Bramson et al (2009) Predictors for loss mortality and loss to follow up among children receiving anti-retroviral therapy in Lilongwi, Malawi. Trop Med Int Health 14:862–869
54. Fathallah I, Parroche P, Gruffat H, Zannetti C, Johansson H et al (2010) EBV latent membrane protein 1 is a negative regulator of TLR9. J Immunol 185:6439–6447
55. Chene A, Donati D, Orem J, Mbidde ER, Kironde F et al (2009) Endemic Burkitt's lymphoma as a polymicrobial disease: new insights on the interaction between Plasmodium falciparum and Epstein-Barr virus. Semin Cancer Biol 19:411–420 (and earlier papers from same sources)
56. Zauner L, Nadal E (2012) Understanding TRP9 action in Epstein-Barr virus infection. Front Biosci 17:1219–1231 (and 4 other papers)
57. Arama C, Giusti P, Bostrom S, Dara V, Traore B et al (2009) Interethnic differences in antigen-presenting cell activation and TLR responses in Malian children during Plasmodium falciparum malaria. PLoS One 6:e18319
58. Orem J, Maganda A, Mbidde EK, Weiderpass E (2009) Clinical characteristics and outcome of children with Burkitt lymphoma in Uganda according to HIV infection. Pediatr Blood Cancer 52:455–458
59. Mutalima N, Molyneux E, Jaffe H, Kamiza S, Borgstein E et al (2008) Associations between Burkitt lymphoma among children in Malawi and infection with HIV, EBV and malaria: results from a case–control-study. PLoS One 3:e2505
60. Mutalima N, Molyneux EM, Johnston WT, Jaffe HW, Kamiza S et al (2010) Impact of infection with human immunodeficiency virus-1 (HIV) on the risk of cancer among children in Malawi – preliminary findings. Infect Agent Cancer 5:5, Feb 12

61. Mantina H, Wiggill TM, Carcoma S, Perner Y, Stevens WS (2010) Characterization of lymphomas in a high prevalence HIV setting. J Acquir Immune Defic Syndr 53:656–660
62. Gormley RP, Madan R, Dulau AE, Xu D, Tamas EF et al (2005) Germinal center and activated B-cell profiles separate Burkitt lymphoma and diffuse large B-cell lymphoma in AIDS and non-AIDS cases. Am J Clin Pathol 124:790–798
63. Watts JM, Dang KK, Gorelick RJ, Leonard CW, Bess JS Jr et al (2009) Architecture and secondary structure of an entire HIV-1 RNA genome. Nature 460:711–716
64. Guech-Ongey M, Simard EP, Anderson WF, Engels EA, Bhatia K et al (2010) AIDS-related Burkitt lymphoma in the United States: what do age and CD4 lymphoma patterns tell us about etiology and/or biology? Blood 116:5600–5604
65. Brower V (2011) AIDS-related cancers increase in Africa. J Natl Cancer Inst 103:918–919
66. Carbone A, Cesarman E, Spina M, Gloghini A, Schulz TF (2009) HIV-associated lymphomas and gamma-herpesviruses. Blood 113:1213–1224
67. Mwanda WO, Orem J, Fu P, Banura C, Kakembo J et al (2009) Dose-modified oral chemotherapy in the treatment of AIDS-related non-Hodgkin's lymphoma in East Africa. J Clin Oncol 27:3480–3488
68. Seto E, Moosmann A, Gromminger S, Walz N, Grundhoff A et al (2010) Micro RNAs of Epstein-Barr virus progression and prevent apoptosis of primary human B cells. PLoS Pathog 6:E1001063
69. De Falco G, Antonicelli G, Onnis A, Lassi S, Bellan C et al (2009) Role of EBV in microRNA dysregulation in Burkitt lymphoma. Semin Cancer Biol 19:401–406
70. Sandhu SK, Croce CM, Garzon R (2011) MicroRNA expression and function in Lymphomas. Adv Hematol 247137
71. Onnis A, De Falco G, Antonicelli G, Onorati M, Bellan C et al (2010) Alteration of microRNAs regulated by c-MYC in Burkitt lymphoma. PLoS One 5:e212960
72. Lenze D, Leoncini L, Hummel M, Volinia S, Liu CG et al (2011) The different epidemiologic subtypes of Burkitt lymphoma share a homogenous micro RNA profile distinct from diffuse large B-cell lymphoma. Leukemia 25(12):1869–1876
73. Akao Y, Nakagawa Y, Kitade Y, Kinoshira T, Naoe T (2007) Downregulation of micro RNAs 143- and -145 in B-cell malignancies. Cancer Sci 98:1914–1920
74. Xue S-A, Griffin BE (2007) Complexities associated with expression of Epstein-Barr virus (EBV) lytic origins of DNA replication. Nucleic Acids Res 35:3391–3406
75. Vrzalikova K, Vockerodt M, Leonard S, Bell A, Wei W et al (2011) Down-regulation of BLIMP1a by the EBV oncogene, LMP-1, disrupts the plasma cell differentiation program and prevents replication in B cells: implications for the pathogenesis of EBV-associated B-cell lymphomas. Blood 117:5907–5917
76. Mandelbaum J, Bhagat G, Tang H, Mo T, Brahmachary M et al (2010) Blimp1 is a tumor suppressor gene frequently disrupted in activated B cell-like diffuse large Bcell lymphoma. Cancer Cell 18:565–579
77. Basso K, Dalla-Favera R (2010) BCL6: master regulator of the germinal center reaction and key oncogene in B cell lymphomageneis. Adv Immunol 105:193–210
78. Basso K, Saito M, Sumazin P, Margoliin AA, Wang K et al (2010) Integrated biochemical and computational approach identified BCL6 direct target genes controlling multiple pathways in normal germinal center B cells. Blood 115:975–984
79. Diehl SA, Schmidlin H, Nagasawa M, van Haren SD, Kwakkenbos MJ et al (2008) Stat3-mediated up-regulation of BLIMP1 is coordinated with BCL6 down-regulation to control human plasma cell differentiation. J Immunol 180:4805–4815
80. Kirano M, Moriyama S, Ando Y, Hikida M, Mori Y et al (2011) Bcl6 protein expression shapes pre-germinal center B cell dynamics and follicular helper T cell heterogeneity. Immunity 34:961–972
81. Johnson NA, Savage KJ, Ludkovski O, Ben-Neriah S, Woods R et al (2009) Lymphomas with concurrent BCL2 and MYC translocations: the critical factors associated with survival. Blood 114:2273–2279

82. Komano J, Takada K (2001) Role of bcl-2 in Epstein-Barr Virus-induced malignant conversion Burkitt's Lymphoma cell line Akata. J Virol 75:1561–1564
83. Srimathandada P, Loomis R, Calbone R, Srimathandada S, Lacy J (2008) Combined protesome and Bcl-2 inhibition stimulates apoptosis and inhibits growth in EBV transformed lymphocytes: a potential therapeutic approach to EBV-associated lymphoproliferative diseases. Eur J Haematol 80:407–418
84. Cohen JI, Fauci AS, Varmus H, Nabel GJ (2011) Epstein-Barr virus: an important vaccine target for cancer prevention. Sci Transl Med 3(107):1–3
85. Kaiser J (2011) Piloting cancer research with a shrinking budget. Science 333:397

Index

DOI 10.1007/978-1-4614-4313-1, © Springer Science+Business Media New York 2013

W

X

Y

MIX
Papier aus verantwortungsvollen Quellen
Paper from responsible sources
FSC® C105338

If you have any concerns about our products,
you can contact us on
ProductSafety@springernature.com

In case Publisher is established outside the EU,
the EU authorized representative is:
Springer Nature Customer Service Center GmbH
Europaplatz 3, 69115 Heidelberg, Germany

Printed by Libri Plureos GmbH
in Hamburg, Germany